Contemporary Management of Esophageal Malignancy

Guest Editors

CHADRICK E. DENLINGER, MD
CAROLYN E. REED, MD

SURGICAL CLINICS
OF NORTH AMERICA

www.surgical.theclinics.com

Consulting Editor
RONALD F. MARTIN, MD

October 2012 • Volume 92 • Number 5

SAUNDERS an imprint of ELSEVIER, Inc.

W.B. SAUNDERS COMPANY

A Division of Elsevier Inc.

1600 John F. Kennedy Blvd., Suite 1800, Philadelphia, PA 19103-2899

http://www.surgical.theclinics.com

SURGICAL CLINICS OF NORTH AMERICA Volume 92, Number 5
October 2012 ISSN 0039–6109, ISBN-13: 978-1-4557-4965-2

Editor: John Vassallo, j.vassallo@elsevier.com

Developmental Editor: Teia Stone

Surgical Clinics of North America (ISSN 0039–6109) is published bimonthly by Elsevier Inc., 360 Park Avenue South, New York, NY 10010-1710. Months of publication are February, April, June, August, October, and December. Business and Editorial Offices: 1600 John F. Kennedy Blvd., Suite 1800, Philadelphia, PA 19103-2899. Periodicals postage paid at New York, NY and additional mailing offices. Subscription prices are $339.00 per year for US individuals, $575.00 per year for US institutions, $166.00 per year for US students and residents, $415.00 per year for Canadian individuals, $714.00 per year for Canadian institutions, $468.00 for international individuals, $714.00 per year for international institutions and $229.00 per year for Canadian and foreign students/residents. To receive student/resident rate, orders must be accompanied by name of affiliated institution, date of term, and the *signature* of program/residency coordinator on institution letterhead. Orders will be billed at individual rate until proof of status is received. Foreign air speed delivery is included in all *Clinics* subscription prices. All prices are subject to change without notice. POSTMASTER: Send address changes to *Surgical Clinics*, Elsevier Health Sciences Division, Subscription Customer Service, 3251 Riverport Lane, Maryland Heights, MO 63043. **Customer Service (orders, claims, online, change of address): Telephone: 1-800-654-2452 (U.S. and Canada); 314-447-8871 (outside U.S. and Canada). Fax: 314-447-8029. E-mail: journalscustomerservice-usa@elsevier.com (for print support); journalsonline support-usa@elsevier.com (for online support).**

Reprints. For copies of 100 or more, of articles in this publication, please contact the Commercial Reprints Department, Elsevier Inc., 360 Park Avenue South, New York, New York 10010-1710. Tel. (212) 633-3812, Fax: (212) 462-1935, e-mail: reprints@elsevier.com.

The Surgical Clinics of North America is also published in Spanish by McGraw-Hill Interamericana Editores S.A., P.O. Box 5-237 06500 Mexico D.F. Mexico; and in Portuguese by Interlivros Edicoes Ltda., Rua Comandante Coelho 1085, CEP 21250, Rio de Janeiro, Brazil; and in Greek by Paschalidis Medical Publications, Athens Greece.

The Surgical Clinics of North America is covered in *MEDLINE/PubMed (Index Medicus)*, *EMBASE/Excerpta Medica*, *Current Contents/Clinical Medicine*, *Current Contents/Life Sciences*, *Science Citation Index*, and *ISI/BIOMED*.

Printed and bound by CPI Group (UK) Ltd, Croydon, CR0 4YY

Transferred to digital print 2012

Contributors

CONSULTING EDITOR

RONALD F. MARTIN, MD
Staff Surgeon, Department of Surgery, Marshfield Clinic, Marshfield, Wisconsin; Clinical Associate Professor, University of Wisconsin School of Medicine and Public Health, Madison, Wisconsin; Colonel, Medical Corps, United States Army Reserve

GUEST EDITORS

CHADRICK E. DENLINGER, MD
Assistant Professor of Surgery, Division of Cardiothoracic Surgery; Surgical Director, Lung Transplant Program, Medical University of South Carolina, Charleston, South Carolina

CAROLYN E. REED, MD
Professor of Surgery, Division of Cardiothoracic Surgery, Medical University of South Carolina, Charleston, South Carolina

AUTHORS

NASSER K. ALTORKI, MD
Professor of Cardiothoracic Surgery; Chief, Division of Thoracic Surgery, Weill Cornell Medical College, New York-Presbyterian Hospital, New York, New York

ANTHONY J. ASCIOTI, MD
Department of Thoracic and Cardiovascular Surgery, St. Vincent Hospital, Indianapolis, Indiana

ANKIT BHARAT, MD
Division of Cardiothoracic Surgery, Washington University School of Medicine, St Louis, Missouri

STEVE CHIN, MD
Director, Neuropsycho-Oncology, Department of Psychiatry and Behavioral Sciences; Assistant Professor of Medicine, Division of Hematology and Oncology, Medical University of South Carolina, Charleston, South Carolina

S. LEWIS COOPER, MD
Resident, Department of Radiation Oncology, Medical University of South Carolina, Charleston, South Carolina

TRAVES CRABTREE, MD
Assistant Professor of Surgery, Division of Cardiothoracic Surgery, Washington University School of Medicine, St Louis, Missouri

STEVEN R. DEMEESTER, MD
Associate Professor, Department of Surgery, Keck School of Medicine, The University of Southern California, Los Angeles, California

TODD L. DEMMY, MD, FACS
Professor of Oncology; Clinical Chair, Department of Thoracic Surgery, Roswell Park
Cancer Institute, University at Buffalo, Buffalo, New York

CHADRICK E. DENLINGER, MD
Assistant Professor of Surgery, Division of Cardiothoracic Surgery; Surgical Director,
Lung Transplant Program, Medical University of South Carolina, Charleston, South
Carolina

FELIX FERNANDEZ, MD
Assistant Professor of Surgery, Division of Cardiothoracic Surgery, Emory University
School of Medicine, Emory University Hospital, Atlanta, Georgia

RICHARD K. FREEMAN, MD
Medical Director of Oncology; Director, Division of Thoracic Surgery, Department of
Thoracic and Cardiovascular Surgery, St. Vincent Hospital, Indianapolis, Indiana

MATTHEW P. FOX, MD
Department of Surgery, School of Medicine, University of Louisville, Louisville, Kentucky

SAMAD HASHIMI, MD
Heart and Lung Institute, St. Joseph's Hospital and Medical Center, Phoenix, Arizona

ROBERT H. HAWES, MD
Center for Interventional Endoscopy, Florida Hospitals, Orlando, Florida

MICHAEL HERMANSSON, MD, PhD
Department of Surgery, Keck School of Medicine, The University of Southern California,
Los Angeles, California

WAYNE L. HOFSTETTER, MD
Associate Professor of Surgery; Director of Esophageal Surgery, Department of Thoracic
and Cardiovascular Surgery, University of Texas MD Anderson Cancer Center, Houston,
Texas

PRASAD G. IYER, MD, MS
Consultant, Associate Professor, Barrett's Esophagus Unit, Division of Gastroenterology
and Hepatology, Mayo Clinic, Rochester, Minnesota

RYAN M. LEVY, MD
Assistant Professor of Cardiothoracic Surgery, Department of Cardiothoracic Surgery,
University of Pittsburgh Medical Center, Pittsburgh, Pennsylvania

ZHIGANG LI, MD, PhD
Assistant Professor of Surgery, Department of Thoracic and Cardiovascular Surgery,
Changhai Hospital, The Second Military Medical University, Shanghai, People's Republic
of China

JAMES D. LUKETICH, MD
Henry Bahnson Professor of Cardiothoracic Surgery and Chairman, Department of
Cardiothoracic Surgery, University of Pittsburgh Medical Center, Pittsburgh,
Pennsylvania

RAJA J. MAHIDHARA, MD
Department of Thoracic and Cardiovascular Surgery, St. Vincent Hospital, Indianapolis,
Indiana

JENIFER L. MARKS, MD
Department of Thoracic and Cardiovascular Surgery, University of Texas MD Anderson Cancer Center, Houston, Texas

ERIC M. NELSEN, MD
Department of Internal Medicine, Mayo Clinic, Rochester, Minnesota

STEVEN J. NURKIN, MD
Assistant Professor of Surgery, Department of Surgical Oncology, Roswell Park Cancer Institute, University at Buffalo, Buffalo, New York

DANIEL RAYMOND, MD, FACS
Thoracic & Cardiovascular Surgery, Cleveland Clinic Foundation, Cleveland, Ohio

CAROLYN E. REED, MD
Professor of Surgery, Division of Cardiothoracic Surgery, Medical University of South Carolina, Charleston, South Carolina

THOMAS W. RICE, MD
Professor of Surgery, Cleveland Clinic Lerner College of Medicine of Case Western Reserve University; The Daniel and Karen Lee Endowed Chair in Thoracic Surgery, Department of Thoracic and Cardiovascular Surgery, Heart and Vascular Institute, Cleveland Clinic, Cleveland, Ohio

J. KYLE RUSSO, MD
Department of Radiation Oncology, Medical University of South Carolina, Charleston, South Carolina

MANU SANCHETI, MD
Resident in Cardiothoracic Surgery, Division of Cardiothoracic Surgery, Emory University School of Medicine, Emory University Hospital, Atlanta, Georgia

SARTAJ S. SANGHERA, MD
Fellow and Assistant Clinical Instructor, Department of Surgical Oncology, Roswell Park Cancer Institute, University at Buffalo, Buffalo, New York

MICHAEL SMITH, MD
Heart and Lung Institute, St. Joseph's Hospital and Medical Center, Phoenix, Arizona

BRENDON M. STILES, MD
Assistant Professor of Cardiothoracic Surgery, Weill Cornell Medical College, New York-Presbyterian Hospital, New York, New York

ROBERT K. THOMPSON, MD
Division of Cardiothoracic Surgery, Medical University of South Carolina, Charleston, South Carolina

DHAVAL TRIVEDI, MD
Assistant Professor of Cardiothoracic Surgery, Department of Cardiothoracic Surgery, University of Pittsburgh Medical Center, Pittsburgh, Pennsylvania

VICTOR VAN BERKEL, MD, PhD
Assistant Professor, Division of Cardiothoracic Surgery, Department of Surgery, School of Medicine, University of Louisville, Louisville, Kentucky

JASON B. WHEELER, MD, MSCR
Department of Surgery, Medical University of South Carolina, Charleston, South Carolina

Contents

Foreword: Contemporary Management of Esophageal Malignancy   xiii

Ronald F. Martin

Preface: Contemporary Management of Esophageal Malignancy   xvii

Chadrick E. Denlinger and Carolyn E. Reed

Epidemiology of Esophageal Cancer   1077

Jason B. Wheeler and Carolyn E. Reed

This article discusses the incidence, geographic differences, and risk factors for the 2 most common cancers of the esophagus: squamous cell and adenocarcinoma.

Molecular Basis of Esophageal Cancer Development and Progression   1089

Chadrick E. Denlinger and Robert K. Thompson

This article discusses the molecular basis of esophageal cancer development and subsequent progression of disease. Differing epidemiologic factors are associated with esophageal adenocarcinoma and squamous cell carcinoma. These 2 different histologic types have differing putative underlying mechanisms of transdifferentiation from normal esophageal mucosa to malignant histologies via gene dysregulation, biochemical modifications, and altered cell signaling pathways. Our developing understanding of the molecular events underlying esophageal cancer is leading to the establishment of identifiable biomarkers and the clinical use of molecularly targeted treatment agents. The identification of driving genetic mutations and altered signaling pathways has also had favorable outcomes.

Diagnosis and Staging of Cancer of the Esophagus and Esophagogastric Junction   1105

Zhigang Li and Thomas W. Rice

Esophageal/esophagogastric junction cancer staging in the 7th edition of the AJCC staging manual is data driven and harmonized with gastric staging. New definitions are Tis, T4, regional lymph node, N, and M. Nonanatomic characteristics (histopathologic cell type, histologic grade, cancer location) and TNM classifications determine stage groupings. Classifications before treatment define clinical stage (cTNM or ycTNM). Current best clinical staging modalities include endoscopic ultrasonography for T and N and CT/PET for M. Classifications at resection define pathologic stage (pTNM or ypTNM). Accurate pathologic stage requires communication/cooperation between surgeon and pathologist. Classifications are defined at retreatment (rTNM) and autopsy (aTNM).

Medical Evaluation of Patients Preparing for an Esophagectomy   1127

Samad Hashimi and Michael Smith

Despite important improvements in the multimodal treatment of upper gastrointestinal tumors in recent years, surgery is still the standard of care and the best way to cure and palliate patients with esophageal cancer. There has been significant improvement in both clinical oncologic staging and functional preoperative evaluation of patients in the last few decades. Despite improvements, esophagectomy is still associated with high operative risk. Diligent perioperative evaluation and risk stratification lead to better outcomes.

Diagnosis and Management of Barrett's Esophagus   1135

Eric M. Nelsen, Robert H. Hawes, and Prasad G. Iyer

Barrett esophagus is characterized by the replacement of squamous mucosa in the esophagus by specialized intestinal metaplasia. Its clinical significance lies in it being the strongest risk factor for and known precursor for esophageal adenocarcinoma. Diagnosis requires endoscopic confirmation of columnar metaplasia in the distal esophagus and histologic confirmation of specialized intestinal metaplasia. Recommendations for the management of subjects diagnosed with Barrett esophagus include periodic endoscopic surveillance to detect the development of high-grade dysplasia or adenocarcinoma. Careful endoscopic evaluation with high-resolution endoscopy and endoscopic resection is recommended in the evaluation of subjects with high-grade dysplasia and early adenocarcinoma.

Management of Stage 1 Esophageal Cancer   1155

Michael Hermansson and Steven R. DeMeester

Barrett esophagus surveillance programs and more liberal use of upper endoscopy are leading to the identification of more patients with high-grade dysplasia or early stage esophageal adenocarcinoma. These patients have several options for therapy, including endoscopic mucosal resection, vagal-sparing esophagectomy, and a combination of endoscopic resection and ablation. Factors that should be considered include the length of the Barrett segment, the presence of a nodule or ulcer within the Barrett segment, and the age and overall physical condition of the patient. Of particular importance will be the incidence of recurrent Barrett esophagus or cancer in the long-term in patients that were initially successfully treated endoscopically.

Management of T2 Esophageal Cancer   1169

Manu Sancheti and Felix Fernandez

Patients with clinically staged T2N0 esophageal cancer are a small subset of patients for whom therapy is not standardized. Current clinical staging modalities are lacking in providing accurate staging for the presumed T2N0 subset. Problems with overstaging and understaging can each have adverse consequences for the patient. Furthermore, the benefit of induction therapy versus esophagectomy followed by adjuvant therapy for upstaged patients is unproven. The management of this challenging group of patients is reviewed.

Management of Advanced-Stage Operable Esophageal Cancer   1179

Ankit Bharat and Traves Crabtree

The incidence of esophageal cancer is increasing in the developed world, with a relative increase in adenocarcinoma compared with squamous cell carcinoma. The distensible nature of the esophagus results in delayed development of symptoms associated with esophageal cancer; hence many patients have locally advanced or metastatic cancer at the time of initial presentation. Although resection remains the treatment of choice for early-stage esophageal cancer, the best treatment strategy for locally advanced esophageal cancer is debatable and, consequently, varies at different centers. This article discusses the published literature on various available therapeutic options for the treatment of locally advanced esophageal cancer.

Management of Gastroesophageal Junction Tumors

Matthew P. Fox and Victor van Berkel

1199

Tumors of the gastroesophageal junction have historically been treated as either gastric or esophageal cancer depending on institutional preferences. The Siewert classification system was designed to provide a more precise means of characterizing these tumors. In general, surgical treatment of Siewert 1 tumors is via esophagectomy. Siewert 2 and 3 tumors may be treated with either esophagectomy with proximal gastrectomy or extended total gastrectomy provided negative margins are obtained. All but the earliest stage tumors should be considered for neoadjuvant chemoradiotherapy.

Definitive Chemoradiotherapy for Esophageal Carcinoma

S. Lewis Cooper, J. Kyle Russo, and Steve Chin

1213

Radiation therapy plays an important role in the treatment of esophageal cancer. Radiation therapy may be combined with chemotherapy, used as a component of induction therapy, used in the adjuvant setting, or used for palliation of advanced disease. Chemotherapy is also occasionally used as a solitary treatment modality for patients with esophageal cancer. Current treatment protocols include multiple agents, and agents directed against specific molecular targets have been investigated in clinical trials. This article discusses future directions related to the selection of radiation treatment protocols, novel targeted chemotherapeutic agents, and the selection of patients for surgery.

Traditional Techniques of Esophagectomy

Brendon M. Stiles and Nasser K. Altorki

1249

Several well described and accepted traditional techniques exist for the performance of an open esophagectomy. The rationale for selecting one of these techniques is determined by the location and histology of the disease being treated and surgeon and institutional preferences. Large retrospective studies and a limited number of prospective studies have comparatively evaluated the operative and long-term oncologic outcomes of transthoracic versus transhiatal surgical approaches, which indicate trends toward higher perioperative complications but improved long-term outcomes among patients treated with a transthoracic approach. Other retrospective studies investigated the extent of a thoracic lympadenectomy that is necessary at the time of an esophagectomy to optimize survival.

Minimally Invasive Esophagectomy   1265

Ryan M. Levy, Dhaval Trivedi, and James D. Luketich

> Minimally invasive esophagectomy (MIE) has become an established approach for the treatment of esophageal carcinoma. In comparison with open esophagectomy MIE reduces blood loss, respiratory complications, and length of hospital stay. At the University of Pittsburgh, the authors now predominantly perform a laparoscopic-thoracoscopic Ivor Lewis esophagectomy. This article details this technique, discusses the recently published series of more than 1000 esophagectomies performed by the authors during the last 15 years, and reviews the current literature on MIE.

Esophageal Reconstruction with Alternative Conduits   1287

Jenifer L. Marks and Wayne L. Hofstetter

> Alternative conduits for esophageal replacement become necessary when the stomach is unavailable for use. Common options for conduit creation include the jejunum and the colon. Prior abdominal operations, inflammatory bowel disease, or other mesenteric or abdominal disorders may limit use of either organ and a thorough history is essential when planning for alternative reconstruction. Most often the jejunum is free of intrinsic disease and provides a long segment for esophageal replacement. Limitations on the length of conduit that can be constructed with the jejunum have largely been overcome. A colonic conduit can also provide adequate length to reach the neck.

Complications of Esophagectomy   1299

Daniel Raymond

> Esophagectomy remains the gold standard curative therapy for the treatment of esophageal cancer. Despite 125 years of evolution, esophagectomy remains a demanding procedure associated with a 5% to 10% mortality and a 50% morbidity rate. Knowledge of the multitude of techniques possible for performing this complex procedure, as well as the host of associated complications, is vital for the practitioner aspiring to treat this challenging disease.

Quality of Life After an Esophagectomy   1315

Sartaj S. Sanghera, Steven J. Nurkin, and Todd L. Demmy

> Specialized centers have reduced the adverse outcomes associated with esophagectomy in the last 2 decades and now report operative mortalities of less than 5%. With the expanding use of screening endoscopy, early invasive esophageal adenocarcinoma is diagnosed more commonly. As a result, more patients enjoy long-term survival after curative resection. Simultaneously, emerging evidence supports the equivalence of competing endoscopic therapies for treatment of very early cancers and benign diseases. Accordingly, surgical resection requires re-evaluation using enhanced parameters to enable more meaningful comparative outcome analyses. This article summarizes the current evidence and examines future directions regarding esophagectomy quality of life.

Palliative Therapy for Patients with Unresectable Esophageal Carcinoma   **1337**

Richard K. Freeman, Anthony J. Ascioti, and Raja J. Mahidhara

Most patients diagnosed with carcinoma of the esophagus do not undergo therapy with curative intent. The focus of treatment for these patients is to maximize their progression-free survival and palliate the most common sequelae of their disease: dysphagia, malnutrition, pain, and intraluminal tumor bleeding. This article discusses the available treatment options for palliation of patients with unresectable esophageal cancer.

Index   **1353**

SURGICAL CLINICS
OF NORTH AMERICA

FORTHCOMING ISSUES

December 2012
Surgical Critical Care
John A. Weigelt, MD, DVM, MMA,
Guest Editor

February 2013
**Complications, Considerations and
Consequences of Colorectal Surgery**
Scott R. Steele, MD, *Guest Editor*

April 2013
**Surgeon's Role in Multidisciplinary Breast
Management**
George M. Fuhrman, MD, and
Tari A. King, MD, *Guest Editors*

June 2013
Pancreatic Surgery
Stephen W. Behrman, MD, FACS, and
Ronald F. Martin, MD, FACS, *Guest Editors*

RECENT ISSUES

August 2012
**Recent Advances and Future Directions in
Trauma Care**
Jeremy W. Cannon, MD, SM, *Guest Editor*

June 2012
Pediatric Surgery
Kenneth S. Azarow, MD, and
Robert A. Cusick, MD, *Guest Editors*

April 2012
**Management of Peri-operative
Complications**
Lewis J. Kaplan, MD, and
Stanley H. Rosenbaum, MD, *Guest Editors*

February 2012
Patient Safety
Juan A. Sanchez, MD, MPA, FACS,
Guest Editor

ISSUE OF RELATED INTEREST

Otolaryngology Clinics August 2012 (Vol. 45, Issue 4)
HPV and Head and Neck Cancer
Sara Pai, MD, *Guest Editor*

DOWNLOAD
Free App!

Review Articles
THE CLINICS

NOW AVAILABLE FOR YOUR iPhone and iPad

Foreword

Contemporary Management of Esophageal Malignancy

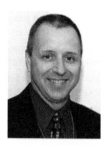

Ronald F. Martin, MD
Consulting Editor

I sometimes wonder how effectively we in medicine disseminate information. Usually, when I wonder this it has been prompted by some strained incredulity on my part that something that I thought should be commonly held knowledge is not. To be fair, I have no idea how many times in a day or month or year someone else feels similarly about my gaps in knowledge. It might even bruise my ego a bit to find out. Feelings put aside though, there remains a fundamental problem with how we disseminate, or fail to disseminate, information.

The *Surgical Clinics of North America* has long been a resource for compiled information for nearly a century now. I have had the privilege of serving as its Consulting Editor since 2004. One of the first issues distributed during my tenure was an issue on esophageal surgery. This current volume is on the same topic but with a slightly different perspective. A great deal of progress has been made since we published the prior issue in 2005 and that progress is excellently captured by Drs Denlinger and Reed and their colleagues. I am optimistic that this volume will serve as a valuable resource for surgeons and other physicians alike. What concerns me though is that some of the information from even the previous volume is still not among the common working knowledge of many.

I suspect there are a multitude of reasons for this: continued specialization to a very narrow range of practice, a generalized increase in desire for "just-in-time" information, a decreased sense of ownership of some patient problems by some physicians, and perhaps a general sense that the information torrent is just too overwhelming to absorb. While I happen to believe that most of those reasons are closer to excuses than explanations, I would bet that I am in the minority opinion on that score.

The reality appears to be that we have fractured health care into discordant elements and there are very few physicians left who feel compelled to desire a comprehensive base set of knowledge. The team approach to medical care has allowed for many to perform a narrow function in the hopes that another team member either

Surg Clin N Am 92 (2012) xiii–xv
http://dx.doi.org/10.1016/j.suc.2012.08.019
0039-6109/12/$ – see front matter © 2012 Elsevier Inc. All rights reserved.

surgical.theclinics.com

will know the other bits of information or will at least take responsibility for finding someone who does know. We have seen this in both the inpatient and the outpatient settings and we have seen this in surgical and nonsurgical disciplines alike.

As I try to understand this process, I keep coming back to the difficulties we collectively, and I would add ironically, have with loss of individual autonomy. It seems the more we try to get physicians to follow guidelines, pathways, processes, algorithms, managed schedules, and managed financial arrangements, the more physicians seem to find a way to limit themselves and reimpose their autonomy by restricting what they will and won't accept responsibility for knowing or doing. This manifests itself by restricting schedules, transferring patients for problems that used to be considered "bread and butter" surgery, obstructing or refusing to accept patients in transfer that used to be welcomed referrals, or decreeing that every problem encountered "belongs" to some other specialty—the last bit occurring more frequently on nights and weekends.

The organization I work for, like many others, struggles mightily with all the above-mentioned problems. If I had a solution, the next volume we produced would be called "The Book of Solutions for Truly Vexing Problems in Health Care," but I don't have those solutions. Sorry. My suspicion is that will take an actual or quasi-existential threat for us to change.

It has been said that as goes General Motors so goes the United States. A number of years ago I referenced that aphorism in a foreword written before what looked like an imminent General Motors collapse and I was hoping it were an untruth. Today, I think I hope it is true. I don't harbor strong feelings one way or another about General Motors. Yet, there may still be an example for us to consider. General Motors appeared to exude an almost irrational arrogance about its future. Faced with significant competition, increasing costs of production and delivery, profound uncertainty as to the costs and availability of fossil fuels for consumers, loss of perceived position in the marketplace, legacy costs to employees, and the costs of paying for health care to those for whom it was responsible—they changed almost nothing. At best they rearranged the deck chairs on the Titanic. It wasn't until the housing market collapse and the subsequent global financial collapse that they found out something very disturbing—durable goods are durable. The cars they made could go a few more years before *needing* to be replaced. The consumer demand for their product could be put on hold for a relatively short while and, figuratively speaking, the wheels would come off the auto industry. Fortunately for General Motors they endured the pain, accepted needed help, revised their mission, reviewed not just the desires of their customers but their needs, and probably came through things as a stronger though humbler company with a better chance of continued survival.

In my opinion, many of the same issues that faced the automotive companies face medicine writ large. Patients and other consumers tell us we are arrogant and that we cost too much. Also, as they shift to higher deductible plans and more out-of-pocket expenses, they are willing to defer maintenance (that may not work out as well for humans as it did for autos in the long run). The biggest difference between medicine as an industry and the auto industry during the recent financial troubles is that along with the banks, the industry of medicine in the United States was too big to fail. We kept the economy on life support by keeping people on life support. Now we need to change. We need to reassess the needs of individual patients and of communities. We need to reduce our cost structure and demand the same from our partners in hospitals, industry, pharma, and insurance companies. We need to explain better to our patients and those who pay their bills why we are spending their money. In short, we need to have a better knowledge of the big picture and we need to take greater ownership of the problems for which we are, or at least should be, best suited to give advice. We need to disseminate quality information that allows us to minimize unjustifiable variation. We need to put the value to and for the patients first.

To do that, we need quality information in a usable format. *Surgical Clinics of North America* will continue to try its best by getting the best people putting the best content we can find in the best context we can in a usable format. We physicians and surgeons as leaders also need to work to find ways to challenge ourselves to stop carrying on business as usual and work to incorporate new ideas into our daily lives. That will require a compromise of our autonomy to some degree—and that will come hard to many physicians.

I was listening to the radio the other night on my way home. The person being interviewed was one of our surgical colleagues, Dr Atul Gawande. He was discussing how a national chain restaurant reconfigured its menu and was achieving not just good but consistent results across the nation with its new offerings. I can't say that I agree with him on the choice of eatery but the ideas expressed in the interview were spot-on. The people who worked in those restaurants were being given standards, held to those standards, and provided with the means to meet those standards. If car builders and cheesecake builders can change to survive and improve under new conditions, one would think that we in medicine could as well.

Ronald F. Martin, MD
Department of Surgery
Marshfield Clinic
1000 North Oak Avenue
Marshfield, WI 54449, USA

E-mail address:
martin.ronald@marshfieldclinic.org

Preface

Contemporary Management of Esophageal Malignancy

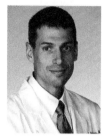 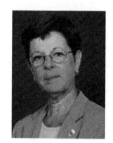

Chadrick E. Denlinger, MD   Carolyn E. Reed, MD
Guest Editors

In this issue of *Surgery Clinics of North America*, we explore a topic that has undergone an impressive evolution in the past several years that will likely continue for the foreseeable future. There has been a dramatic shift in the incidence of the 2 primary histological subtypes of esophageal cancer, with the incidence of adenocarcinoma rising at least 4-fold in the past 3 decades. Ongoing investigations are seeking to determine the reasons for this dramatic increase. Collectively, we are gaining a better understanding of the molecular events underlying the progression from normal esophageal mucosa to malignant growth. These studies may eventually indicate the precise reasons for the observed differences in disease occurrence and provide direction for novel therapies.

The greatest recent changes in the management of esophageal diseases relate to the treatment of Barrett's esophagus and early stage esophageal cancers. These changes are the result of an improved esophageal staging system discussed by Dr. Rice, who has played an instrumental role in the development of the most recent AJCC staging manual for esophageal cancers. The subdivision of the mucosa and submucosa of the esophagus into 6 separate strata in the new staging system correlates with the risk of regional lymph node metastases. As the result of our improved understanding of the risks for metastases, combined with the known immediate and long-term risks associated with an esophagectomy, novel therapies have become available and acceptable for the treatment of Barrett's esophagitis and early stage esophageal cancers. The management options and indications for early stage diseases are discussed in articles 5 and 6 of this publication. The decision to recommend a less invasive therapy other than an esophagectomy must be considered in the context of the overall medical condition of the patient and the risks associated with both endoscopic and surgical therapies. An emerging role for minimally invasive esophagectomy is also discussed by Dr. Luketich, who is one of the nation's pioneers

Surg Clin N Am 92 (2012) xvii–xviii
http://dx.doi.org/10.1016/j.suc.2012.08.002
0039-6109/12/$ – see front matter © 2012 Elsevier Inc. All rights reserved.

surgical.theclinics.com

in the development of this operation, which has at least equivalent oncologic outcomes and a lower incidence of perioperative complications.

Patients with more advanced stages of esophageal cancer are traditionally treated with induction chemotherapy and radiation followed by surgical resection. There are several areas of controversy related to the management of advanced diseases. Our current inability to stage T2 tumors reliably prior to surgery contributes to differing opinions of whether T2N0 tumors are best treated surgically with or without chemotherapy or if they should be treated with neoadjuvant chemotherapy and radiation followed by surgical resection. Another area of controversy regards the management of tumors located at the gastroesophageal junction and whether these tumors should be treated as esophageal cancers or as gastric cancers. Differences in the management of these 2 diseases include the use of neoadjuvant chemotherapy with or without the addition of radiation, the extent of resection, and regional lymph nodes excised. Separate articles discussing the management of T2 tumors and gastroesophageal junction tumors are included in this text to highlight their importance and to provide a balanced review of the controversy.

Finally, many patients present with advanced diseases and only palliative treatments are appropriate. The final article of this text discusses palliative treatment options available to improve the quality of life for patients suffering from advanced disease. The guest editors of this text hope that you enjoy reading this work and that you find it to be a useful reference as you treat patients with esophageal malignancies in your practice.

Chadrick E. Denlinger, MD
Assistant Professor of Surgery
Division of Cardiothoracic Surgery
Surgical Director
Lung Transplant Program
Medical University of South Carolina
25 Courtenay Drive, Suite 7018
Charleston, SC 29425, USA

Carolyn E. Reed, MD
Professor of Surgery
Division of Cardiothoracic Surgery
Medical University of South Carolina
25 Courtenay Drive, Suite 7024
Charleston, SC 29425, USA

E-mail addresses:
denlinge@musc.edu (C.E. Denlinger)
reedce@musc.edu (C.E. Reed)

Epidemiology of Esophageal Cancer

Jason B. Wheeler, MD, MSCR, Carolyn E. Reed, MD*

KEYWORDS

- Epidemiology squamous cell carcinoma of the esophagus
- Epidemiology adenocarcinoma of the esophagus
- Risk factors for esophageal cancer

KEY POINTS

- Esophageal cancer is the eighth most common cancer worldwide; 484,000 new cases were diagnosed in 2008.
- Adenocarcinoma is predominantly a disease of Western Europe, Australia, and North America; squamous cell carcinoma predominates in Southeastern Africa, Southern Russia, and Asia.
- Esophageal adenocarcinoma is predominantly a cancer of white males in the Western world.
- The incidence of adenocarcinoma of the esophagus in the United States increased sevenfold between 1973 (3.6 cases per million) and 2006 (25.6 per million); however, from 1996 to 2006, the annual increase declined from 8.2% to 1.3%.
- The incidence of squamous cell carcinoma in the United States is decreasing, but this histology remains the most common in black males.

INTRODUCTION

This article will discusses the epidemiology of the most common cancers of the esophagus: squamous cell carcinoma and adenocarcinoma. Although the treatment for these 2 histologies is often the same, the epidemiology is quite different. Although an oversimplification, the obese white male with reflux typical of adenocarcinoma contrasted with the poorly nourished African American male smoker with a history of alcohol abuse typical of squamous cell carcinoma, emphasizes this disparity. The differences are highlighted in **Table 1**. As more is learned about the molecular characteristics of the 2 histologies, it is hoped that preventive strategies (avoidance or manipulation of risk factors) and ultimately treatment will be more tailored.

Incidence and Geographic Considerations

Esophageal cancer is the eighth most common cancer worldwide; 484,000 new cases were diagnosed in 2008.[1] Adenocarcinoma is predominantly a disease of Western

Department of Surgery, Medical University of South Carolina, 25 Courtenay Drive, Charleston, SC 29425, USA
* Corresponding author.
E-mail address: reedce@musc.edu

Surg Clin N Am 92 (2012) 1077–1087
http://dx.doi.org/10.1016/j.suc.2012.07.008
0039-6109/12/$ – see front matter © 2012 Elsevier Inc. All rights reserved.

Table 1
Risk factors for squamous cell carcinoma and adenocarcinoma of the esophagus

Risk Factor	Squamous Cell Carcinoma	Adenocarcinoma
Geography	Southeastern Africa, Iran, Asia	Western Europe, North America
Race	B > W	W > B
Gender	M > F	M > F
Alcohol	↑↑↑↑	–
Tobacco	↑↑↑↑	↑↑
Obesity	–	↑↑↑
GERD	–	↑↑↑↑
Diet		
Low fruits and vegetables	↑↑	↑↑
Pickled vegetables	↑↑	–
Hot beverages	↑↑	–
Socioeconomic conditions	Low, nonurban	High, urban, industrialized

Abbreviations: B, black; F, female; GERD, gastroesophageal reflux disease; M, male; W, white; ↑, associated risk; –, no risk associated.

Europe, Australia, and North America. Squamous cell carcinoma predominates in southeastern Africa, and an area that extends from the border of the Caspian Sea and Turkey through the southern republics of the former Soviet Union and into northern China ("esophageal cancer belt"). There are focal "hot spots" of squamous cell carcinoma in industrialized countries, including northwestern France, Iceland, Scotland, and Finland, and in the United States in coastal South Carolina and metropolitan Washington, DC/Baltimore. In the squamous cell "esophageal cancer belt," the incidence rate in males reaches 23 per 100,000 and about 16 per 100,000 in females. For males in South Africa, the rate reaches 23.6.[1]

The incidence of adenocarcinoma of the esophagus in the United States increased sevenfold between 1973 (3.6 cases per million) and 2006 (25.6 per million); however, from 1996 to 2006, the annual increase declined from 8.2% to 1.3%.[2] Whether the incidence of adenocarcinoma has peaked will require further observation. Both detection bias and misclassification bias could account for part of the rising incidence of adenocarcinoma in the United States; however, careful review supports a true increase in occurrence.[3] Although adenocarcinoma has the fastest increasing incidence of any solid tumor in the United States for the past 30 years, the disease is still rare. An estimated 16,980 cases of esophageal cancer (including both squamous and adenocarcinoma) were diagnosed in 2011.[4]

The incidence of squamous cell carcinoma in the United States is decreasing, but this histology remains the most common in black males. The incidence trends in US males are shown in (**Fig. 1**).[5] Worldwide squamous cell cancer is the most common histology, reaching 90% in the "esophageal cancer belt."

Squamous Cell Carcinoma

Race and gender
The incidence of squamous cell carcinoma is higher in males than females in most countries and higher in black men than white men in the United States. The incidence of squamous cell carcinoma in the United States peaked in the 1970s and early 1980s

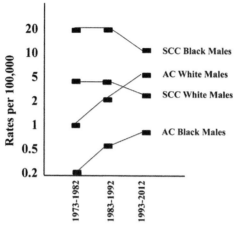

Fig. 1. Esophageal cancer incidence trends in US males. AC, adenocarcinoma; SCC, squamous cell carcinoma. (*Data from* Holmes RS, Vaughan TL. Epidemiology and pathogenesis of esophageal cancer. Semin Radiat Oncol 2006;17:2–9.)

at about 21 per 100,000 and has decreased by more than 60% since then to 7.6 per 100,000 in 2002.[5] The disease incidence peaks in both males and females between 70 and 74 years of age. **Box 1** lists the major risk factors for squamous cell carcinoma.

Tobacco

The 2 major risk factors for squamous cell carcinoma in the United States are tobacco and alcohol. Case control studies have shown both independent and synergistic effects of alcohol and smoking. Smokers have a 5-fold higher risk than nonsmokers with excess risk increasing to nearly 10-fold among heavy cigarette smokers.[6] The risk of cancer decreases significantly within a decade of smoking cessation.

The major carcinogenic activity of tobacco smoke is contained in the tar fraction. The primary initiators are presumably the polynuclear aromatic hydrocarbons and volatile nitrosamines.

In other parts of the world, smoking is a less important risk factor. In a prospective study of risk factors for esophageal cancer in the Linxian province of China, smoking only modestly increased the risk of squamous cell carcinoma.[7] Dietary factors are much more important (discussed in a subsequent section). A study from Taiwan revealed an OR of 4.2 and 3.4 for current and former smokers, respectively, compared

Box 1
Squamous cell cancer risk factors

- Race and gender
- Tobacco
- Alcohol
- Diet and Nutrients
- Hereditary factors
- Preexisting conditions

with nonsmokers.[8] A positive dose response was found for both duration and intensity of tobacco consumption. In contrast to alcohol, duration rather than intensity of smoking was more important.

Alcohol

Alcohol consumption is a consistent risk factor for squamous cell carcinoma of the esophagus. The relative risk increases with the amount of alcohol consumed, being approximately 1.8 for 5 to 11 drinks per week and increasing to 7.4 for more than 30 drinks per week.[6] The mechanism of effect of alcohol is uncertain. Theories include its irritant effect on esophageal mucosa, role in increased susceptibility to other carcinogens, or its contribution to dietary deficiencies that could play a role in the development of squamous cell carcinoma.

As noted previously, alcohol has a synergistic effect with smoking on risk. Both intensity and duration of alcohol use effects risk, but unlike smoking, intensity is more important.

Drinking specific alcoholic beverages has been implicated in focal "hot spots" of esophageal squamous cell cancer: the intake of apple brandies in northern France, the consumption of maize beer in South African Transkei, the drinking of sugar-distilled beverages in Puerto Rico, and intake of moonshine whiskeys in South Carolina.[6] In the northern China "esophageal cancer belt," alcohol use is rare, and therefore, there is no significant risk association.

Diet and nutrients

Recurrent thermal injury to the esophageal mucosa caused by the consumption of large amounts of hot beverages has been consistently speculated to be a risk factor for squamous cell carcinoma. This potential causative factor would explain a large number of cases occurring in populations in which drinking tea, coffee, or maté (an herbal infusion of *Ilex paraguariensis*, commonly consumed in South American countries) and hot foods are common. In a systematic review of 59 studies,[9] most publications showed an increased risk of squamous cell carcinoma with higher drinking temperature. There was little evidence that the amount of coffee or tea (unrelated to temperature) had any significant risk. For maté drinking, the cancer risk was increased for both amount consumed and temperature. The investigators concluded that available studies strongly support an association between esophageal squamous cell carcinoma and high-temperature beverage drinking.

Foods containing N-nitroso compounds have long been implicated in the development of squamous cell carcinoma of the esophagus. In high-risk areas of China, pickled vegetables are a common food staple. Pickling allows the fermentation and growth of fungi and yeasts that can generate potentially carcinogenic N-nitroso compounds and mycotoxins. A meta-analysis suggested a twofold increased risk of cancer associated with the intake of pickled vegetables.[10] Nitrates and their conversion products are by-products of the smoking process for meats and fish that remains common in select populations worldwide.

Chewing betel quid, consisting of areca nut and other ingredients (sometimes including tobacco), is common is Southeast Asia and India and has been implicated in the development of esophageal squamous cell carcinoma. In Taiwan, where tobacco is not included in betel quid, the OR for current betel nut chewers versus never chewers was 2.3.[8] There was a positive dose response with duration and intensity of use.

In underdeveloped areas, vitamin and mineral deficiencies may play a role in the development of esophageal squamous cell carcinoma. Deficiencies in molybdenum, B-carotene, vitamin A, vitamin E, selenium, and zinc have all been implicated.[10]

Intake of both fruits and vegetables probably contributes to the risk of both squamous cell carcinoma and adenocarcinoma of the esophagus. Studies suggest that low intake of these 2 food groups after adjusting for smoking and alcohol consumption increase cancer risk twofold.[6]

Hereditary factors
Tylosis is a rare disorder associated with hyperkeratosis of the palms of the hands and soles of the feet and a high rate of squamous cell carcinoma of the esophagus. The inherited type of tylosis (Howell-Evans syndrome) is an autosomal dominant disease with a gene locus mapped to 17q 25.1.

Familial aggregation of esophageal cancer has been described in high-incidence regions such as China.[11]

Preexisting conditions
There are several preexisting conditions that increase the risk of developing squamous cell carcinoma of the esophagus. These include the following:

- Caustic injury[12]
- Achalasia[13]
- Current or past history of squamous cell carcinoma of the head and neck[14–17]
- Plummer Vinson syndrome[14]
- Zenker diverticulum[14]

Other possible risks
Low socioeconomic status is associated with a higher risk of squamous cell carcinoma of the esophagus.[7,18] Although a Swedish study[19] showed significant associations between esophageal squamous cell carcinoma and 3 occupational groups (concrete and construction [OR 2.2], food and tobacco processing [OR 5.1], and hotel and restaurant work OR 3.9]), a case-control study in the United States did not confirm these findings.[20]

Summary
It is clear that specific risk factors for squamous cell carcinoma of the esophagus vary widely in different parts of the world. In the United States, it has been estimated that a history of smoking, alcohol consumption, and diets low in fruits and vegetables account for almost 90% of cases.[21] Major risk factors in the "esophageal cancer belt" of Iran and Asia remain less well understood **Box 2**.

Adenocarcinoma

Gender, race, and age
The incidence of esophageal adenocarcinoma is 8 times higher in males than females and 5 times higher in white males than black males in the United States.[22] As mentioned previously, adenocarcinoma has the fastest increasing incidence of any solid tumor in the United States, and this increase has occurred predominantly in white males.[23]

Box 2
Squamous cell cancer summary

- Risk factors vary worldwide
- Tobacco, alcohol consumption, and diet low in fruits and vegetable account for 90% of US cases
- Factors in the "esophageal cancer belt" are not well understood

Adenocarcinoma, rather than squamous cell carcinoma, is now the major histologic type of esophageal cancer in the United States. It is not known what factors have contributed to the alarming increase of this emerging disease. Adenocarcinomas, either in the distal esophagus or at the gastroesophageal junction (GEJ), generally affect patients older than 50 years, with the peak between 55 and 65 years (**Box 3**).[24]

Gastroesophageal reflux disease

Gastroesophageal reflux is a key mechanism of esophageal mucosal inflammation. The prevalence of gastroesophageal reflux disease (GERD) in the Western world is 10% to 20%: approximately 30 to 60 million people in the United States.[25] GERD is the strongest individual risk factor for both esophageal adenocarcinoma and Barrett's esophagus (BE), a precursor lesion of adenocarcinoma. Several risk factors exist for GERD, including family history, hiatal hernia, diet, and obesity. Gender is not a risk factor for GERD. GERD is equally, if not more, prevalent in blacks than whites in the United States.[25]

Reflux symptoms were associated with adenocarcinoma risk (OR 7.7) in a large Swedish case control study.[26] The risk was greatest in those with more than 20 years of severe reflux symptoms (OR 43.5). Adenocarcinoma risk is associated with symptom frequency (sevenfold for daily vs fivefold for weekly).[27] Oddly, it has been reported that more than 50% of adenocarcinoma cases have no symptomatic reflux history.[28] Thus, whereas reflux plays a major role in the development of adenocarcinoma, other etiologic factors demand further attention and research.

Barrett's esophagus

Most adenocarcinomas arise from a region of Barrett's metaplasia. BE occurs as an adaptive response to injury from refluxed acid and bile, as intestinal columnar epithelium is protected by mucus secretion.[29] The increase in BE incidence over the past 30 years parallels that seen with adenocarcinoma. BE develops in 6.0% to 14.0% of individuals with GERD, and approximately 0.5% to 1.0% of patients with BE develop adenocarcinoma.[30] Relative to the general population, BE increases adenocarcinoma risk 30-fold, and the presence of BE is associated with a 0.12% annual risk of developing adenocarcinoma.[31] BE, which is most commonly attributable to GERD, is therefore the most important risk factor for adenocarcinoma.

Obesity

Obesity, which has been linked by several studies to adenocarcinoma of the esophagus, is rapidly increasing in the United States. By 2015, it is estimated that 75% of

---

Box 3
Adenocarcinoma risk factors

- White race and male gender
- Gastroesophageal reflux disease/Barrett's esophagus
- Obesity
- Smoking
- Diet and nutrients
- Absence of *Helicobacter pylori*
- Lower esophageal sphincter tone lowering agents
- Hereditary factors
- Preexisting conditions

US adults will be at least overweight, with 41% being obese.[32] Given rising obesity rates, it is reasonable to expect that obesity-associated comorbidities, like adenocarcinoma, will also continue to increase.

ORs increase for adenocarcinoma beginning at a body mass index (BMI) of 25, the upper limit of normal, and increase with BMI. Pooled adjusted ORs from a meta-analysis of 8 studies showed those with a BMI of 25 to 30 had an OR of 1.52 and 2.00 for BMI of greater than 30 or an OR of 2.78, respectively, compared with normal BMI.[33]

Interestingly, obesity-associated adenocarcinoma risk was found to be higher among men than women (OR 2.6 vs 1.4).[34] This may explain some of the gender disparity associated with adenocarcinoma. Those with obesity and reflux had significantly higher risk of adenocarcinoma (OR 16.5) than obesity without reflux (OR 2.2) and reflux without obesity (OR 5.6), suggesting a synergism between obesity and reflux.

Central adiposity is more strongly associated with adenocarcinoma than BMI. Central adiposity is thought to contribute to GERD and thus BE by compressing the stomach and increasing hiatal hernias.[35]

Tobacco and alcohol

Similar to squamous cell carcinoma, several studies have reported that smoking is a risk factor for adenocarcinoma, especially in the presence of BE. Adenocarcinoma risk appears to double with ever smoking and appears dose dependent.[36,37] Smoking cessation reduces this risk, but it does not return to the level of those who have never smoked.

In contrast to squamous cell carcinoma, alcohol consumption has not been found to be associated with adenocarcinoma in population-based studies. In fact, consumption of wine may even be protective (OR 0.6), whereas consumption of liquor or beer was unrelated in a large population-based study.[38]

Diet and nutrients

Diets high in fiber, antioxidants, fruits, and vegetables have been associated with a decreased risk of adenocarcinoma, whereas high protein and cholesterol diets have been associated with an increased risk of adenocarcinoma.[39–41] A Swedish population-based study found an inverse association between total dietary cereal fiber intake and gastric cardia adenocarcinoma risk (OR 0.3 for the highest vs lowest quartile).[39] An American case-control study also found that diets high in vitamins, fruits, and vegetables were protective against BE.[41]

Dietary nitroso compounds have been associated with carcinogenesis. A mechanism for nitrosative stress-inducing adenocarcinoma development has been proposed and supported by in vitro, animal model, and human studies. The mechanisms of nitrosative stress and their attributable risks for esophageal adenocarcinoma are poorly understood.[42]

Absence of Helicobacter pylori infection

Helicobacter pylori infection of the stomach reduces gastric acid secretion. The absence of *H pylori* infection may be a risk factor for adenocarcinoma, although conflicting studies exist. Significant inverse associations were found between the presence of *H pylori* infection and adenocarcinoma (OR 0.52) and BE (OR 0.64), suggesting a protective role for *H pylori* in contrast to its carcinogenic role in malignancies of the stomach.[43]

Use of nonsteroidal anti-inflammatory drugs, proton pump inhibitors, and statins

Chronic inflammation predisposes to the development of gastrointestinal malignancies. Data from several studies suggest that aspirin and other nonsteroidal

---

Box 4
Adenocarcinoma summary

- Primarily a cancer of white males in Western world
- Reasons for this gender and race disparity are not well understood
- Reflux, obesity, smoking, and diet low in fruits and vegetable account for 80% of US cases
- Prevention and early detection are goals for clinicians

---

anti-inflammatory drugs (NSAIDs), which inhibit cyclo-oxygenase (COX) enzymes and reduce inflammation, might protect against the development of esophageal adenocarcinoma, particularly in the setting of BE.[44] However, results from one clinical trial did not find COX-2 inhibitors useful in preventing the progression from BE to adenocarcinoma.[45] A large observational study found that the use of NSAIDs, proton pump inhibitors, and statins in patients with BE was associated with a reduced progression to adenocarcinoma.[46]

Use of drugs decreasing lower esophageal sphincter tone
Decreasing the tone of the lower esophageal sphincter (LES) may contribute to increased acid exposure of the distal esophagus. Therefore, medications that may lower LES pressure may contribute to the development of BE and adenocarcinoma. A case-control study found that prior use of drugs known to relax the LES (eg, nitroglycerin, anticholinergics, beta agonists, and benzodiazepines) for more than 5 years increased the risk of esophageal adenocarcinoma (OR 3.8).[47] This association may account for up to 10% of adenocarcinomas occurring in men older than 60.

Hereditary factors
Inherited polymorphisms of the epidermal growth factor (EGF) gene causing increased serum EGF have been associated with increased adenocarcinoma risk, especially in patients with BE.[48]

In addition to the previously discussed BE risk factors, BE also aggregates in families. Familial BE can be confirmed in 7.3% of persons presenting with BE or adenocarcinoma of the distal esophagus or GEJ.[49] A first-degree or second-degree relative with BE or adenocarcinoma of the distal esophagus or GEJ was significantly higher among case subjects compared with controls (OR 12.23).

Multiple endocrine neoplasia Type 1 is an autosomal dominant disorder associated with 25% of cases of Zollinger-Ellison syndrome, a gastric acid hypersecretory state secondary to gastrinoma. Increased acid exposure from this and other heritable conditions may increase risk for adenocarcinoma.

Preexisting conditions
Many preexisting conditions may increase the risk of developing esophageal adenocarcinoma secondary to increasing gastric acid production or increasing esophageal exposure to refluxed gastric acid or bile. These include the following:

- Myotomy or dilation of the LES
- Scleroderma
- Zollinger-Ellison syndrome
- Any condition requiring medications known to relax the LES

Summary
Esophageal adenocarcinoma is predominantly a cancer of white males in the Western world. Little is known about the causes of the significant racial and gender disparity

seen with this cancer. A history of a GERD/BE, BMI higher than the lowest quartile, smoking, and a diet low in fruits and vegetables accounts for almost 80% of cases of esophageal adenocarcinoma in the United States.[21]

Given the dismal survival rate of patients with esophageal adenocarcinoma with current therapies, prevention of this emerging disease is of paramount importance. A significant impact in the incidence of adenocarcinoma may be made through mitigating exposure to the previously mentioned major modifiable risk factors. Risk factor reduction and early detection should be the ultimate goals of clinicians (**Box 4**).

REFERENCES

1. Cancer Statistics, World Cancer Research Fund International. Available at: www. werf.org/cancer_statistics/index/php. Accessed August 12, 2012.
2. Pohl H, Sirovich B, Welch HG. Esophageal adenocarcinoma incidence: are we reaching the peak? Cancer Epidemiol Biomarkers Prev 2010;19:1468–70.
3. Wei JT, Shaheen NJ. The changing epidemiology of esophageal adenocarcinoma. Semin Gastrointest Dis 2003;14:112–27.
4. Sampliner RE, Gibson MK. Epidemiology, pathobiology, and clinical manifestations of esophageal cancer. Up To Date; 2011. Available at: www.uptodate.com. Accessed August 12, 2012.
5. Holmes RS, Vaughan TL. Epidemiology and pathogenesis of esophageal cancer. Semin Radiat Oncol 2006;17:2–9.
6. Blot WJ, McLaughlin JK. The changing epidemiology of esophageal cancer. Semin Oncol 1999;26:2–8.
7. Tran GD, Sun XD, Abnet CC, et al. Prospective study of risk factors for esophageal and gastric cancers in the Linxian general population trial cohort in China. Int J Cancer 2005;113:456–63.
8. Lee CH, Lee JM, Wu DC, et al. Independent and combined effects of alcohol intake, tobacco smoking and betel quid chewing on the risk of esophageal cancer in Taiwan. Int J Cancer 2005;113:475–82.
9. Islami F, Boffetta P, Ren JS, et al. High-temperature beverages and foods and esophageal cancer risk—a systematic review. Int J Cancer 2009;125:491–524.
10. Lukanich JM. Section I: epidemiologic review. Semin Thorac Cardiovasc Surg 2003;15:158–66.
11. Chang-Claude J, Becher H, Blettner M, et al. Familial aggregation of oesophageal cancer in a high incidence area in China. Int J Epidemiol 1997;26:1159–65.
12. Appelqvist P, Salmo M. Lye corrosion carcinomas of the esophagus: a review of 63 cases. Cancer 1980;45:2655–8.
13. Sandler RS, Nyrén O, Ekbom A, et al. The risk of esophageal cancer in patients with achalasia: a population-based study. J Am Med Assoc 1995;274:1359–62.
14. Ribeiro U, Rosner MC, Safatle-Ribeiro AV, et al. Risk factors for squamous cell carcinoma of the oesophagus. Br J Surg 1996;83:1174–85.
15. Cooper JS, Pajak TF, Rubin P, et al. Second malignancies in patients who have head and neck cancer: incidence, effect on survival and implications based on the RTOG experience. Int J Radiat Oncol Biol Phys 1989;17:449–56.
16. Erkal HS, Mendenhall WM, Amdur RJ, et al. Synchronous and metachronous squamous cell carcinomas of the head and neck mucosal sites. J Clin Oncol 2001;19:1358–62.
17. Muto M, Hironaka S, Nakane M, et al. Association of multiple Lugol-voiding lesions with synchronous and metachronous esophageal squamous cell

carcinoma in patients with head and neck cancer. Gastrointest Endosc 2002;56: 517–21.

18. Brown LM, Devesa SS. Epidemiologic trends in esophageal and gastric cancer in the United States. Surg Oncol Clin N Am 2002;11:235–56.

19. Jansson C, Plato N, Johansson AL, et al. Airborne occupational exposures and risk of oesophageal and cardia adenocarcinoma. Occup Environ Med 2006;63: 107–12.

20. Engel LS, Vaughan TL, Gammon MD, et al. Occupation and risk of esophageal and gastric cardia adenocarcinoma. Am J Ind Med 2002;42:11–22.

21. Engel LS, Chow WH, Vaughan TL, et al. Population attributable risks of esophageal and gastric cancers. J Natl Cancer Inst 2003;95:1404–13.

22. El-Serag HB, Mason AC, Petersen N, et al. Epidemiological differences between adenocarcinoma of the oesophagus and adenocarcinoma of the gastric cardia in the USA. Gut 2002;50:368–72.

23. Pera M, Manterola C, Vidal O, et al. Epidemiology of esophageal adenocarcinoma. J Surg Oncol 2005;92:151–9.

24. Pera M. Recent changes in the epidemiology of esophageal cancer. Surg Oncol 2001;10:81–90.

25. Dent J, El-Serag HB, Wallander MA, et al. Epidemiology of gastro-oesophageal reflux disease: a systematic review. Gut 2005;54:710–7.

26. Lagergren J, Bergström R, Lindgren A, et al. Symptomatic gastroesophageal reflux as a risk factor for esophageal adenocarcinoma. N Engl J Med 1999; 340:825–31.

27. Rubenstein JH, Taylor JB. Meta-analysis: the association of oesophageal adenocarcinoma with symptoms of gastro-oesophageal reflux. Aliment Pharmacol Ther 2010;32:1222–7.

28. Bytzer P, Christensen PB, Damkier P, et al. Adenocarcinoma of the esophagus and Barrett's esophagus: a population-based study. Am J Gastroenterol 1999; 94:86–91.

29. Shalauta MD, Saad R. Barrett's esophagus. Am Fam Physician 2004;69:2113–8.

30. Reynolds JC, Waronker M, Pacquing MS, et al. Barrett's esophagus: reducing the risk of progression to adenocarcinoma. Gastroenterol Clin North Am 1999;28: 917–45.

31. Hvid-Jensen F, Pedersen L, Drewes AM, et al. Incidence of adenocarcinoma among patients with Barrett's esophagus. N Engl J Med 2011;365:1375–83.

32. Wang Y, Beydoun MA. The obesity epidemic in the United States—gender, age, socioeconomic, racial/ethnic, and geographic characteristics: a systematic review and meta-regression analysis. Epidemiol Rev 2007;29:6–28.

33. Hampel H, Abraham NS, El-Serag HB. Meta-analysis: obesity and the risk for gastroesophageal reflux disease and its complications. Ann Intern Med 2005; 143:199–211.

34. Whiteman DC, Sadeghi S, Pandeya N, et al. Combined effects of obesity, acid reflux and smoking on the risk of adenocarcinomas of the oesophagus. Gut 2008;57:173–80.

35. Corley DA, Kubo A, Levin TR, et al. Abdominal obesity and body mass index as risk factors for Barrett's esophagus. Gastroenterologist 2007;133:34–41.

36. Gray MR, Donnelly RJ, Kingsnorth AN. The role of smoking and alcohol in metaplasia and cancer risk in Barrett's columnar lined oesophagus. Gut 1993;34: 727–31.

37. Cook MB, Kamangar F, Whiteman DC, et al. Cigarette smoking and adenocarcinoma of the esophagus and esophagogastric junction: a pooled analysis

from the international BEACON consortium. J Natl Cancer Inst 2010;102: 1344–53.
38. Anderson LA, Cantwell MM, Watson RG, et al. The association between alcohol and reflux esophagitis, Barrett's esophagus, and esophageal adenocarcinoma. Gastroenterologist 2009;136:799–805.
39. Terry P, Lagergren J, Ye W, et al. Inverse association between intake of cereal fiber and risk of gastric cardia cancer. Gastroenterologist 2001;120:387–91.
40. Mayne ST, Risch HA, Dubrow R, et al. Nutrient intake and risk of subtypes of esophageal and gastric cancer. Cancer Epidemiol Biomarkers Prev 2001;10: 1055–62.
41. Kubo A, Levin TR, Block G, et al. Dietary antioxidants, fruits, and vegetables and the risk of Barrett's esophagus. Am J Gastroenterol 2008;103:1614–23.
42. Iijima K, Grant J, McElroy K, et al. Novel mechanism of nitrosative stress from dietary nitrate with relevance to gastro-oesophageal junction cancers. Carcinogenesis 2003;24:1951–60.
43. Rokkas T, Pistiolas D, Sechopoulos P, et al. Relationship between *Helicobacter pylori* infection and esophageal neoplasia: a meta-analysis. Clin Gastroenterol Hepatol 2007;5:1413–7.
44. Anderson LA, Johnston BT, Watson RG, et al. Nonsteroidal anti-inflammatory drugs and the esophageal inflammation-metaplasia-adenocarcinoma sequence. Cancer Res 2006;66:4975–82.
45. Heath EI, Canto MI, Piantadosi S, et al. Secondary chemoprevention of Barrett's esophagus with celecoxib: results of a randomized trial. J Natl Cancer Inst 2007; 99:545–57.
46. Nguyen DM, Richardson P, El-Serag HB. Medications (NSAIDs, statins, proton pump inhibitors) and the risk of esophageal adenocarcinoma in patients with Barrett's esophagus. Gastroenterologist 2010;138:2260–6.
47. Lagergren J, Bergström R, Adami HO, et al. Association between medications that relax the lower esophageal sphincter and risk for esophageal adenocarcinoma. Ann Intern Med 2000;133:165–75.
48. Lanuti M, Liu G, Goodwin JM, et al. A functional epidermal growth factor (EGF) polymorphism, EGF serum levels, and esophageal adenocarcinoma risk and outcome. Clin Cancer Res 2008;14:3216–22.
49. Chak A, Ochs-Balcom H, Falk G, et al. Familiality in Barrett's esophagus, adenocarcinoma of the esophagus, and adenocarcinoma of the gastroesophageal junction. Cancer Epidemiol Biomarkers Prev 2006;15:1668–73.

Molecular Basis of Esophageal Cancer Development and Progression

Chadrick E. Denlinger, MD*, Robert K. Thompson, MD

KEYWORDS

- Esophageal cancer • Barrett esophagus • Adenocarcinoma
- Squamous cell carcinoma • Molecular biology • Targeted therapy

KEY POINTS

- Bile salts in an acidic environment promote esophageal mucosa dysplasia and progression to adenocarcinoma.
  - Bile salts upregulate the transcriptional activity of CDX-2 in an epidermal growth factor receptor (EGFR)-dependent manner.
  - CDX-2 promotes intestinal cell differentiation.
  - Bile salt promotes cellular proliferation of Barrett esophagus.
- Progression of Barrett esophagus to adenocarcinoma is associated with inflammation, cyclooxygenase 2 activation, and epigenetic modifications.
- The development of clinically relevant molecular targeted agents relates to their use in other forms of carcinoma rather than the current understanding of molecular events specific to esophageal carcinoma:
  - EGFR antibodies and tyrosine kinase inhibitors
  - Her2/neu inhibitors
  - Vascular endothelial growth factor antibodies
- Squamous cell cancers seem more sensitive to epithelial growth factor receptor inhibition than adenocarcinomas.
- Alcohol and smoking act synergistically to induce gene mutations and epigenetic modifications related to esophageal cancer initiation.

INTRODUCTION

This article is divided into 2 separate, but parallel, sections regarding the molecular mechanisms underlying the development and progression of esophageal neoplasms. Adenocarcinomas and squamous cell carcinomas are known to have differing risk

Division of Cardiothoracic Surgery, Medical University of South Carolina, 25 Courtenay Drive, Charleston, SC 29425, USA
* Corresponding author.
E-mail address: denlinge@musc.edu

Surg Clin N Am 92 (2012) 1089–1103
http://dx.doi.org/10.1016/j.suc.2012.07.002
0039-6109/12/$ – see front matter © 2012 Elsevier Inc. All rights reserved.

factors and characteristic demographic factors, suggesting that the molecular events that lead to each of these cancers are distinct. In addition, our developing understanding of the molecular biology of these diseases confirms this assumption. Therefore, the first section of the article describes the current understanding of molecular events leading to esophageal adenocarcinomas and the second section relates to the development of esophageal squamous cell carcinomas.

ADENOCARCINOMA
Epidemiology

The overall epidemiology of esophageal cancers is more thoroughly described elsewhere in this issue by Reed and colleagues. The incidence of esophageal adenocarcinoma has increased by 400% over the past decade, which is greater than any other malignancy in the same period. This phenomenon has been observed primarily in Western nations, whereas squamous cell cancers remain the predominant histology in most of Asia and other nations.

The most notable risk factors for adenocarcinoma are gastroesophageal (GE) acid and nonacid reflux, as well as obesity, which is a major contributing factor. Studies have shown that the presence of alkaline reflux and bilirubin were more strongly correlated with the presence of Barrett metaplasia than acid reflux.[1] In addition, the presence of Barrett esophagus and the use of proton pump inhibitors and other acid-suppressing medications are more common among populations afflicted with the rapidly increasing incidence of adenocarcinoma.

Barrett Esophagus

The development of Barrett esophagus is closely linked with chronic exposure to acid reflux. There are theoretically 2 possible pathway mechanisms through which squamous epithelium could undergo metaplasia and differentiate into intestinalized columnar epithelium. The first mechanism involves the transdifferentiation of mature squamous cells directly into intestinal cells. Alternatively, esophageal intestinal mucosal cells may be the result of altered differentiation of stem cells within the esophageal mucosa.[2] There are at least 4 putative origins of stem cells that develop into Barrett esophagus, each with their respective camps of supporters backed with experimental evidence. The 4 cellular origins are: (1) stem cells in the basal cell layer of squamous epithelium undergo de novo metaplasia, producing stem cells that differentiate into intestinal cells; (2) stem cells at the GE junction or transitional zone may colonize the distal esophagus in response to noxious stimuli, (3) stem cells in the neck of the esophageal submucosal gland ducts may colonize the esophagus after damage of the squamous cell epithelium; (4) bone marrow-derived stem cells may migrate to the esophagus in the presence of inflammation or damage and undergo metaplasia.

Barrett Esophagus by Transdifferentiation

The development of intestinalized epithelium from resident esophageal stem cells that normally produce squamous cells has been experimentally shown. Clinically derived evidence and in vitro studies suggest that the caudal related homeobox gene, CDX-2, is likely a significant causative factor in the establishment of Barrett esophagus. CDX-2 is a transcription factor that is markedly upregulated in the intestinal cells of Barrett esophagus.[3] This transcription factor is known to drive intestinal differentiation in the caudal region of the gut. CDX-2 knockout studies have shown that CDX-2 null mice die in utero, but histologic examination of the colon mucosa shows a squamous rather than columnar differentiation. The role of CDX-2 in driving intestinal differentiation in the esophagus is further supported by in vitro studies showing that it drives transcription of MUC2, villin, and human guanylyl cyclase 2, which are genes tightly linked with an intestinal phenotype.[4–6] Furthermore, the causative role of CDX-2 is further supported by the fact that exposure of either immortalized nontransformed esophageal squamous cells or esophageal squamous cancer cells to deoxycholic, chenodeoxycholic, or glycocholic acids in cell culture drives the expression of CDX-2.[7] Collectively, these data indicate that bile salt exposure to the distal esophagus likely induces intestinal differentiation and this process is mediated through the transcription factor CDX-2 (**Fig. 1**).

Although the intracellular mechanism linking the exposure of bile salts to transcription of CDX-2 has not been thoroughly investigated, some evidence has indicated that this phenomenon is mediated through the epidermal growth factor receptor (EGFR) receptor.[8] In this study, mucosal epithelial cells were exposed to bile salts at either a normal pH or under acidic conditions. In either case, the bile salts led to increased CDX-2 transcriptional activity, and this effect was abrogated by Mab528, a small molecule EGFR inhibitor. Furthermore this study confirmed the autophosphorylation of EGFRs after treatment with bile salts, which is the well-described first step in activation on binding with a ligand. This study indicates that bile acids function as EGFR ligands and likely contribute to cellular proliferation. Bile salts also induce other changes in cellular physiology, including the activation of protein kinase C, cyclooxygenase 2 (COX-2), and the transcription factor FXR, which are known to enhance cellular proliferation.[9,10]

Analysis of differentially expressed genes in Barrett esophagus has shown upregulation of 19 different known CDX-1 or CDX-2 target genes, indicating that these transcription factors likely play a role in the development of Barrett esophagus.[2] In a culture of immortalized esophageal keratinocytes, the expression of CDX-2 was not sufficient alone to establish the differentiation of cells into an intestinal morphology. Others have shown that this may be related to the fact that gene targets of CDX-2 are hypermethylated in squamous epithelial stem cells, and are therefore strongly suppressed. The addition of 5-AzaC, a demethylating agent, in combination with overexpression of CDX-2, does lead to intestinal differentiation.[2] This finding suggests that silencing of epigenetic gene targets of CDX-2 prevents the intestinal differentiation of esophageal stem cells, and these epigenetic modifications are reversible.

The molecular events leading to the development of Barrett from squamous stem cells are a multistep process. Expression of bone morphogenetic protein 4 (BMP-4) in squamous epithelium leads to cellular dedifferentiation into nonspecialized

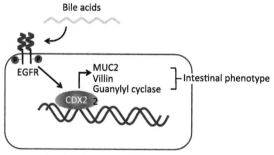

Fig. 1. Bile acids promote the development of Barrett esophagus by activating the transcription factor CDX-2 by signals mediated through EGFR. CDX-2 promotes transcription of villin, MUC2, and guanylyl cyclase 2, which are characteristic of intestinal epithelium.

columnar epithelium.[11] This process is mediated by interactions with the SMAD proteins 1, 5, and 8, and the influence of BMP-4 was abrogated by the addition of noggin, a known BMP inhibitor. Genetic analysis of cells treated with BMP-4, compared with squamous cells and Barrett epithelium, showed that the genetic profile of BMP-4–treated cells had migrated toward the expression profile of Barrett cells. Furthermore, incubation of cells overexpressing CDX-2 with BMP-4 leads to the step-wise dedifferentiation into nonspecialized columnar epithelium and subsequent differentiation into intestinal epithelium.[2] Collectively, these data map a putative pathway explaining the transdifferentiation of squamous epithelium into intestinal epithelium.

Chronic Acid Exposure

Chronic intracellular acidification leads to genetic mutations through the hydrolysis of DNA, leading to the loss of purines and pyrimidines, and imperfect base excision repair. The intracellular pH is normally regulated by a ubiquitous Na^+/H^+ exchange pump, and the expression of this cell surface protein is increased in the esophagus among patients with chronic GE reflux.[12] In addition to the damaging effects of intra-luminal acid, refluxed gastric contents also contain bile acids with carcinogenic effects mediated through the activation of different cellular pathways such as EGFR, p38, and mitogen-activated protein (MAP) kinase.[13,14] Bile acids also induce the production of reactive oxygen species and nitric oxide by enhancing the activity of inducible nitric oxide synthase.[15] Each of these factors has been associated with DNA damage. Furthermore, as cellular nitric oxide levels increase, the activity of the cellular membrane Na^+/H^+ exchange pump is inhibited. In this way, the reflux of bile salts and gastric acid synergistically increases the intracellular acid content. The associated role of this process in the development of cancer has been supported by the observation that nitric oxide synthase is increased in the esophageal epithelium as cells progress from nondysplastic Barrett to esophageal cancers.[15]

The Role of Bone Marrow-Derived Cells in Barrett Esophagus

The role of chronic inflammation and the development of cancer is a well-described phenomenon. Bone marrow-derived cells are recruited to areas of inflammation and are believed to play roles in the reparative process. Most of these bone marrow-derived cells are terminally differentiated when they arrive and therefore have a short half-life, with little potential for directly contributing to the metaplasia of Barrett esophagus. However, there is clinical and experimental evidence supporting a significant role.

In a mouse model, transplantation of bone marrow cells expressing β-galactosidase into wild-type mice with surgically induced Barrett esophagus allowed the tracking of bone marrow-derived cells. Barrett esophagus lesions were identified and characterized by islands of columnar cells with distorted glands surrounded by normal squamous epithelium. Immunohistochemical stains confirmed the presence of β-galactosidase within the columnar epithelium cells of approximately 50% glands. The β-galactosidase was confined to small clusters of cells and was never found throughout entire glands.[16] Furthermore, the development of Barrett esophagus and esophageal adenocarcinoma in a male patient who had previously received a bone marrow transplant from a female patient showed similar findings. Fluorescence in situ hybridization analysis of the 23rd chromosome from the malignant cells confirmed the presence of bone marrow-derived cells expressing the X/X phenotype, and some comprised epithelial and stromal components of the esophageal cancer. Although the evidence is limited, this study does provide convincing evidence that the bone marrow is likely an important contributor to the development of both Barrett esophagus and adenocarcinoma of the esophagus in some patients.[17]

Ongoing research will likely broaden our understanding of molecular mechanisms involved in the transformation of normal esophageal squamous epithelium into the intestinal epithelium of Barrett esophagus. These studies will likely focus on the relevance of transcription factors that are differentially expressed in the intestinal mucosa relative to squamous mucosa such as p63, Sox2, and Pax9, which are strongly downregulated in Barrett mucosa and CDX1, CDX2, HNF1α, HFN3α, HFN3β, HNF3γ, HFN4α, GATA4, GATA6, Sox9, and Math1.[18] The downregulated transcription factors are normally expressed in the proximal foregut, where they facilitate epithelial differentiation into squamous mucosa, and transcription factors upregulated in Barrett esophagus are normally expressed in the distal gut, where they normally drive columnar cell differentiation of the epithelium.

Progression from Barrett Esophagus to Adenocarcinoma

Patients with Barrett esophagus have a 30-fold to 150-fold greater risk of developing esophageal adenocarcinoma compared with those without Barrett. The risk of cancer progression among patients with Barrett esophagus is 0.5% to 1.0% each year. An understanding of the molecular events responsible for the malignant transformation of the metaplastic cells continues to develop.

In vitro experiments have supported the hypothesis of a causative role of gastric and bile reflux. Immortalized nontransformed esophageal Barrett cells grown in cell culture recapitulate the histologic changes of the distal esophageal mucosa progressing to cancer when repetitively exposed to bile salts in an acid environment over an extended period.[19] In this model, cells were exposed to glycochenodeoxycholic acid at a pH of 4 for 5 minutes each day. Phenotypic changes were observed as early as 2 weeks by identifying the expression of colon-specific antigen Das-1. After 30 weeks of daily exposure, the observed histologic changes revealed that the cells had become rounded and began to organize into glandlike units. More than 65 weeks later, more aggressive growth patterns were recognized, and the cells became tumorigenic in a nude mouse model.

Analysis of the molecular events occurring in parallel with the morphologic changes identified several genes that became activated. The most pronounced change was a 10-fold to 20-fold increase in COX-2 expression between weeks 22 and 62. The expression of p53 and TC22 were also increased 2-fold and 3-fold, respectively. In addition, numerous factors implicated in cell cycle regulation were upregulated as cells progressed to a more aggressive phenotype. ATM (ataxia telangiectasia, mutated) and ATR (ATM and Rad3-related), which are important cell cycle checkpoint regulators that prevent cells from exiting the G_1 phase in the presence of DNA damage, were induced after 20 weeks of daily exposure to bile acids. In addition, the following genes were upregulated, relative to untreated control cells, by the indicated values at 20 weeks: RB1 (2.18), E2F1 (5.55), CCNE1 (6.56), CDC25A (8.24), BRCA1 (3.82), TP53 (2.2), CHEK2 (2.13).[20] It remains unclear whether these gene products play a causative role in promoting rapid progression through the cell cycle or if they are secondarily upregulated as the result of tumor progression.

Role of Reactive Oxygen Species in Acid-Induced Progression to Adenocarcinoma

High levels of reactive oxygen species have been identified in both Barrett esophagus cells and esophageal adenocarcinoma, indicating that they incite tumor progression. Phagocytic cells are the prototypical cell type responsible for the generation of reactive oxygen species, and their formation is catalyzed by the enzyme NADPH (nicotinamide adenine dinucleotide phosphate) oxidase. Recently, homologs (NOX isoforms) of this enzyme have been identified in nonphagocytic cell types and function in signal transduction. NOX5-S has been shown to be a predominant isoform in esophageal adenocarcinoma, and a stepwise increased expression of this enzyme has been noted when comparing messenger RNA isolated from normal squamous mucosa, Barrett mucosal cells, and adenocarcinoma.[20,21] The physiologic importance of NOX5-S in the progression of esophageal cancer has been supported by showing that repetitive acid exposure of esophageal squamous cells results in the production of H_2O_2 and that this response is attenuated by NOX5-S depletion using small interfering (siRNA).[21] Similarly, cellular depletion of Ca^{2+} or the knockdown cyclic adenosine monophosphate (cAMP) response element binding protein levels with siRNA also attenuated the NOX5-S expression and H_2O_2 generation typically induced by acid exposure[22] The downstream effects of H_2O_2 generation leading to the progression to cancer are likely multifactorial, but they have been most strongly linked to COX-2 activation and hypermethylation of the p16 promoter.[21,23] Collectively, these effects would be expected to increase cellular proliferation and resistance to apoptosis.

Identification of Biomarkers for Barrett Progression to Adenocarcinoma

Early identification of patients with Barrett esophagus who are at the greatest risk for progression to adenocarcinoma or those who have early-stage disease could be expected to have a meaningful impact on the clinical outcomes of these patients. As a more thorough understanding of the mechanism underlying disease progression is developed, putative biomarkers have been investigated. Because inactivation of p16 is frequently found in Barrett esophagus as it progresses to cancer, it has been studied as a putative biomarker. p16 is also frequently silenced in nonneoplastic tissue, thus limiting its usefulness as a biomarker. In a retrospective double-blind study of biomarkers for esophageal adenocarcinoma using 8 different promoter methylation markers (p16, HPP1, RUNX3, CDH13, TAC1, NELL1, AKAP12, and SST), only methylation of p16, HPP1, and RUNX3 was found more frequently among patients who progressed to cancer compared with those who did not. Maintaining a specificity of 0.9 or 0.8, the sensitivity of the biomarkers were 0.443 and 0.629, respectively.[24] These findings need to be confirmed through independent studies, and the results are less than robust. However, they do provide hope that we are capable of developing tests to stratify patients according to their risks for progression.

Esophageal Cancer Targeted Therapy

Another important clinical application resulting from an improved understanding of the molecular events responsible for malignant degeneration in the esophagus is the development of targeted agents. In the past decade, this topic has become increasingly popular and relevant for different types of carcinoma, including esophageal adenocarcinoma. Targeted agents in the clinical arena for esophageal cancer are largely taken from the understanding of carcinomas in general, which also seems relevant to esophageal cancer. The molecular understanding of the progression of esophageal cancer has not led to the development of specific agents likely to be efficacious for this disease. Specifically, great interest has been directed toward the use of agents targeting the similar cell surface receptors EGFR and Her2/neu. In addition, the vascular endothelial growth factor (VEGF) is also being targeted with selective agents.

Epidermal Growth Factor Receptor

Epithelial growth factor receptor (EGFR) is a cell surface receptor tyrosine kinase, which is bound by several different ligands, including epidermal growth factor, transforming growth factor α, and other members of the ErbB family. When activated, EFGR autophosphorylates, dimerizes, and then phosphorylates intracellular targets involved in at least 3 different oncogenic pathways, including phosphatidylinositol (PIP_2), JAK/STAT, and Ras/Raf. EGFR belongs to a family of closely related cell surface tyrosine kinases, which are popular targets in several different types of carcinoma. The EGFR family includes EGFR (ErbB-1), Her2/neu (ErbB-2), Her 3 (ErbB-3), and Her 4 (ErbB-4). Activating mutations of EGFR have been identified in which the mutant receptor no longer requires ligand binding to constitutively phosphorylate intracellular targets. These mutations have also been identified in esophageal cancers.[25] EGFR is upregulated in Barrett high-grade dysplasia and esophageal adenocarcinoma, suggesting that it may play some role in disease progression.[26,27] In addition, increased expression of EGFR correlates with higher tumor stages and worse overall survival compared with tumors with lower EGFR expression.[28]

Given the prevalence of EFGR overexpression and mutations in numerous types of cancers, the development of agents targeting this protein has received significant attention. Two monoclonal antibodies targeting the extracellular domain of EGFR have been developed and studied clinically. In addition, 2 small molecule drugs targeting the intracellular tyrosine kinase activity have been investigated (**Fig. 2**). Two antibodies that have already received approval by the US Food and Drug Administration for the treatment of colorectal cancer are cetuximab and panitumumab. Cetuximab has been clinically evaluated among patients with advanced gastric and GE junction cancers and is used in conjunction with irinotecan and 5-fluorouracil in a single-arm phase II trial.[29] In this study, most patients had gastric cancer rather than GE junction tumors, but the results are encouraging because the median time to progression and estimated overall survival were 8 and 16 months, respectively. These values compare favorably with several similar phase II trials in which the time to progression and median survival times were 4.5 and 10.8 months, respectively.[30] These 2 trials enrolled patients of similar age and performance status. Collectively, these studies suggest that EGFR inhibition may effectively treat esophageal and gastric cancers. Panitumumab in

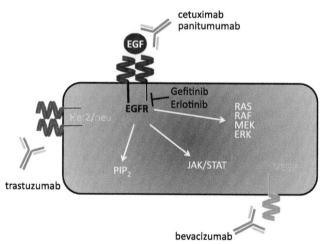

Fig. 2. The molecules most relevant for targeted therapy for esophageal cancer pictured with their respective targeted agents. Cetuximab and panitumumab are antibodies that target the extracellular domain of EFGR. Tratuzumab and bevacizumab are antibodies targeting Her2/neu and VEGF, respectively. Gefitinib and erlotinib are small molecule inhibitors of the EGFR tyrosine kinase.

conjunction with docetaxel, cisplatin, and radiation has recently been investigated as neoadjuvant treatment of patients with operative esophageal cancer, and this study recently completed accruing patients (ACOSOG Z4051). The results are not yet available.

Several small molecule tyrosine kinase inhibitors that compete for the aspartate aminotransferase-binding site on the intracellular domain of EGFR have been investigated in preclinical and clinical trials. This group of molecules includes gefitinib and erlotinib. Gefitinib has been evaluated in conjunction with oxaliplatin and radiation therapy in a phase II study of patients with either gastric or GE junction tumors.[31] The study included only 3 patients with GE junction tumors, and the clinical response was complete, partial, and stable disease in 1 case each. Gefitinib has also been evaluated as a single agent in 27 patients with inoperable esophageal cancer. Three patients had a partial response and 10 patients had stable disease (37%), but this was observed over a median of only 1.9 months.[32] Similarly, erlotinib has been shown to have a modest 9% response rate among patients with advanced GE junction adenocarcinomas.[33]

The clinical response and survival rates to EGFR antibodies and small molecule tyrosine kinase inhibitors have been limited. This finding likely relates to the fact that patient eligibility for these trials did not require the presence of EGFR mutations in the tumor specimens. Similar studies of EGFR inhibition in lung cancer have clearly shown superior response rates among patients with EGFR gene mutations rather than simple overexpression of the protein. Furthermore, clinical studies in patients with lung cancer have also shown that that k-RAS mutations predicts resistance to EGFR inhibition because this mutant protein is constitutively active and no longer requires phosphorylation by EGFR. The clinical studies investigating the use of EGFR inhibitors in patients with esophageal or gastric cancer did not evaluate or exclude patients with k-RAS mutations. Perhaps with a more stringent enrollment criteria base on EGFR or k-RAS mutations, a meaningful clinical response could be observed.

VEGF Receptor Inhibitors

Studies conducted in tissue culture indicate that exposure of esophageal intestinal cells to bile salts transcriptionally upregulated VEGF expression.[34] Data supporting the role of VEGF in the development or progression of esophageal adenocarcinoma are also limited, although angiogenesis is understood to be a necessary component to support the growth of any malignancy. A recent nonrandomized phase II study of patients with gastric (n = 42) and esophageal (n = 2) cancer treated with bevacizumab in addition to docetaxel, cisplatin, and fluorouracil has been performed.[35] The 6-month progression-free survival was 79% and the median overall survival in this study was 16.8 months. This finding compares favorably with a historical progression-free survival rate of 43% among patients treated with the same 3 cytotoxic agents without the addition of bevacizumab. Other ongoing clinical investigations continue to evaluate the efficacy of VEGF inhibition in esophageal cancers.

Her2/Neu (ErbB2) Inhibitors

The Her2/neu receptor is enhanced in 17% to 43% of esophageal adenocarcinomas through gene amplification.[36,37] Conflicting data regarding the prognostic implications of Her2/neu amplification exist. The presence of Her2/neu gene amplification was found more frequently among patients with adjacent Barrett esophagus compared with those without, and Her2/neu was associated with improved overall and disease-free survival in a series of 344 patients.[36] In addition, Her2/neu amplification was found more frequently among patients with lower T stage (T1-2 vs T3-4), absence of lymph node metastases (N0 vs N1), and lower tumor grades (G1-3 vs G4). Conversely, Brien and colleagues[38] reported in a smaller study of 54 patients that Her2/neu amplification was associated with a decreased overall survival rate. Despite the conflicting prognostic implications of Her2/neu expression, it remains an attractive molecular target for therapy. Activation of this transmembrane receptor tyrosine kinase activates MAP kinase and phosphitidyl-inosite-3 kinase/Akt pathways, resulting in cellular resistance to apoptosis.

Trastuzumab is a monoclonal antibody against the Her2/neu receptor that was initially evaluated clinically in breast cancer. Its efficacy has also been evaluated among patients with esophageal cancer. A phase I/II trial of trastuzumab with cisplatin, paclitaxel, and radiation in locally advanced esophageal adenocarcinoma strongly expressing the Her2/neu receptor showed a median overall survival of 24 months, which is slightly better than historical control patients treated with only cytotoxic chemotherapy and radiation.[37] Trastuzumab has also been evaluated in a prospective randomized phase III trial of patients with advanced Her2/neu gastric or GE junction cancers and showed improved survival compared with chemotherapy alone. In this study, patients were treated with 6 cycles of cisplatin and fluorouracil, or capecitibin with or without trastuzumab. The median survival in the trastuzumab plus chemotherapy group was 13.8 months versus 11.1 months for chemotherapy alone ($P = .0046$).[39] A preplanned subgroup analysis of the 106 patients in this study with GE junction tumors showed improved survival after treatment with trastuzumab in addition to chemotherapy with a hazard ratio of 0.67. Patients with GE junction tumors in this study may have responded slightly better to trastuzumab than patients with gastric cancer. An ongoing randomized phase III clinical trial (RTOG-1010) is evaluating the efficacy of trastuzumab in addition to standard chemotherapy for the neoadjuvant setting in patients with locally advanced esophageal cancer with Her2/neu overexpression.

Because the activation mechanism of Her2/neu is most frequently through gene amplification, it is important to evaluate additional genes located on the same amplicon of chromosome 17q. DARPP and its truncated cancer-specific isoform t-DARPP is located in the same region on chromosome 17q and is also upregulated. t-DARPP is known to activate Akt, resulting in enhanced cell survival, and may bypass the inhibitory effects of Her2/neu inhibition.[40] This gene is not under clinical investigation, but may be targeted in the future.

SUMMARY

The most clinically relevant molecular targets in esophageal cancer are those targets previously identified in other more common types of carcinomas, and the importance of these proteins in esophageal cancer was later established. Previous clinical studies of targeted agents in the treatment of other cancers has established clinical safety profiles, which has facilitated the adoption of agents such as inhibitors of EFGR, Her2/neu, and VEGF for the treatment of esophageal cancer. Ongoing investigations of the specific pathophysiology related to the development of esophageal adenocarcinomas and Barrett esophagus may lead to the development of agents uniquely suited for the treatment of these diseases.

SQUAMOUS CELL CARCINOMA

Worldwide, squamous cell carcinoma of the esophagus is more common than adenocarcinoma. In America, squamous cell cancers comprise only 20% of all esophageal cancers, and this incidence is declining. Smoking and alcohol consumption are considered the major risk factors for the development of squamous cell cancers, and the molecular pathways leading from these environmental exposures to carcinogenesis are still being established. Both alcohol and smoking are known to have numerous carcinogenic compounds, which are discussed later. In addition, genetic evaluation of esophageal squamous cell cancers has revealed common genetic abnormalities, although the direct links between the carcinogen and cancer have not been proved conclusively.

The Toxicity of Alcohol

The molecular events resulting from chronic ethanol exposure to the mucosa of the upper digestive tract are complex, and several parallel and redundant carcinogenic pathways have been described. Ethanol is metabolized through a 2-step pathway that involves the oxidation of ethanol to acetaldehyde by alcohol dehydrogenase, which is then further oxidized by aldehyde dehydrogenase 2 (ALDH2) to acetic acid. Acetaldehyde is known to induce genetic mutations by inhibiting DNA methylation and interfering with retinoid metabolism. In addition, epidemiologic studies show that inactivation of ALDH2 in humans causes an increased accumulation of acetaldehyde, which is associated with the development of aerodigestive tract cancers, including esophageal squamous cell carcinoma.[41,42] Although ethanol is normally metabolized in the liver, bacteria in the oral cavity possess alcohol dehydrogenase and are capable of oxidizing ethanol, resulting in the accumulation of acetaldehyde levels in the saliva, which exceed blood levels by 100-fold.[43] Acetaldehyde intercalates into the DNA and forms stable adducts, leading to miscoding and point mutations. This finding represents the first pathway through which ethanol is believed to contribute to carcinogenesis of the esophagus.

Alcohol consumption may also contribute to carcinogenesis through the local generation of reactive oxygen species. Chronic exposure to ethanol induces marked expression of the cytochrome P450 2E1 (CYP2E1) enzyme in the liver. CYP2E1 has also been shown to be upregulated in the mucosa of animals with chronic oral exposure to ethanol.[44] CYP2E1 is responsible for the local generation of reactive oxygen species, which include superoxide anions (O_2^-) and H_2O_2. Chronic ethanol consumption also induces nitric oxide synthase, which generates peroxynitrite ($ONOO^-$).[41] The oxidative stress resulting from reactive oxygen species is a well-accepted mechanism of carcinogenesis in numerous types of cancer and is also believed to contribute to esophageal cancer.

A third mechanism through which ethanol contributes to carcinogenesis is by the inhibition of DNA methylation. An important mechanism of epigenetic regulation is gene silencing through DNA histone methylation in which S-adenosyl-L-methionine (SAM) serves as the universal methyl group donor. Ethanol inhibits SAM generation and has been shown to lead to global hypomethylation, which facilitates expression of oncogenes.[45]

Smoking and Esophageal Squamous Cell Cancers

Cigarette smoke contains at least 60 different carcinogens, and there are strong links between smoking and several cancers, including lung, esophageal, pancreatic and laryngeal cancers. Polycyclic aromatic hydrocarbons (PAH) and N-nitrosamines are likely the most important carcinogens in cigarette smoke, which create DNA adducts, alter gene methylation, and induce mutations.[46] Benzo[a]pyrene is believed to be one of the most harmful PAH and has been shown to cause cancer by local exposure in lung, skin, and bladder tissues. Although a direct causal link has not been established in esophageal cancer, it is likely a contributor to the disease process. The most established pathway between toxins in cigarette smoke and cancer is the formation of adducts within DNA that can result in gene mutations if they are not recognized by DNA excision repair mechanisms.

Alcohol and Smoking Synergism

The synergistic effects of smoking and alcohol are likely multifactorial, and experimental evidence does support several specific mechanisms. Local production of acetaldehyde by bacteria in the oral cavity is known to have carcinogenic effects. Heavy smoking and drinking are frequently associated with poor oral hygiene, which alters the normal bacterial flora of the mouth, leading to a greater population of bacteria and yeast capable of metabolizing ethanol into acetaldehyde.[43] This problem is exacerbated by a depletion of bacteria capable of further metabolizing acetaldehyde into acetic acid.[47] Collectively, these 2 modifications in the oral flora increase the local concentration of acetaldehyde. A second described mechanism is the induction of P450 enzymes in the proximal digestive tract by chronic exposure to alcohol. This process is known to enhance the conversion of procarcinogens in cigarette smoke to carcinogens.[48]

Gene Mutations Frequently Recognized in Esophageal Squamous Cell Cancers

Numerous different genetic mutations have been identified in esophageal squamous cell cancers and many are associated with cell cycle regulation, apoptosis, DNA repair mechanisms, growth factors, and their receptors. Although coherent links between specific mutations and the development of malignancies have not been established, several genes are discussed later with their approximate incidence in cancers. A basic understanding of these mutations will be important as our knowledge continues to evolve, and more targeted therapies become available. Several known mutated or dysregulated genes in esophageal cancers are listed in **Table 1**. This may be a starting point for the development of targeted agents. However, most genetic abnormalities identified in esophageal cancer have also been identified in other forms of malignancies and have yet to become the focus of targeted therapies.

Targeted Therapy for Esophageal Squamous Cell Cancer

The use of targeted agents for squamous cell cancers has evolved in a similar manner to that for adenocarcinomas. Gefitinib and erlotinib are agents that have been extensively evaluated in other types of cancer and have established safety profiles. Because esophageal squamous cell cancers are known to overexpress EGFR, it seems

Table 1	
Gene mutations identified in esophageal squamous cell cancers	
Gene Mutation	**Function**
p53	Tumor suppressor
p21	G1 arrest in response to DNA damage
p16	Blocks G1-S progression
Cyclin D	Promotes G1-S progression
EGFR	Regulates proliferation and apoptosis
COX-2	Regulates proliferation and apoptosis
E-cadherin	Inhibits cell migration
BRCA1	Tumor suppressor

reasonable to determine whether the EGFR inhibitors exert a clinical response. Although there are no clinical studies that have specifically enrolled patients with squamous cell cancers, subgroup analyses of studies that have included both adenocarcinoma and squamous cell cancers of the esophagus indicate that squamous cell cancers may have a more significant response to EGFR inhibition.

In a single-arm phase II clinical trial using gefitinib as a second-line agent for patients with recurrent esophageal cancers, the partial response rate was only 2.8% and stable disease was observed in 27%. A higher disease control rate was found among patients with squamous cell cancers compared with adenocarcinoma (55% vs 19%).[49] In this study, the number of patients overexpressing EGFR was also higher among patients with squamous cell cancers. In a similar study, erlotinib was also found to be more efficacious among patients with squamous cell cancers when used as a second-line agent. The time to progression was 3.3 months among patients with squamous histology compared with 1.6 months for patients with adenocarcinoma.[50]

Erlotinib has also been used along with concurrent radiation and cisplatin/paclitaxel as definitive therapy for advanced stage III/IV esophageal squamous cell cancer. The 2-year local regional control in this study was 87.5% and the disease-free survival at 2 years was 57.4%. These results seem more favorable considering that the inclusion criteria for this study allowed patients to have a Karnofsky performance status as low as 60. These results compare favorably with previous studies in which the local control rate for esophageal cancers treated with radiation and cisplatin/paclitaxel was only 75%.[51]

SUMMARY

Our understanding of the molecular events responsible for the development of esophageal adenocarcinoma and squamous cell carcinoma continues to evolve. As further knowledge is gained, more options for targeted molecular therapy are anticipated. Currently, targeted agents in clinical trials are those agents previously investigated for the treatment of other diseases that are more prevalent in America. Early results from several nonrandomized trials that include these agents are encouraging, but the clinical responses are modest.

REFERENCES

1. Oberg S, Peters JH, DeMeester TR, et al. Determinates of intestinal metaplasia within the columnar lined esophagus. Arch Surg 2000;135:651–6.
2. Dvorak K, Goldman A, Kong J, et al. Molecular mechanisms of Barrett's esophagus and adenocarcinoma. Ann N Y Acad Sci 2011;1232:381–91.
3. Groisman GM, Amar M, Meir A. Expression of the intestinal marker Cdx2 in the columnar-lined esophagus with and without intestinal (Barrett's) metaplasia. Mod Pathol 2004;17:1282–8.
4. Steininger H, Pfofe DA, Muller H, et al. Expression of CDX2 and MUC2 in Barrett's mucosa. Pathol Res Pract 2005;2018:573–7.
5. Braunstein EM, Qiao XT, Madison B, et al. Villin: a marker for development of the epithelial pyloric border. Dev Dyn 2002;224:90–102.
6. Park J, Schulz S, Waldman SA. Intestine-specific activity of the human guanylyl cyclase C promoter is regulated by Cdx2. Gastroenterology 2000;119:89–96.
7. Hu Y, Williams VA, Gellerson O, et al. The pathogenesis of Barrett's esophagus: secondary bile acids upregulates intestinal differentiation factor CDX2 expression in esophageal cells. J Gastrointest Surg 2007;142:540–5.

8. Avissar NE, Toia L, Hu Y, et al. Bile acid alone, or in combination with acid, induces CDX2 expression through activation of the epidermal growth factor receptor (EGFR). J Gastrointest Surg 2009;13:212–22.

9. Anisfeld AM, Kast-Woelbern HR, Lee H, et al. Activation of the nuclear factor receptor FXR induces fibrinogen expression: a new role for bile acid signaling. J Lipid Res 2005;46:458–68.

10. Kaur BS, Triadafelopoulos G. Acid and bile-induced PGE(2) release and hyper-proliferation in Barrett's esophagus are COX-2 and PKC-epsilon dependent. Am J Physiol Gastrointest Liver Physiol 2002;283:G327–34.

11. Milano F, van Baal JW, Buttat NS, et al. Bone morphogenetic protein 4 expressed in esophagitis induces a columnar phenotype in esophageal squamous cells. Gastroenterology 2007;132:2412–21.

12. LeBoeuf RA, Kerckaert GA. The induction of transformed-like morphology and enhanced growth in Syrian hamster embryo cells grown at acid pH. Carcinogenesis 1986;7:1431–40.

13. Merchant NP, Rogers CM, Trivedi B, et al. Ligand-dependent activation of the epithelial growth factor receptor by secondary bile acids in polarizing colon cancer cells. Surgery 2005;138:415–21.

14. Jaiswal K, Lopez-Guzman C, Souza RF, et al. Bile salt exposure increases proliferation through p38 and ERK MAPK pathways in a non-neoplastic Barrett's cell line. Am J Physiol Gastrointest Liver Physiol 2006;290:G335–42.

15. Goldman A, Shahidullah M, Goldman D, et al. A novel mechanism of acid and bile acid-induced DNA damage involving Na^+/H^+ exchanger: implication for Barrett's oesophagus. Gut 2010;59:1606–16.

16. Hutchinson L, Stenstrom B, Chen D, et al. Human Barrett's adenocarcinoma of the esophagus, associated myofibroblasts, and endothelium can arise from bone marrow-derived cells after allogeneic stem cell transplant. Stem Cells Dev 2011;20:11–7.

17. Korbling M, Katz RL, Khanna A, et al. Hepatocytes and epithelial cells of donor origin in recipients of peripheral-blood stem cells. N Engl J Med 2002;346:738–46.

18. Chen H, Fang Y, Tevebaugh W, et al. Molecular mechanisms of Barrett's esophagus. Dig Dis Sci 2011;56:3405–20.

19. Das KM, Kong Y, Bajpai M, et al. Transformation of benign Barrett's epithelium by repeated acid and bile exposure over 65 weeks: a novel in vitro model. Int J Cancer 2011;128:274–82.

20. Fang D, Kas KM, Cao W, et al. Barrett's esophagus: progression to adenocarcinoma and markers. Ann N Y Acad Sci 2011;1232:210–29.

21. Hong H, Resnick M, Behar J, et al. Acid-induced p16 hypermethylation contributes to development of esophageal adenocarcinoma via activation of NADPH oxidase NOS5-S. Am J Physiol Gastrointest Liver Physiol 2010;299:G697–706.

22. Fu X, Beer DG, Behar J, et al. cAMP-response element-binding protein mediates acid-induced NADPH oxidase NOX5-S expression in Barrett's esophageal adenocarcinoma cells. J Biol Chem 2006;281:20368–82.

23. Si J, Fu X, Behar J, et al. NADPH oxidase NOX5-S mediates acid induced cyclooxygenase-2 expression via activation of NF-κB in Barrett's esophageal adenocarcinoma cells. J Biol Chem 2007;282:16244–55.

24. Jin Z, Cheng Y, Gu W, et al. A multicenter, double-blinded validation study of methylation biomarkers for progression prediction of Barrett's esophagus. Cancer Res 2009;69:4112–5.

25. Kwak EL, Jankowski J, Thayer SP, et al. Epidermal growth factor receptor kinase domain mutations in esophageal and pancreatic adenocarcinomas. Clin Cancer Res 2006;12:4283–7.

26. Rygiel AM, Milano F, Ten Kate FJ, et al. Gains and amplifications of c-myc, EGFR, and 20.Q13 loci in the no dysplasia-dysplasia-adenocarcinoma sequence of Barrett's esophagus. Cancer Epidemiol Biomarkers Prev 2008;17:1380–5.

27. Friess H, Fukuda A, Tang WH, et al. Concomitant analysis of the epidermal growth factor receptor family in esophageal cancer: overexpression of epidermal growth factor receptor mRNA but not of c-erbb-2 and c-erbb-3. World J Surg 1999;23:1010–8.

28. Wilkinson NW, Black JD, Roukhadze E, et al. Epidermal growth factor receptor expression correlates with histologic grade in resected esophageal adenocarcinoma. J Gastrointest Surg 2004;8:448–53.

29. Pinto C, Di Fabio F, Siena S, et al. Phase II study of cetuximab in combination with FOLFIRI in patients with untreated advanced gastric or gastroesophageal junction adenocarcinoma. Ann Oncol 2007;18:510–7.

30. Moehler M, Eimermacher A, Siebler J, et al. Randomized phase II evaluation of irinotecan plus high-dose 5-fluorouracil and leucovorin (ILP) vs. 5-fluorouracil, leucovorin and etoposide (ELF) in untreated gastric cancer. Br J Cancer 2005;92:2122–8.

31. Javle M, Pande A, Iyer R, et al. Pilot study of gefitinib, oxaliplatin, and radiotherapy for esophageal adenocarcinoma: tissue effect predicts clinical response. Am J Clin Oncol 2008;31:329–34.

32. Ferry DR, Anderson M, Beddard K, et al. A phase II study of gefitinib monotherapy in advanced esophageal adenocarcinoma: evidence of gene expression, cellular, and clinical response. Clin Cancer Res 2007;13:5869–75.

33. Dragovich T, McCoy S, Fenoglio-Preiser CM, et al. Phase II trial of erlotinib in gastroesophageal junction and gastric adenocarcinomas: SWOG 0127. J Clin Oncol 2006;24:4922–7.

34. Burnat G, Rau T, Elshimi E, et al. Bile acids induce overexpression of homeobox gene CDX-2 and vascular endothelial growth factor (VEGF) in human Barrett's esophageal mucosa and adenocarcinoma cell line. Scand J Gastroenterol 2007;42:1460–5.

35. Shah MA, Jhawer M, Ilson DH, et al. Phase II study of modified docetaxel, cisplatin and fluorouracil with bevacizumab in patients with metastatic gastroesophageal adenocarcinoma. J Clin Oncol 2011;29:868–74.

36. Yoon HH, Shi Q, Sukov WR, et al. Association of her2/erbb2 expression and gene amplification with pathologic features and prognosis in esophageal adenocarcinomas. Clin Cancer Res 2012;18:546–54.

37. Safran H, Dipetrillo T, Akerman P, et al. Phase I/II study of trastuzumab, paclitaxel, cisplatin and radiation for locally advanced, HER2 overexpressing, esophageal adenocarcinoma. Int J Radiat Oncol Biol Phys 2007;67:405–9.

38. Brien TP, Odze RD, Sheehan CE, et al. Her-2/neu gene amplification by FISH predicts poor survival in Barrett's esophagus-associated adenocarcinoma. Hum Pathol 2000;31:35–9.

39. Bang YJ, van Cutsem E, Feyereislova A, et al. Trastuzumab in combination with chemotherapy versus chemotherapy alone for treatment of HER2-positive gastric or gastro-oesophageal junction cancer (toGA): a phase 3, open-label, randomized controlled trial. Lancet 2010;28:687–97.

40. Belkhiri A, Zaika A, Pidkovka N, et al. DARPP-32: a novel antiapoptotic gene in upper gastrointestinal carcinomas. Cancer Res 2005;65:6583–92.

41. Seitz HK, Stickel F. Molecular mechanisms of alcohol mediated carcinogenesis. Nat Rev Cancer 2007;7:599–612.
42. Yokoyama A, Kumagai Y, Yokoyama T, et al. Health risk appraisal models for mass screening for esophageal and pharyngeal cancer: an endoscopic follow-up study of cancer-free Japanese men. Cancer Epidemiol Biomarkers Prev 2009;18:651–5.
43. Homann N, Tillonen J, Meurman JH, et al. Increased salivary acetaldehyde levels in heavy drinkers and smokers: a microbiological approach to oral cavity cancer. Carcinogenesis 2000;21:663–8.
44. Shimizu M, Lasker JM, Tsutsumi M, et al. Immunohistochemical localization of ethanol-induced P450IIE1 in the rat alimentary tract. Gastroenterology 1990;99: 1044–53.
45. Choi SW, Stickel F, Baik HW, et al. Chronic alcohol consumption induces genomic but not p53-specific DNA hypomethylation in rat colon. J Nutr 1999;129:1945–50.
46. Toh Y, Oki E, Ohgaki K, et al. Alcohol drinking, cigarette smoking, and the development of squamous cell carcinoma of the esophagus; molecular mechanisms of carcinogenesis. Int J Clin Oncol 2010;15:135–44.
47. Salaspuro V, Salaspuro M. Synergistic effect of alcohol drinking and smoking on in vivo acetaldehyde concentration in saliva. Int J Cancer 2004;111:480–3.
48. Pfeifer GP, Denissenko MF, Olivier M, et al. Tobacco smoke carcinogens, DNA damage and p53 mutations in smoking-associated cancers. Oncogene 2002; 21:7435–51.
49. Janmaat ML, Gallegos-Ruiz MI, Rodriguez JA, et al. Predictive factors for outcomes in a phase II study of gefitinib in second-line treatment of advanced esophageal cancer patients. J Clin Oncol 2006;24:1612–9.
50. Ilson DH, Kelsen D, Shah M, et al. A phase 2 trial of erlotinib in patients with previously treated squamous cell and adenocarcinoma of the esophagus. Cancer 2011;117:1409–14.
51. Cooper JS, Gui MD, Herskovic A, et al. Chemoradiotherapy of locally advanced esophageal cancer: long-term follow up of a prospective randomized trial (RTOG 85-01). JAMA 1999;281:1623–7.

Diagnosis and Staging of Cancer of the Esophagus and Esophagogastric Junction

Zhigang Li, MD, PhD[a], Thomas W. Rice, MD[b,c],*

KEYWORDS

- Clinical stage • Pathologic stage • Retreatment stage • Autopsy stage
- Endoscopic esophageal ultrasound • Computed tomography
- Positron emission tomography

KEY POINTS

- The seventh edition esophagus and esophagogastric junction cancer staging is data driven and harmonized with gastric cancer staging.
- Changes include new definitions for Tis, T4, regional lymph node, and N and M classifications.
- Nonanatomic characteristics, histopathologic cell type, histologic grade, and cancer location are included with TNM classifications to determine stage groupings.
- Clinical stage (cTNM and ycTNM) is best determined by combinations of staging tools including endoscopic ultrasonography (EUS), EUS fine-needle aspiration, and computed tomography/positron emission tomography.
- Pathologic stage (pTNM and ypTNM) is ascertained at resection and requires communication and cooperation of the surgeon and pathologist.
- Classifications and stage groupings may also be defined at retreatment (rTNM) and autopsy (aTNM).

INTRODUCTION

TNM staging of esophageal cancer was introduced in 1977.[1] This inaugural system had only 3 T classifications (T1, cancer length $\leq$5 cm; T2, cancer length >5 cm; and T3, extraesophageal cancer spread), 2 N classifications (N0 and N1), 2 M classifications (M0 and M1), and 3 stage groupings (no Stage0 or IV). Barium esophagram

Dr Li is the 2011-2012 AATS Evart Graham Traveling Fellow.
[a] Department of Thoracic and Cardiovascular Surgery, The Second Military Medical University, Changhai Hospital, Shanghai, People's Republic of China; [b] Cleveland Clinic Lerner College of Medicine of Case Western Reserve University; [c] Department of Thoracic and Cardiovascular Surgery, Heart and Vascular Institute, Cleveland Clinic, 9500 Euclid Avenue / Desk J4-1, Cleveland, OH 44195, USA
* Corresponding author. Department of Thoracic and Cardiovascular Surgery, Cleveland Clinic, 9500 Euclid Avenue / Desk J4-1, Cleveland, OH 44195.
E-mail address: ricet@ccf.org

was the primary tool for both diagnosis and staging. Flexible fiberoptic esophago-scopy had just entered the commercial market, thus rigid esophagoscopy was still the procedure of choice for biopsy, but it was not freely available or always used. In the ensuing 35 years, advances in imaging, esophagoscopy, and TNM staging and introduction of minimally invasive staging procedures have produced an invaluable, sophisticated process for diagnosing and staging esophageal cancer.

DIAGNOSIS

Diagnosis of esophageal cancer requires a history, physical examination, and esoph-agoscopy with biopsy. Solid dysphagia in a middle-aged to older white man with a long-standing history of gastroesophageal reflux disease (GERD) and a known hiatal hernia is the classic presentation in the western hemisphere. Increasingly seen is a second presentation: that of a middle-aged white male with sudden onset of solid dysphagia without GERD or hiatal hernia. The clinical diagnoses of these patients are adenocarcinoma of the distal esophagus (classic presentation) or esophagogas-tric junction (EGJ)/gastric cardia (second presentation). Typically, physical examina-tion reveals a robust middle-aged to older white man with potential lifestyle-related comorbidities, without weight loss or clinically detectable metastases to nonregional lymph nodes (supraclavicular) or distant sites (eg, liver, pleura). In contradistinction, squamous cell carcinoma is found in the midthoracic or upper thoracic esophagus in middle-aged nonwhite men, usually from an endemic area and a lower socioeco-nomic class. History is typically of dysphagia, weight loss, and heavy smoking and drinking, and examination usually reveals an advanced-stage cancer.

For many outside the western world, barium esophagram remains the principal diag-nostic test for esophageal cancer. The principal finding is a stricture. The radiographic appearance is an asymmetric, abrupt, irregular narrowing with shelflike margins and a nodular or ulcerated surface within the stricture. In esophageal patients who have cancer, modern barium esophagram detects a lesion in 98% of studies, is suggestive or diagnostic of esophageal cancer in 96%, and has an estimated positive predictive value of 42%.[2] However, today the clinical diagnosis of cancer of the esophagus and EGJ requires tissue confirmation, not obtained by barium esophagram. In most centers, esophagoscopy has replaced barium esophagography as the first investiga-tion in the evaluation of dysphagia and clinical diagnosis of esophageal cancer.

For pathologic diagnosis of esophageal carcinoma, flexible fiberoptic video esoph-agoscopy is the procedure of choice. Cytology brushings followed by at least 6 biopsies are diagnostic in most patients; however, this protocol is rarely followed.[3–6] Useful in the diagnosis of malignant strictures that are not endoscopically accessible are endoscopic esophageal ultrasonography (EUS) and EUS fine-needle aspiration (EUS FNA) of the abnormal esophageal wall.[7] FNA or open biopsy of distant metas-tases can provide both a pathologic diagnosis and crucial staging.

In North America, it is suggested that patients with a columnar-lined (Barrett) esoph-agus should have esophagoscopy and biopsy (4 quadrant biopsies every 2 cm) every 3 years. Surveillance of these high-risk groups allows diagnosis of early-stage cancer in asymptomatic patients and is cost-effective compared with other cancer surveillance programs.[8,9]

STAGING

Staging of cancer of the esophagus and EGJ has been extensively changed and improved in the seventh edition of the American Joint Committee on Cancer (AJCC)/Union for International Cancer Control (UICC) Cancer Staging Manuals.[10,11]

Changes address problems of empiric stage grouping and lack of harmonization with stomach cancer. This goal was accomplished by assembling worldwide data and using modern machine learning techniques for data-driven staging.[12–15] Improvements include new definitions of Tis, T4, regional lymph node, N classification, and M classification, and addition of nonanatomic cancer characteristics: histopathologic cell type, histologic grade, and cancer location. Stage groupings were constructed by adherence to principles of staging, including monotonic decreasing survival with increasing stage group, distinct survival between groups, and homogeneous survival within groups.

Depth of cancer invasion classifies the primary cancer (T) (**Box 1, Fig. 1**). Tis tumors are intraepithelial malignancies confined to the epithelium without invasion of the basement membrane and are now termed high-grade dysplasia. Tis includes all noninvasive neoplastic epithelium that was previously called carcinoma in situ. T1 cancers breach the basement membrane to invade the lamina propria, muscularis mucosa, or the submucosa, but do not invade beyond the submucosa. T1 cancers may be subclassified into T1a, cancers that invade only the mucosa, and T1b, cancers that invade the submucosa.[16] T2 cancers invade into but not beyond the muscularis propria. T3 cancers invade beyond the esophageal wall into the periesophageal tissue, but do not invade adjacent structures. T4 cancers invade structures in the vicinity of the esophagus. T4 has been subclassified as T4a and T4b; T4a cancers are resectable cancers invading adjacent structures, such as pleura, pericardium, or diaphragm. T4b cancers are unresectable cancers invading other adjacent structures, such as aorta, vertebral body, or trachea.

A regional lymph node has been redefined to include any paraesophageal lymph node extending from cervical nodes to celiac nodes (see **Box 1**, see **Fig. 1**). Data analyses support convenient coarse groupings of number of cancer-positive nodes.[12–14] Regional lymph node (N) classification comprises N0 (no cancer-positive nodes), N1 (1 or 2), N2 (3–6), and N3 (7 or more). These classifications are identical to those of stomach cancer.

The subclassifications M1a and M1b have been eliminated, as has MX (see **Box 1**). Distant metastases are designated M0, no distant metastasis, and M1, distant metastasis.

Three nonanatomic cancer characteristics (histopathologic cell type, histologic grade, and cancer location) are necessary for staging (see **Box 1**). Because the AJCC/UICC seventh edition staging of cancer of the esophagus and EGJ is based on cancers arising from the epithelium, histopathologic cell type is either adenocarcinoma or squamous cell carcinoma. Because the data indicate that squamous cell carcinoma has a poorer prognosis than adenocarcinoma, a cancer of mixed histopathologic type is staged as squamous cell carcinoma. Nonmucosal cancers arising in the wall are classified according to their cell of origin.

The nonanatomic cancer characteristic histologic grade is categorized as G1, well differentiated; G2, moderately differentiated; G3, poorly differentiated; or G4, undifferentiated (see **Box 1**). Because the data indicate that squamous cell carcinoma has a poorer prognosis than adenocarcinoma, G4, undifferentiated cancers, are staged similar to G3 squamous cell carcinoma.

Cancer location is defined by position of the upper end of the cancer in the esophagus (**Fig. 2**). It is best expressed as distance from incisors to proximal edge of the cancer, and conventionally by its location within broad regions of the esophagus. Typical esophagoscopy measurements of cervical esophageal cancer measured from the incisors is from 15 to less than 20 cm. In the absence of esophagoscopy, location can be assessed by computed tomography (CT). If thickening of the esophageal

Box 1
Seventh edition AJCC/UICC staging of cancer of the esophagus and esophagogastric junction

T: Primary Tumor

TX Tumor cannot be assessed

T0 No evidence of tumor

Tis High-grade dysplasia

T1 Tumor invades the lamina propria, muscularis mucosa, or submucosa. It does not breach the submucosa

T2 Tumor invades into but not beyond the muscularis propria

T3 Tumor invades the paraesophageal tissue, but does not invade adjacent structures

T4

    T4a Resectable tumor invades adjacent structures, such as pleura, pericardium, diaphragm

    T4b Unresectable tumor invades other adjacent structures, such as aorta, vertebral body, trachea

N: Regional Lymph Nodes

Any periesophageal lymph node from cervical lymph nodes to celiac node

    N0 No regional lymph node metastases

    N1 1 to 2 positive regional lymph nodes

    N2 3 to 6 positive regional lymph nodes

    N3 7 or more positive regional lymph nodes

M: Distant Metastasis

M0 No distant metastases

M1 Distant metastases

Nonanatomic Cancer Characteristics

Histopathologic cell type

    Adenocarcinoma

    Squamous cell carcinoma

Histologic grade

    G1 Well differentiated

    G2 Moderately differentiated

    G3 Poorly differentiated

    G4 Undifferentiated

Tumor location

    Upper thoracic 20–25 cm from incisors

    Middle thoracic >25–30 cm from incisors

    Lower thoracic >30–40 cm from incisors

    Esophagogastric junction includes cancers with an epicenter in the distal thoracic esophagus, esophagogastric junction, or within the proximal 5 cm of the stomach (cardia) that extend into the esophagogastric junction or esophagus and are stage grouped similar to adenocarcinoma of the esophagus

From Edge SB, Byrd DR, Compton CC, ediotrs. American Joint Committee on Cancer staging manual. TNM staging of esophageal cancer. 7th edition. New York: Springer; 2010; with permission

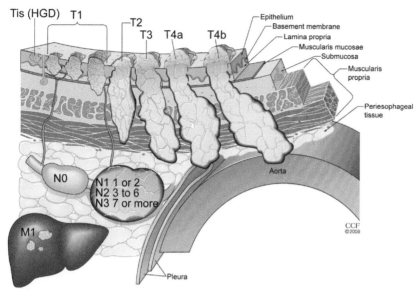

Fig. 1. Seventh edition TNM classifications. T is classified as Tis: high-grade dysplasia; T1: cancer invades lamina propria, muscularis mucosae, or submucosa; T2: cancer invades into but not beyond the muscularis propria; T3: cancer invades the paraesophageal tissue, but does not invade adjacent structures; T4a: resectable cancer invades adjacent structures, such as pleura, pericardium, or diaphragm; and T4b: unresectable cancer invades other adjacent structures, such as aorta, vertebral body, or trachea. N is classified as N0: no regional lymph node metastasis; N1: regional lymph node metastases involving 1 to 2 nodes; N2: regional lymph node metastases involving 3 to 6 nodes; and N3: regional lymph node metastases involving 7 or more nodes. M is classified as M0: no distant metastasis; and M1: distant metastasis. (*Reprinted* with permission, Cleveland Clinic Center for Medical Art & Photography © 2001–2012. All Rights Reserved.)

wall begins above the sternal notch, location is cervical. Typical esophagoscopy measurements of upper thoracic esophageal cancer from the incisors are from 20 to less than 25 cm. CT location of an upper thoracic cancer is esophageal wall thickening that begins between the sternal notch and azygos vein. Typical esophagoscopy measurements of middle thoracic esophageal cancer from the incisors are from 25 to less than 30 cm. CT location is wall thickening that begins between the azygos vein and inferior pulmonary vein. Typical esophagoscopy measurements of lower thoracic esophageal cancer from the incisors are from 30 to 40 cm. CT location is wall thickening that begins below the inferior pulmonary vein. The abdominal esophagus is included in the lower thoracic esophagus. Cancers with an epicenter in the lower thoracic esophagus, EGJ, or within the proximal 5 cm of the stomach (cardia) that extend into the EGJ or esophagus (Siewert III) are staged as adenocarcinoma of the esophagus. All other cancers with an epicenter in the stomach greater than 5 cm distal to the EGJ, or those within 5 cm of the EGJ but not extending into the EGJ or esophagus, are stage grouped using the gastric (non-EGJ) cancer staging system.[9]

TNM classifications are grouped into stages to assemble subgroups with similar behavior and prognosis. Stages 0 and IV are by definition (not data driven) TisN0M0 and Tany Nany M1, respectively. Stage groupings for M0 adenocarcinoma are shown in **Fig. 3**. For T1N0M0 and T2N0M0 adenocarcinoma, subgrouping is by histologic grade, G1 and G2 (not G3) versus G3. The difference in survival between

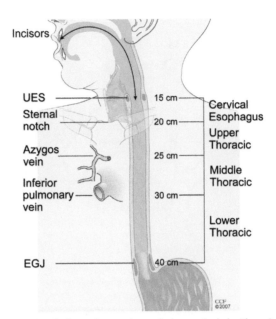

Fig. 2. Cancer location. Cervical esophagus, bounded superiorly by the cricopharyngeus and inferiorly by the sternal notch, is typically 15 to 20 cm from the incisors at esophagoscopy. Upper thoracic esophagus, bounded superiorly by the sternal notch and inferiorly by the azygos arch, is typically more than 20 to 25 cm from the incisors at esophagoscopy. Middle thoracic esophagus, bounded superiorly by the azygos arch and inferiorly by the inferior pulmonary vein, is typically more than 25 to 30 cm from the incisors at esophagoscopy. Lower thoracic esophagus, bounded superiorly by the inferior pulmonary vein and inferiorly by the lower esophageal sphincter, is typically more than 30 to 40 cm from the incisors at esophagoscopy; it includes cancers with an epicenter within the proximal 5 cm of the stomach that extend into the esophagogastric junction or lower thoracic esophagus. (*Reprinted* with permission, Cleveland Clinic Center for Medical Art & Photography © 2001–2012. All Rights Reserved.)

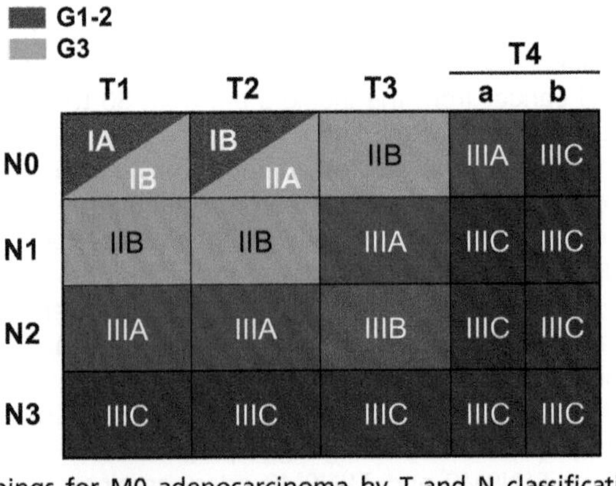

■ G1-2
■ G3

	T1	T2	T3	T4 a	T4 b
N0	IA / IB	IB / IIA	IIB	IIIA	IIIC
N1	IIB	IIB	IIIA	IIIC	IIIC
N2	IIIA	IIIA	IIIB	IIIC	IIIC
N3	IIIC	IIIC	IIIC	IIIC	IIIC

Fig. 3. Stage groupings for M0 adenocarcinoma by T and N classification and histologic grade (G).

adenocarcinoma and squamous cell carcinoma was best managed by separate stage groupings for stages I and II.

Stage groupings for M0 squamous cell carcinoma are shown in **Fig. 4**. For T1N0M0 squamous cell carcinoma, subgrouping is by histologic grade: G1 versus all other G (see **Fig. 4**A). For T2N0M0 and T3N0M0 squamous cell carcinoma, stage grouping is by histologic grade and location (see **Fig. 4**A). The 4 combinations range from G1 lower thoracic squamous cell carcinoma (stage IB), which has the best survival, to G2 to G4 upper and middle thoracic squamous cell carcinomas (stage IIB), which have the worst. G2 to G4 lower thoracic squamous cell carcinomas and G1 upper and middle thoracic squamous cell carcinomas are grouped together (stage IIA) with intermediate survival.

Stage 0, III, and IV adenocarcinoma (see **Fig. 3**) and squamous cell carcinoma (see **Fig. 4**B) are stage grouped identically. Adenosquamous carcinomas are staged as squamous cell carcinoma.

CLINICAL STAGE (cSTAGE)

Clinical stage (cStage) is based on evidence before primary therapy, and requires determination of T, N, M classifications, histologicgrade (G), histopathologic type, and cancer location. Clinical staging tools include esophagoscopy with biopsy, EUS, EUS FNA, CT, 2[^{18}F]fluoro-2-deoxy-D-glucose (FDG) positron emission tomography (PET). These investigations may be supplemented by cervical lymph node biopsy, bronchoscopy, endoscopic bronchial ultrasonography (EBUS) and EBUS-FNA, mediastinoscopy, thoracoscopy, laparoscopy, and ultrasound-directed or CT-directed percutaneous biopsy. Clinical stage provides the baseline for rational treatment decisions and treatment evaluation. The seventh edition AJCC staging form for cancer of the esophagus and esophagogastric junction requires description of clinical staging used in treatment planning.

DETERMINATION OF NONANATOMIC CANCER CHARACTERISTICS

Esophagoscopy and biopsy are necessary to determine nonanatomic cancer characteristics. Location, which is defined as the distance from incisors to the proximal edge of the cancer, is assessed at esophagoscopy (see **Fig. 2**). The seventh edition staging form requires that the site-specific factor distance from incisors to the distal edge of

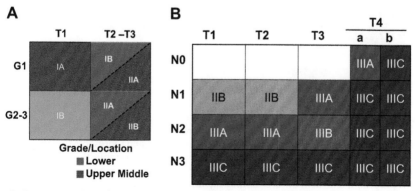

Fig. 4. Stage groupings for M0 squamous cell carcinoma. (*A*) Stage groupings for T1N0M0 and T2-3N0M0 squamous cell carcinomas by histologic grade (G) and cancer location. (*B*) Stage groupings for all other M0 squamous cell carcinomas.

the cancer be recorded.[10] This strategy allows esophageal cancer length (determined by esophagoscopy) to be calculated. Histopathologic cell type and histologic grade are obtained from pathologic assessment of biopsy specimens. The reported accuracy of clinical determination of histologic grade was 73%.[17] For T1-T2N0 cancers, cancers for which histologic grade affects stage grouping, accuracy of clinical determination of histologic grade was 79%. In this subgroup, most grading discordance was reported for G3 cancers, with 57% being understaged.

DETERMINATION OF cT

EUS is the only clinical tool that provides sufficient, detailed examination of the esophageal wall necessary to determine cT. The muscularis propria (fourth ultrasound layer) defines T1, T2, and T3 cancers (**Fig. 5**). cT1 cancer invasion is superficial to the muscularis propria (fourth ultrasound layer); cT2 cancer invasion is confined to the muscularis propria; and cT3 cancer invasion is beyond. EUS evaluates the interfaces between the primary cancer and adjacent structures. If invasion is detected, the cancer is cT4.

In a review of 21 series of early EUS experience, accuracy of EUS in determination of T classification was 84%.[18] This report confirmed that accuracy of T classification varied with T; accuracy was 84% for T1, with 16% of cancers overstaged; 73% for T2, with 10% understaged and 17% overstaged; 89% for T3, with 5% understaged and 6% overstaged; and 89% for T4, with 11% understaged. This review also showed variation in accuracy within T classifications: 75% to 82% for T1, 64% to 85% for T2, 89% to 94% for T3, and 88% to 100% for T4. It has been reported that cT2 is the most unreliable of cT EUS determinations.[19–22] However, a recent meta-analysis of 49 publications reported pooled sensitivity and specificity to be 81.6% and 99.4%, respectively, for T1 classification; 81.4% and 96.3% for T2; 91.4% and 94.4% for T3; and 92.4% and 97.4% for T4.[23] Over time, there was improved EUS determination of T classification, and the investigators speculated that this was due to new technology and increasing operator experience. The analysis also confirmed that EUS

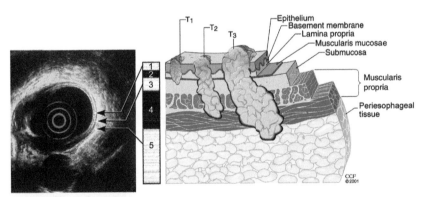

Fig. 5. The esophageal wall is visualized as 5 alternating layers of differing echogenicity by EUS. The first layer is hyperechoic (*white*) and represents the superficial mucosa (epithelium and lamina propria). The second layer is hypoechoic (*black*) and represents the deep mucosa (muscularis mucosa). The third layer is hyperechoic and represents the submucosa. The fourth ultrasound layer is hypoechoic and represents the muscularis mucosa. This layer (muscularis propria) is critical in differentiating T1, T2, and T3 cancers. The fifth ultrasound layer is hyperechoic and represents the periesophageal tissue. The thickness of the EUS layers is not equal to the thickness of anatomic layers. (*Reprinted* with permission, Cleveland Clinic Center for Medical Art & Photography © 2001–2012. All Rights Reserved.)

performed better for T classification of advanced than early cancers. A meta-analysis of 27 publications showed EUS as being highly effective in the differentiation of T1 and T2 cancers from T3 and T4 cancers, with a performance index of 0.89 for esophageal cancer and 0.91 for EGJ cancer.[24] EUS was not accurate in distinguishing Tis from T1 cancers, and other examinations such as pathologic examination of endoscopic mucosal resection specimens are necessary for this distinction.[25]

Esophagoscopy and EUS are complementary and should be performed as a single examination (**Fig. 6**). A cancer length greater than 5 cm is predictive of T3 cancer, with 89% sensitivity, 92% specificity, 89% positive predictive value, and 92% negative predictive value.[26] A malignant stricture prohibiting passage of the EUS probe is highly predictive of advanced stage cancer.[26–28]

CT requires contiguous soft tissues to provide radiographic contrast necessary to define the esophagus and provide clinical staging information. Physiologic absence of fat planes complicates the assessment of invasion of adjacent structures. These planes may be absent in cachectic patients, but fat between an esophageal cancer and aorta, trachea, left main bronchus, or pericardium may be absent in normal weight patients. The preservation of fat planes between an esophageal cancer and adjacent structures at CT excludes cT4 cancers and is the only cT determination provided by this examination.

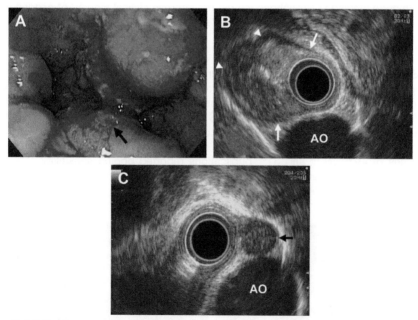

Fig. 6. (*A*) Esophagoscopy shows an EGJ cancer. The 2.5-cm-long adenocarcinoma occupies 25% of the circumference of the esophageal wall from 12 o'clock to 3 o'clock. It arises at the squamocolumnar junction (*white arrow*) above rugal folds (*black arrow*). (*B*) EUS of this cancer. The fourth ultrasound layer (*arrows*) is critical in differentiating T1, T2, and T3 cancers. This cT3 cancer breaches the fourth ultrasound layer (*arrowheads*) to invade the fifth ultrasound layer. (*C*) EUS shows, at 3 o'clock, a round, 1-cm-diameter, well-demarcated, hypo-echoic, periaortic, regional lymph node. This node is situated just above the cT3 cancer and has findings of a positive regional lymph node. Metastases to this lymph node were confirmed by cytologic review of an EUS FNA specimen. AO, aorta.

Alternative CT criteria have been proposed to identify cT4 cancers. Aortic invasion is suggested by an arc of contact between the cancer and the aorta greater than 90°, although this is not an absolute confirmation of a T4 cancer. Thickening or indentation of the normally flat or slightly convex posterior membranous wall of the intrathoracic trachea or left main bronchus is suggestive of airway invasion. On occasion, cancer in the airway lumen or a fistula between the esophagus and airway may be visualized; however, bronchoscopic confirmation with biopsy is necessary. Pericardial invasion is suspected if pericardial thickening, pericardial effusion, or indentation of the heart with loss of the pericardial fat plane at the level of the cancer is seen. Routine magnetic resonance imaging (MRI) offers no significant advantage over CT. However, high-resolution T2-weighted MRI may be helpful in differentiating T2 from T3 cancers and classifying T4 cancers.[29]

2 [^{18}F]fluoro-2-deoxy-D-glucose used in FDG PET is reported to accumulate in 92% to 100% of esophageal cancers.[30,31] However, PET and PET/CT do not provide definition of the esophageal wall or paraesophageal tissue sufficient to accurately determine cT (Fig. 7). With a reported accuracy of 43%, this imaging modality is of no value in determination of cT.[32]

Theoretically, thoracoscopy could exclude cT4 cancer but requires dissection of the cancer and adjacent structure believed to be invaded. Although mentioned as a possible staging tool for cT4 detection,[33,34] the only documentation of cT4 cancer staging is in 14% of patients undergoing thoracoscopy and laparoscopy for regional lymph node staging.[35] Bronchoscopy did not improve clinical staging of esophageal cancers at or above the tracheal carina after EUS determination of cT.[36]

DETERMINATION OF cN

EUS evaluates nodal size, shape, border, and internal echo characteristics in regional lymph node classification (see Fig. 6). In a retrospective review of 100 EUS examinations, determination of N classification was 89% sensitive, 75% specific, and 84% accurate.[37] Positive predictive value of EUS for N+ cancer was 86%; negative predictive value was 79%. A review of 21 series of early EUS experience reported EUS as being 77% accurate for N, 69% for N0, and 89% for N+.[18] Three recent meta-analyses of 49,[23] 39,[38] and 31[39] publications reported pooled sensitivity of 84%, 76%, and 80% and specificity of 85%, 72%, and 70%, respectively, for EUS determination of N classification.

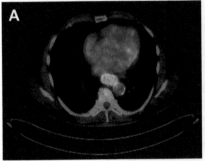 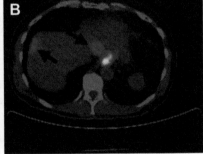

Fig. 7. (A) CT PET of a distal esophageal cancer with a standardized uptake value of 18.2. The lack of anatomic detail, such as fat planes, and the intense hypermetabolism make assessment of cT4 and cN classifications impossible. (B) CT PET of an EGJ cancer with multiple hepatic metastases (arrows).

EUS FNA further refines clinical staging by adding tissue sampling to endosonography findings (**Fig. 8**). A selective sampling guided by EUS finding is recommended.[40] In a multicenter study, 171 patients had EUS FNA of 192 lymph nodes.[41] EUS FNA for determination of lymph node classification was 92% sensitive, 93% specific, 100% positively predictive, and 86% negatively predictive. Compared with EUS classification alone, EUS FNA improved pooled sensitivity and specificity from 84.7% to 96.7% and 84.6% to 95.5%, respectively.[23] Combined EUS and EUS FNA assessment of celiac lymph nodes was 72% sensitive, 97% specific, 95% positively predictive, and 82% negatively predictive.[42] FNA confirmed positive EUS celiac lymph nodes in 88% of patients. More recent experience of this group reported 98% accuracy of EUS FNA detection of malignant celiac lymph nodes.[43]

Subclassification of N+ requires determination of number of regional lymph nodes containing metastases (positive nodes). EUS can accurately determine number of positive regional lymph nodes, and this clinical assessment is predictive of survival.[44–46]

An enlarged lymph node measured at CT suggests nodal metastasis. The short axis of lymph nodes is easily measured; intrathoracic and abdominal lymph nodes greater than 1 cm are enlarged. Supraclavicular lymph nodes with a short axis greater than

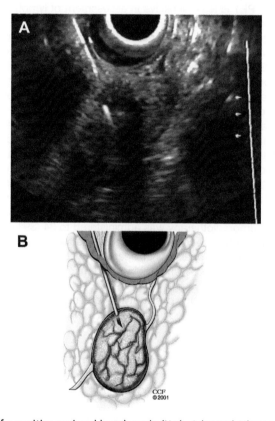

Fig. 8. EUS FNA of a positive regional lymph node (N+). *A (upper)* Ultrasonographic image with a needle passed through the esophageal wall and into the positive regional lymph node. *B (lower)* A positive regional lymph node undergoing FNA under curvilinear electronic endoscopic examination. (*Reprinted* with permission, Cleveland Clinic Center for Medical Art & Photography © 2001–2012. All Rights Reserved.)

0.5 cm and retrocrural lymph nodes greater than 0.6 cm are radiographically patho-logic.[47] However, the probability is small that cN classification can be determined by lymph node size alone.[48] Normal-sized nodes that contain metastatic deposits and metastatic nodes in direct contact with the cancer may be indistinguishable from the primary cancer. These nodes result in false-negative examinations and influ-ence the sensitivity and negative predictive value. All enlarged lymph nodes may not be malignant. Inflammatory nodes are the most common cause of a false-positive examination and of lower specificity and positive predictive value. CT assessment of lymph nodes varies with anatomic site; accuracies of 61% to 96%, sensitivities of 8% to 75%, and specificities of 60% to 98% were reported for cervical, mediastinal, and abdominal nodes.[49] A recent meta-analysis of 20 publications[38] reported a pooled sensitivity and specificity for CT determination of cN classification to be 59% and 81%, respectively. Routine MRI offers no important advantage over CT.

Physiologic evaluation of esophageal carcinoma provided by FDG PET relies not only on size of the metastatic deposit but also on the intensity of FDG uptake and decay. Theoretically, it is possible to identify microscopic metastases if glucose metabolism is sufficient to concentrate large quantities of FDG. FDG PET cannot differentiate adjacent positive regional lymph nodes (N+) from the primary cancer (see **Fig. 7**).[30] FDG PET is least sensitive in assessment of lymph nodes in the mid-thoracic and lower thoracic esophagus.[50] The accuracy of FDG PET in the detection of lymph node metastases from esophageal carcinomas is variable, ranging from 37% to 90%.[31,51–54] A meta-analysis of 12 publications reported a pooled sensitivity and specificity for FDG PET in determination of cN classification to be 59% and 81%, respectively.[38] Compared with detection of lymph node metastases in lung cancer, FDG PET is less accurate in esophageal carcinoma.[55] The addition of FDG PET to EUS FNA did not change cN classification.[56]

Thoracoscopic and laparoscopic staging have been used to evaluate regional lymph node classification. A combination of thoracoscopic and laparoscopic staging was 94% accurate in detecting regional lymph node metastases.[35] For thoracic lymph nodes, sensitivity, specificity, and positive predictive value were 63%, 100%, and 100%, respectively. For abdominal lymph nodes, sensitivity, specificity, and positive predictive value were 85%, 100%, and 100%, respectively. Of 88 patients entered into the study, thoracoscopy was performed in 82 (93%), laparoscopy in 55 (63%), and both in 49 (57%). Induction chemoradiotherapy was administered to 34 (39%) patients. Only 47 (53%) patients underwent resection, making comparative pathologic stage available in only 13 (15%) patients. Compared with laparoscopy, EUS FNA was 90% accurate, overall staging accuracy was 76%, and staging differences were reflected not by N clas-sification but by EUS FNA understaging of M classification.[57] These procedures are not without serious morbidity[58] and the possibility of port site metastasis.[59] The best oper-ative time and hospital stay reported were 3.6 hours and 1.8 days, respectively.[60]

DETERMINATION OF cM

In patients with recently diagnosed esophageal cancer, metastases were found in the liver in 35%, lung in 20%, bone in 9%, gland in 2%, brain in 2%, and 1% each in the peri-cardium, pleura, soft tissues, stomach, pancreas, and spleen.[61] Except for the brain, CT scanning of the esophagus includes all or a portion of all other sites. Contrast-enhanced CT scanning with imaging during the portal venous phases of contrast distribution provides both screening for and diagnosis of masses in these areas.

Hepatic metastases appear as ill-defined, low-density lesions of variable size. Conventional CT imaging with intravenous bolus contrast enhancement is excellent in the detection of hepatic metastases greater than 2 cm.[62] Sensitivity is 70% to 80%.[47] CT frequently does not recognize subcentimeter metastases; the main cause of false-negative examinations and low sensitivity of CT in the detection of liver metastases. To distinguish benign from malignant nodules, ultrasonography is used for diagnosis of benign cysts and MRI for hemangiomas. Adrenal metastases cause heterogeneous focal enlargement of adrenal glands. Contrast-enhanced CT is a sensitive but nonspecific screening tool for adrenal masses. Noncontrast CT, MRI, percutaneous FNA, or laparoscopy may be required to confirm the nature of these nodules.

In a cohort of patients with predominantly squamous cell carcinoma of the esophagus, solitary lung metastases were rare at diagnosis of the primary cancer and were likely to be benign nodules or synchronous primary lung cancer.[63] Although multiple lung metastases were uncommon at diagnosis, they became more common during late stages of cancer. Many were not visualized by chest radiograph. CT is very sensitive in detection of pulmonary nodules; however, histologic confirmation of these abnormalities is required if their presence alone determines therapy.

Presence of ascites, pleural effusion, or nodules in omentum or pleura suggests metastases to these mesothelial-lined surfaces. Laparoscopy or thoracoscopy confirms these findings.

Brain metastases are reported in 2% to 4% of patients presenting with esophageal carcinoma.[61,64] They tend to occur in patients with large EGJ adenocarcinomas with local invasion or positive regional lymph nodes. Pretreatment CT of the brain may be reasonable in these patients.

Despite improved technology, CT is only 37% to 66% sensitive in screening for distant metastases in patients with esophageal cancer.[51,52,55,65] FDG PET is superior to CT in detecting M1 cancers. In 91 patients undergoing 100 FDG PET studies, distant metastatic cancer was detected in 27 scans at 51 sites.[55] Seventy distant metastases were confirmed in 39 patients by biopsy or at resection. Thus, sensitivity of FDG PET was 69%, specificity 93%, and overall accuracy 84%. In this series, the sensitivity of CT was 46%, specificity 74%, and accuracy 63%. FDG PET failed to diagnose distant metastases in the liver in 10 patients, pleura in 4 patients, lung in 2 patients, and peritoneum in 1 patient. All metastases were less than 1 cm in diameter. Of 21 false-negative CT scans, FDG PET identified distant metastases in 11 (62%); of 12 false-negative FDG PET scans, CT was accurate in 4 (33%). These results are less favorable than in an earlier report by the same group in which sensitivity of FDG PET in detection of distant metastases was 88%, specificity 93%, and accuracy 91%.[53]

Of 7 patients with distant metastatic cancer, 5 (71%) were diagnosed by FDG PET.[30] The 2 false-negative examinations were a liver metastasis less than 1 cm in diameter and a pancreatic metastasis misinterpreted as a left gastric lymph node metastasis. There were no false-positive examinations in 36 patients. Over a similar period, the same group reported 17 distant metastases in 59 patients with FDG PET. There were no false-negative examinations; however, transhiatal esophagectomy was commonly used to obtain pathologic stage.[51]

FDG PET detected radiographically occult distant metastatic cancer in 10% to 20% of patients with esophageal cancer.[51–53,55] The combination of FDG PET and CT has a diagnostic accuracy of 80% to 92%[51,52] and avoids unnecessary surgery in 90%.[48]

A meta-analysis has shown FDG PET to be a superior imaging modality for liver metastases from gastrointestinal cancers.[66] In another meta-analysis, the sensitivity and specificity of FDG PET and CT in detecting distant metastases from esophageal cancer were 71% and 93% and 52% and 91%, respectively. These results were not statistically different, but the investigators speculated that the combination of CT and FDG PET would be superior to either examination alone.[38]

Laparoscopy was reported to change therapy in 10% of patients, allowing resection in 2% who are overstaged and avoiding resection in 8% with undetected M1 cancer.[67] The sensitivities of laparoscopy in detecting peritoneal and liver metastases are 71% and 86%, respectively. Laparoscopy was reported to change treatment in 17%.[68] Laparoscopic ultrasonography does not improve staging by laparoscopy alone.[69,70]

EUS has limited value in detecting distant metastases. The distant organ must be in direct contact with the upper gastrointestinal tract for EUS to be useful (eg, the left lateral segment of the liver and retroperitoneum).

Selection Of Examinations For Clinical Staging

Esophagoscopy with biopsy, EUS, EUS FNA, and CT PET are mainstays in clinical staging of esophageal carcinoma. No single test is sufficient to determine clinical stage, and these investigations are complimentary.[71–74] This finding is well illustrated by EUS and CT staging of cT1-2N0M0 cancers. Unanticipated pathologic nodal cancer was reported in 24% of cT1N0 patients and 39% of cT2N0.[75] Intense cancer uptake on staging PET was predictive of upstaging of cT1-2N0 cancers.

Results of these studies determine the necessity for invasive staging techniques such as thoracoscopy and laparoscopy and direct their use. Clinical stage is highly predictive of pathologic stage and outcome and is key in determining therapy.

CLINICAL STAGE AFTER NEOADJUVANT THERAPY (ycSTAGE)

Clinical stage after chemotherapy, radiotherapy, or chemoradiotherapy as primary therapy or before surgery is termed ycStage. It uses evidence acquired before treatment, supplemented or modified by additional clinical and pathologic staging information obtained after therapy. The same staging modalities used for clinical staging are available for staging in this setting. However, effective therapy reduces clinical staging accuracy and makes response (downstaging) prediction difficult.

Repeat esophagoscopy and rebiopsy may not identify residual mucosal cancer after aggressive therapy. Residual cancer at biopsy after chemoradiotherapy had a sensitivity and negative predictive value of 23% and a specificity and positive predictive value of 92% for cancer in the esophagectomy specimen.[76] Biopsy-positive patients were more likely to have residual positive regional lymph nodes compared with biopsy-negative patients. Endoscopy and rebiopsy had 60% and 36% sensitivity, 34% and 100% specificity, 49% and 100% positive predictive value, and 44% and 24% negative predictive value, in predicting histomorphologic regression after chemoradiotherapy.[77]

EUS is inaccurate in determining T classification after therapy, with reported accuracies of 27% to 47%.[78–81] The most common error was overstaging, because EUS is unable to distinguish cancer from inflammation and fibrosis produced by chemoradiotherapy. Similar difficulties with this differentiation have also been reported with EUS staging of rectal cancer.[82]

EUS accuracy for N classification after chemoradiotherapy ranged from 49% to 71%.[78–81,83] The primary reasons for this reduced accuracy are alterations in the ultrasonographic appearance of lymph nodes after chemoradiotherapy such that established EUS criteria do not apply and residual foci of cancer within the nodes that are too small for detection by any modality other than pathologic analysis.

Change in maximal cross-sectional area before and after chemoradiotherapy seems to be a more useful means of assessing the response of esophageal cancer to preoperative therapy.[79,84] A response has been defined as a 50% or greater reduction in cancer area. Improved survival was reported in patients who responded and had surgery after chemoradiotherapy, patients with adenocarcinoma, and patients who had cT3N+M0 cancer before treatment.[84] Identification of persistent cancer in lymph nodes by EUS FNA has been used to modify treatment of patients receiving preoperative chemoradiotherapy.[85] Despite these shortcomings, in a systematic literature review,[86] EUS and FDG PET had similar diagnostic accuracy in assessment of response to neoadjuvant therapy.

The main role of FDG PET in ycStaging is to rule out development of distant metastases after therapy and before surgery (interval metastases). Single-institution studies have found various measures, including change in maximal standardized uptake value, metabolic cancer length, metabolic cancer volume, and total lesion glycolysis, to be useful in assessing response to therapy. However, 3 reviews[87–89] confirm that further studies are needed to define the role of FDG PET in measuring response to therapy.

PATHOLOGIC STAGE (pSTAGE)

Pathologic stage (pStage) uses evidence acquired before treatment, supplemented or modified by additional evidence acquired during and from surgery, particularly from pathologic evaluation of the surgical specimen. pT classification requires resection (primary cancer mobilization and biopsy in the case of pT4 cancers) sufficient in extent to evaluate highest pT category. pN classification entails removal of a sufficient number of lymph nodes to evaluate highest pN category. Only 1 study has examined the number of resected lymph nodes necessary to adequately predict positive lymph node classification (pN+).[90] Although the sensitivity of classifying pN+ continued to improve up to 100 nodes examined, maximum increase of sensitivity occurred from 0 to 6 nodes, and more than 90% sensitivity was reached at 12. Based on worldwide data, adequacy of lymphadenectomy depends on T classification: For pT1, approximately 10 nodes must be resected to maximize survival; for pT2, 20 nodes; and for pT3 or pT4, 30 nodes or more.[10,91] This number is greater than the typical US experience of 13 ± 9 nodes resected, as recently reported by the American College of Surgeons study group.[92] This study recommended that the surgeon prepare all esophagectomy specimens to maximize number of regional lymph nodes available for pathologic review. This recommendation requires careful dissection about the primary cancer to both maximize nodal analysis and maintain of radial resection margins. Biopsy of distant metastasis without removal of the primary cancer is necessary to confirm pM.

Although recommendations are available for the handling of esophageal resection specimens, no uniform criteria for the examination of the resection specimen exist.[93–95] The histologic determination of pT and pN is subject to sampling error.

PATHOLOGIC STAGE AFTER NEOADJUVANT THERAPY (ypSTAGE)

Pathologic stage after neoadjuvant therapy uses evidence acquired before treatment, supplemented or modified by additional evidence acquired during and from surgery, particularly from pathologic evaluation of the surgical specimen. The considerations and guidelines for determining pStage apply to ypStage.

RETREATMENT STAGE (rSTAGE)

Stage of a recurrent cancer after a disease-free interval is designated retreatment stage (rStage). Biopsy or FNA cytology determines retreatment stage. Local recurrence rT can usually be established by endoscopy and biopsy. Determination of rN and rM may require mediastinoscopy, thoracoscopy, or laparoscopy. Open biopsy may sometimes be necessary. Imaging, although less accurate in the retreatment staging, directs these biopsy procedures.

From the experience of staging after induction chemoradiotherapy (yc Stage), EUS is not accurate in the determination of rT and rN after effective therapy. EUS has been useful in restaging patients with anastomotic recurrences that are not endoscopically visible.[96,97] CT is inaccurate in determining rT and rN after chemoradiotherpy.[98] CT detection of a mass in the field of resection or a distant metastasis is helpful in determining retreatment stage. The role of FDG PET in restaging is still being defined. It may not differentiate anastomosis recurrence from stricture. However, it is valuable in detecting regional and distant recurrences.[99–101] Compared with conventional imaging, it provided additional information in 11 of 41 (27%) patients and had a major impact on staging in 5 of these patients, with equivocal findings after other extensive diagnostic testing before PET.[101]

AUTOPSY STAGE (aSTAGE)

Every effort should be made to obtain a postmortem examination to determine autopsy stage (aStage). Therapeutic assessment in treated patients and natural history in untreated patients provide valuable information.[102–111]

SUMMARY

The diagnosis and staging of cancer of the esophagus and EGJ require determination of histopathologic cell type, histologic grade, cancer location, and T, N, and M classifications. Diagnostic and staging modalities are specific for each of these determinations. Stage should be determined at each milestone in a patient's battle against cancer of the esophagus.

REFERENCES

1. Rice TW. Staging of esophageal cancer: TNM and beyond. Esophagus 2010;7: 189–95.
2. Levine MS, Chu P, Furth EE, et al. Carcinoma of the esophagus and esophagogastric junction: sensitivity of radiographic diagnosis. Am J Roentgenol 1997; 168:1423–6.
3. Jacobson BC, Hirota W, Baron TH, et al. The role of endoscopy in the assessment and treatment of esophageal cancer. Gastrointest Endosc 2003;57: 817–22.
4. Zagar SA, Khurro MS, Jan GM, et al. Prospective comparison of the value of brushings before and after biopsy in endoscopic diagnosis of gastroesophageal malignancy. Acta Cytol 1991;35:549–52.
5. Graham DY, Schwartz JT, Cain GD, et al. Prospective evaluation of biopsy number in the diagnosis of esophageal and gastric carcinoma. Gastroenterology 1982;82:228–31.
6. Lal N, Bhasin DK, Malik AK, et al. Optimal number of biopsy specimens in the diagnosis of carcinoma of the esophagus. Gut 1992;33:724–6.
7. Faigel DO, Deveney C, Phillips D, et al. Biopsy-negative malignant esophageal stricture: diagnosis by endoscopic ultrasound. Am J Gastroenterol 1998;93: 2257–60.
8. Provenzale D, Schmitt C, Wong JB. Barrett's esophagus: a new look at surveillance based on emerging estimates of cancer risk. Am J Gastroenterol 1999;94: 2043–53.

9. Streitz JM Jr, Ellis FH Jr, Tilden RL, et al. Endoscopic surveillance of Barrett's esophagus: a cost-effectiveness comparison with mammographic surveillance for breast cancer. Am J Gastroenterol 1998;93:911–5.

10. American Joint Committee on Cancer. AJCC cancer staging manual. 7th edition. New York: Springer; 2010.

11. International Union Against Cancer. TNM classification of malignant tumors. 7th edition. Oxford (United Kingdom): Wiley-Blackwell; 2009.

12. Rice TW, Rusch VW, Apperson-Hansen C, et al. Worldwide esophageal cancer collaboration. Dis Esophagus 2009;22:1–8.

13. Ishwaran H, Blackstone EH, Apperson-Hansen C, et al. A novel approach to cancer staging: application to esophageal cancer. Biostatistics 2009;10:603–20.

14. Rice TW, Rusch VW, Ishwaran H, et al. Cancer of the esophagus and esophagogastric junction: data-driven staging for the 7th edition of the AJCC cancer staging manual. Cancer 2010;16:3763–73.

15. Rice TW, Blackstone EH, Rusch VW. A cancer staging primer: esophagus and esophagogastric junction. J Thorac Cardiovasc Surg 2010;139:527–9.

16. Rice TW, Blackstone EH, Rybicki LA, et al. Refining esophageal cancer staging. J Thorac Cardiovasc Surg 2003;125:1103–13.

17. Dikken JL, Coit DG, Klimstra DS, et al. Prospective impact of tumor grade assessment in biopsies on tumor stage and prognostic grouping in gastroesophageal adenocarcinoma. Cancer 2012;118:349–57.

18. Rosch T. Endosonographic staging of esophageal cancer: a review of literature results. Gastrointest Endosc Clin North Am 1995;5:537–47.

19. Rice TW, Blackstone EH, Adelstein DJ, et al. Role of clinically determined depth of tumor invasion in the treatment of esophageal carcinoma. J Thorac Cardiovasc Surg 2003;125:1091–102.

20. Heidemann J, Schilling MK, Schmassmann A, et al. Accuracy of endoscopic ultrasonography in preoperative staging of esophageal carcinoma. Dig Surg 2000;17:219–24.

21. Rice TW, Mason DP, Murthy SC, et al. T2N0M0 esophageal cancer. J Thorac Cardiovasc Surg 2007;133:317–24.

22. Pech O, Günter E, Dusemund F, et al. Accuracy of endoscopic ultrasound in preoperative staging of esophageal cancer: results from a referral center for early esophageal cancer. Endoscopy 2010;42:456–61.

23. Puli SR, Reddy JBK, Bechtold ML, et al. Staging accuracy of esophageal cancer by endoscopic ultrasound: a meta-analysis and systematic review. World J Gastroenterol 2008;14:1479–90.

24. Kelly S, Harris KM, Berry E, et al. A systematic review of the staging performance of endoscopic ultrasound in gastrooesophageal carcinoma. Gut 2001;49:534–9.

25. Young PE, Gentry AB, Acosta RD, et al. Endoscopic ultrasound does not accurately stage early adenocarcinoma or high-grade dysplasia of the esophagus. Clin Gastroenterol Hepatol 2010;8:1037–41.

26. Bhutani MS, Barde CJ, Markert RJ, et al. Length of esophageal cancer and degree of luminal stenosis during upper endoscopy predict T stage by endoscopic ultrasound. Endoscopy 2002;34:461–3.

27. Van Dam J, Rice TW, Catalano MF, et al. High-grade malignant stricture is predictive of esophageal tumor stage. Risks of endosonographic evaluation. Cancer 1993;71:2910–7.

28. Pfau PR, Ginsberg GG, Lew RJ, et al. Esophageal dilation for endosonographic evaluation of malignant esophageal strictures is safe and effective. Am J Gastroenterol 2000;95:2813–5.

29. Riddell AM, Allum WH, Thompson JN, et al. The appearance of esophageal carcinoma demonstrated on high-resolution, T2-weighted MRI, with histopathological correlation. Eur Radiol 2007;17:391–9.

30. Flanagan FL, Dehdashti F, Siegel BA, et al. Staging of esophageal cancer with 18F-fluorodeoxyglucose positron emission tomography. Am J Roentgenol 1997; 168:417–24.

31. Rankin SC, Taylor H, Cook GJ, et al. Computed tomography and positron emission tomography in the pre-operative staging of oesophageal carcinoma. Clin Radiol 1998;53:659–65.

32. Lowe VJ, Booya F, Fletcher JG, et al. Comparison of positron emission tomography, computed tomography, and endoscopic ultrasound in the initial staging of patients with esophageal cancer. Mol Imaging Biol 2005;7:422–30.

33. Krasna MJ. Minimally invasive staging for esophageal cancer. Chest 1997;112: 191S–4S.

34. Buenaventura P, Luketich JD. Surgical staging of esophageal cancer. Chest Surg Clin North Am 2000;10:487–97.

35. Krasna MJ, Mao YS, Sonett J, et al. The role of thoracoscopic staging of esophageal cancer patients. Eur J Cardiothorac Surg 1999;16(Suppl 1):S31–3.

36. Omloo JM, van Heijl M, Bergman JJ, et al. Value of bronchoscopy after EUS in the preoperative assessment of patients with esophageal cancer at or above the carina. J Gastrointest Surg 2008;12:1874–9.

37. Catalano MF, Sivak MV Jr, Rice T, et al. Endosonographic features predictive of lymph node metastasis. Gastrointest Endosc 1994;40:442–6.

38. Sgourakis G, Gockel I, Lyros O, et al. Detection of lymph node metastases in esophageal cancer. Expert Rev Anticancer Ther 2011;11:601–12.

39. van Vilet EP, Heijenbrok-Kal MH, Hunik MG, et al. Staging investigations for oesophageal cancer: a meta-analysis. Br J Cancer 2008;98:547–57.

40. Vazquez-Sequerios E, Levy MJ, Cain JE, et al. Routine vs. selective EUS-guided FNA approach for preoperative nodal staging of esophageal carcinoma. Gastrointest Endosc 2006;63:204–11.

41. Wiersema MJ, Vilmann P, Giovannini M, et al. Endosonography-guided fine-needle aspiration biopsy: diagnostic accuracy and complication assessment. Gastroenterology 1997;112:1087–95.

42. Reed CE, Mishra G, Sahai AV, et al. Esophageal cancer staging: improved accuracy by endoscopic ultrasound of celiac lymph nodes. Ann Thorac Surg 1999;67:319–21.

43. Eloubeidi MA, Wallace MB, Reed CE, et al. The utility of EUS and EUS-guided fine needle aspiration in detecting celiac lymph node metastasis in patients with esophageal cancer: a single-center experience. Gastrointest Endosc 2001;54:714–9.

44. Natsugoe S, Yoshinaka H, Shimada M, et al. Number of lymph node metastases determined by presurgical ultrasound and endoscopic ultrasound is related to prognosis in patients with esophageal carcinoma. Ann Surg 2001;234:613–8.

45. Chen J, Xu R, Hunt GC, et al. Influence of the number of malignant regional lymph nodes detected by endoscopic ultrasonography on survival stratification in esophageal adenocarcinoma. Clin Gastroenterol Hepatol 2006;4:573–9.

46. Twine CP, Roberts SA, Rawlinson CE, et al. Prognostic significance of the endoscopic ultrasound defined lymph node metastasis count in esophageal cancer. Dis Esophagus 2010;23:652–9.

47. van Overhagen H, Becker CD. Diagnosis and staging of carcinoma of the esophagus and gastroesophageal junction, and detection of postoperative

recurrence, by computed tomography. In: Meyers M, editor. Neoplasms of the digestive tract. Imaging, staging and management. Philadelphia: Lippincott-Raven; 1998. p. 31–48.

48. Doi N, Aoyama N, Tokunaga M, et al. Possibility of preoperative diagnosis of lymph node metastasis based on morphology. Hepatogastroenterology 1999;46:977–80.

49. Chandawarkar RY, Kakegawa T, Fujita H, et al. Comparative analysis of imaging modalities in the preoperative assessment of nodal metastasis in esophageal cancer. J Surg Oncol 1996;61:214–7.

50. Kato H, Kuwano H, Nakajima M, et al. Comparison between positron emission tomography and computed tomography in the use of the assessment of esophageal carcinoma. Cancer 2002;94:921–8.

51. Block MI, Patterson GA, Sundaresan RS, et al. Improvement in staging of esophageal cancer with the addition of positron emission tomography. Ann Thorac Surg 1997;64:770–6 [discussion: 776–77].

52. Kole AC, Plukker JT, Nieweg OE, et al. Positron emission tomography for staging of oesophageal and gastroesophageal malignancy. Br J Cancer 1998;78:521–7.

53. Luketich JD, Schauer PR, Meltzer CC, et al. Role of positron emission tomography in staging esophageal cancer. Ann Thorac Surg 1997;64:765–9.

54. Lerut T, Flamen P, Ectors N, et al. Histopathologic validation of lymph node staging with FDG-PET scan in cancer of the esophagus and gastroesophageal junction: a prospective study based on primary surgery with extensive lymphadenectomy. Ann Surg 2000;232:743–52.

55. Luketich JD, Friedman DM, Weigel TL, et al. Evaluation of distant metastases in esophageal cancer: 100 consecutive positron emission tomography scans. Ann Thorac Surg 1999;68:1133–6.

56. Keswani RN, Early DS, Edmundowicz SA, et al. Routine positron emission tomography does not alter nodal staging in patients undergoing EUS-guided FNA for esophageal cancer. Gastrointest Endosc 2009;69:1210–7.

57. Kaushik N, Khalid A, Brody D, et al. Endoscopic ultrasound compared with laparoscopy for staging esophageal cancer. Ann Thorac Surg 2007;83:2000–2.

58. Gilbert TB, Goodsell CW, Krasna MJ. Bronchial rupture by a double-lumen endobronchial tube during staging thoracoscopy. Anesth Analg 1999;88:1252–3.

59. Freeman RK, Wait MA. Port site metastasis after laparoscopic staging of esophageal carcinoma. Ann Thorac Surg 2001;71:1032–4.

60. Luketich JD, Schauer P, Landreneau R, et al. Minimally invasive surgical staging is superior to endoscopic ultrasound in detecting lymph node metastasis in esophageal cancer. J Thorac Cardiovasc Surg 1997;114:817–21.

61. Quint LE, Hepburn LM, Francis IR, et al. Incidence and distribution of distant metastases from newly diagnosed esophageal carcinoma. Cancer 1995;76:1120–5.

62. Wernecke K, Rummeny E, Bongartz G, et al. Detection of hepatic masses in patients with carcinoma: comparative sensitivities of sonography CT, and MR imaging. Am J Roentgenol 1991;157:731–9.

63. Margolis ML, Howlett P, Bubanj R. Pulmonary nodules in patients with esophageal carcinoma. J Clin Gastroenterol 1998;26:245–8.

64. Gabrielsen TO, Eldevik OP, Orringer MB, et al. Esophageal carcinoma metastatic to the brain: clinical value and cost-effectiveness of routine enhanced head CT before esophagectomy. AJNR Am J Neuroradiol 1995;16:1915–21.

65. O'Brien MG, Fitzgerald EF, Lee G, et al. A prospective comparison of laparoscopy and imaging in the staging of esophagogastric cancer before surgery. Am J Gastroenterol 1995;90:2191–4.

66. Kinkel K, Lu Y, Both M, et al. Detection of hepatic metastasis from cancers of the gastrointestinal tract by non-invasive imaging methods (US, CT, MR imaging, PET): a meta-analysis. Radiology 2002;224:748–56.

67. Bonavina L, Incarbone R, Lattuada E, et al. Preoperative laparoscopy in management of patients with carcinoma of the esophagus and of the esophago-gastric junction. J Surg Oncol 1997;65:171–4.

68. Heath EI, Kaufman HS, Talamini MA, et al. The role of laparoscopy in preoperative staging of esophageal cancer. Surg Endosc 2000;14:495–9.

69. Bemelman WA, van Delden OM, van Lanschot JJ, et al. Laparoscopy and laparoscopic ultrasonography in staging of carcinoma of the esophagus and gastric cardia. J Am Coll Surg 1995;181:421–5.

70. Romijn MG, van Overhagen H, Spillenaar Bilgen EJ, et al. Laparoscopy and laparoscopic ultrasonography in staging of oesophageal and cardial carcinoma. Br J Surg 1998;85:1010–2.

71. Wakelin SJ, Deans C, Crofts TJ, et al. A comparison of computerised tomography, laparoscopic ultrasound and endoscopic ultrasound in the preoperative staging of oesophago-gastric carcinoma. Eur J Radiol 2002;41:161–7.

72. Weaver SR, Blackshaw GR, Lewis WG, et al. Comparison of special interest computed tomography, endosonography and histopathological stage of oesophageal cancer. Clin Radiol 2004;59:499–504.

73. Blackshaw G, Lewis WG, Hopper AN, et al. Prospective comparison of endosonography, computed tomography, and histopathological stage of junctional oesophagogastric cancer. Clin Radiol 2008;63:1092–8.

74. Walker AJ, Spier BJ, Perlman SB, et al. Integrated PET/CT fusion imaging and endoscopic ultrasound in the pre-operative staging and evaluation of esophageal cancer. Mol Imaging Biol 2011;13:166–71.

75. Crabtree TD, Yacoub WN, Puri V, et al. Endoscopic ultrasound for early stage esophageal adenocarcinoma: implications for staging and survival. Ann Thorac Surg 2011;91:1509–15.

76. Yang Q, Cleary KR, Yao JC, et al. Significance of post-chemoradiation biopsy in predicting residual esophageal carcinoma in the surgical specimen. Dis Esophagus 2004;17:38–43.

77. Schneider PM, Metzger R, Schafer H, et al. Response evaluation by endoscopy, rebiopsy and endoscopic ultrasound does not accurately predict histopathologic regression after neoadjuvant chemoradiation for esophageal cancer. Ann Surg 2008;248:902–8.

78. Isenberg G, Chak A, Canto MI, et al. Endoscopic ultrasound in restaging of esophageal cancer after neoadjuvant chemoradiation. Gastrointest Endosc 1998;48:158–63.

79. Laterza E, de Manzoni G, Guglielmi A, et al. Endoscopic ultrasonography in the staging of esophageal carcinoma after preoperative radiotherapy and chemotherapy. Ann Thorac Surg 1999;67:1466–9.

80. Kalha I, Kaw M, Fukami N, et al. The accuracy of endoscopic ultrasound for restaging esophageal carcinoma after chemoradiation therapy. Cancer 2004;101:940–7.

81. Beseth BD, Bedford R, Isacoff WH, et al. Endoscopic ultrasound does not accurately assess pathologic stage of esophageal cancer after neoadjuvant chemoradiotherapy. Am Surg 2000;66:827–31.

82. Fleshman JW, Myerson RJ, Fry RD, et al. Accuracy of transrectal ultrasound in predicting pathologic stage of rectal cancer before and after preoperative radiation therapy. Dis Colon Rectum 1992;35:823–9.

83. Zuccaro G Jr, Rice TW, Goldblum JR, et al. Endoscopic ultrasound cannot determine suitability for esophagectomy after aggressive chemoradiotherapy in patients with esophageal cancer. Gastroenterol 1999;94:906–12.

84. Chak A, Canto MI, Cooper GS, et al. Endosonographic assessment of multimodality therapy predicts survival of esophageal carcinoma patients. Cancer 2000; 88:1788–95.

85. Agarwal B, Swisher S, Ajani J, et al. Endoscopic ultrasound after preoperative chemoradiation can help identify patients who benefit maximally after surgical esophageal resection. Am J Gastroenterol 2004;99:1258–66.

86. Ngamruengphong S, Sharma VK, Nguyen B, et al. Assessment of response to neoadjuvant therapy in esophageal cancer: an updated systematic review of diagnostic accuracy of endoscopic ultrasonography and fluorodeoxyglucose positron emission tomography. Dis Esophagus 2010;3:216–31.

87. Robello Aguirre AC, Ramos-Font C, Portero RV, et al. 18F-fluorodeoxiglucose positron emission tomography for the evaluation of neoadjuvant therapy response in esophageal cancer. Systematic review of the literature. Ann Surg 2009;250:247–54.

88. Kwee RM. Prediction of tumor response to neoadjuvant therapy in patients with esophageal cancer with use of [18]FDG PET: a systematic review. Radiology 2010;254:707–17.

89. Chen Y, Pan X, Tong L, et al. Can ^{18}F-fluorodeoxyglucose positron emission tomography predict responses to neoadjuvant therapy in oesophageal cancer patients? A meta-analysis. Nucl Med Commun 2011;32:1005–10.

90. Dutkowski P, Hommel G, Böttger T, et al. How many lymph nodes are needed for an accurate pN classification in esophageal cancer? Evidence for a new threshold value. Hepatogastroenterology 2002;49:176–80.

91. Rizk NP, Ishwaran H, Rice TW, et al. Optimum lymphadenectomy for esophageal cancer. Ann Surg 2009;250:1–5.

92. Veeramachaneni NK, Zoole JB, Decker PA, et al. Lymph node analysis in esophageal resection: American College of Surgeons Oncology Group Z0060 trial. Ann Thorac Surg 2008;86:418–21.

93. Haggitt RC, Appelman HD, Lewin KJ, et al. Recommendations for the reporting of resected esophageal carcinomas. Associations of Directors of Anatomic Surgical Pathology. Hum Pathol 2000;31:1188–90.

94. Ibrahim NB. ACP. Best Practice No 155. Guidelines for handling oesophageal biopsies and resection specimens and their reporting. J Clin Pathol 2000;53: 89–94.

95. Lee RG, Compton CC. Protocol for the examination of specimens removed from patients with esophageal carcinoma. A basis for checklists. The Cancer Committee, College of American Pathologists, and the Task Force on the Examination of Specimens from Patients with Esophageal Cancer. Arch Pathol Lab Med 1997;121:925–9.

96. Catalano MF, Sivak MV Jr, Rice TW, et al. Postoperative screening for anastomotic recurrence of esophageal carcinoma by endoscopic ultrasonography. Gastrointest Endosc 1995;42:540–4.

97. Lightdale CJ, Botet JF, Kelson DP, et al. Diagnosis of recurrent upper gastrointestinal cancer at the surgical anastomosis by endoscopic ultrasound. Gastrointest Endosc 1989;35:407–12.

98. Jones DR, Parker LA Jr, Detterbeck FC, et al. Inadequacy of computed tomography in assessing patients with esophageal carcinoma after induction chemoradiotherapy. Cancer 1999;85:1026–32.

99. Paulus P, Hustinx R, Daenen F, et al. Usefulness of 18FDG positron emission tomography in detection and follow-up of digestive cancers. Acta Gastroenterol Belg 1997;60:278–80.

100. Skehan SJ, Brown AL, Thompson M, et al. Imaging features of primary and recurrent esophageal cancer at FDG PET. Radiographics 2000;20:713–23.

101. Flamen P, Lerut A, Van Cutsem E, et al. The utility of positron emission tomography for the diagnosis and staging of recurrent esophageal cancer. J Thorac Cardiovasc Surg 2000;120:1085–92.

102. Attah EB, Hajdu SI. Benign and malignant tumors of the esophagus at autopsy. J Thorac Cardiovasc Surg 1968;55:396–404.

103. Mandard AM, Chasle J, Marnay J, et al. Autopsy findings in 111 cases of esophageal cancer. Cancer 1981;48:329–35.

104. Anderson LL, Lad TE. Autopsy findings in squamous cell carcinoma of the esophagus. Cancer 1982;50:1587–90.

105. Chan KW, Chan EY, Chan CW. Carcinoma of the esophagus. An autopsy study of 231 cases. Pathology 1986;18:400–5.

106. Chan CK, Josephy BR, Wells CK, et al. An analysis of gastric and oesophageal cancers found with 'epidemiological necropsy' during 1953-1982. Int J Epidemiol 1989;18:315–9.

107. Soares FA, Landell GA, de Olivera JA. Pulmonary tumor embolism from squamous cell carcinoma of the oesophagus. Eur J Cancer 1991;27:495–8.

108. Jaskiewicz K, Banach L, Mafungo V, et al. Oesophageal mucosa in a population at risk of oesophageal cancer: post-mortem studies. Int J Cancer 1992;50:32–5.

109. Mafune KI, Tanaka Y, Takubo K. Autopsy findings in patients with esophageal carcinoma: comparison between resection and nonresection groups. J Surg Oncol 2000;74:196–200.

110. Katayama A, Mafune K, Tanaka Y, et al. Autopsy findings in patients alter curative esophagectomy for esophageal cancer. J Am Coll Surg 2003;196:866–73.

111. Lam KY, Law S, Wong J. Low prevalence of incidentally discovered and early-stage esophageal cancers in a 30-year autopsy study. Dis Esophagus 2003; 16:1–3.

Medical Evaluation of Patients Preparing for an Esophagectomy

Samad Hashimi, MD*, Michael Smith, MD

KEYWORDS

- Esophageal cancer • Esophagectomy • Medical work-up of esophageal cancer

KEY POINTS

- Despite important improvement in the multimodal treatment of upper gastrointestinal tumors, in recent years, surgery is still the standard of care and the best way to cure and palliate patients with esophageal cancer.
- There has been significant improvements in both clinical oncologic staging and functional preoperative evaluation of patients in the last few decades.
- Despite improvements in perioperative treatment, esophagectomy can be associated with high morbidity and mortality in poorly selected candidates.
- Diligent perioperative evaluation and risk stratification leads to better outcome.

Surgery is the primary curative therapy for esophageal cancer. Although mortality from esophageal surgery has significantly decreased in the last few decades, it is still associated with substantial morbidity. In high-volume centers, the mortality is currently less than 5%[1,2] but postoperative morbidity can significantly affect a patient's quality of life. Several studies have shown that both perioperative mortality and morbidity are lower for esophageal resection when the procedure is performed in high-volume centers.[3,4] The procedure is complex, is physiologically taxing to the patient, and requires careful perioperative management for optimal results. To ensure favorable outcomes, proper patient selection by means of accurate staging and preoperative risk assessment must be undertaken. This article discusses the proper medical work-up of a patient for esophagectomy.

Several studies have focused on predisposing risk factors for complications after esophagectomy.[5–9] Advanced age, poor preoperative performance, pulmonary condition, cardiovascular status, nutritional status, and neoadjuvant chemotherapy/radiotherapy have all been named as potential risk factors for poor outcome. This article discusses these potential risk factors and potential preoperative optimization.

Disclosures: The authors have nothing to disclose.
Heart and Lung Institute, St Joseph's Hospital and Medical Center, 500 West Thomas Toad, Suite 500, Phoenix, AZ 85013, USA
* Corresponding author.
E-mail address: palang76kabul@gmail.com

Surg Clin N Am 92 (2012) 1127–1133
http://dx.doi.org/10.1016/j.suc.2012.07.005
0039-6109/12/$ – see front matter © 2012 Elsevier Inc. All rights reserved.

surgical.theclinics.com

AGE

The aging population and a longer life expectancy have led to more patients with esophageal carcinoma being referred for surgical treatment. Advanced age has been considered a relative contraindication for surgery secondary to the high operative mortality and also poor physiologic status of older patients. Several studies have shown age to be an independent risk factor for poor outcomes.[5–7] However, recent studies have shown good outcomes with older patients (70 years and older) with mortality of 2% to 8% and morbidity of 24% to 49%, which is comparable with the younger cohorts.[10–13] Others have published their experience with esophagectomy in octogenarians.[12,14,15] Even in this highly selected group, morbidity (33%–45%) and mortality (0%–11%) are comparable with younger cohorts, although the quality of life offered in this age group is uncertain. With current surgical management, esophagectomy for carcinoma of the esophagus can be performed with acceptable risk in the elderly, but intensive perioperative support is required. Long-term survival for cancer in selective small studies seems to be similar to the survival rates among younger cohorts.[16] Therefore, advanced age in itself is not a contraindication to surgery. Coexisting diseases and overall functional capacity are more likely to affect perioperative morbidity more than age alone.

PULMONARY CONDITION

Pulmonary complications are the most common cause of postoperative morbidity and mortality.[17–19] These complications can range from atelectasis and pneumonia to respiratory insufficiency requiring prolonged ventilatory support. Several factors may contribute to these problems. Patients who require surgical exploration in 2 or 3 body compartments (neck, chest, abdomen) are at highest risk for pulmonary complications. Patients' preoperative status can significantly affect their postoperative recovery and preoperative pulmonary function tests are recommended for any patients undergoing esophagectomy. Poor pulmonary status (forced vital capacity [FVC] of less than 80% and forced expiratory volume in 1 second [FEV_1] less than 70% of predicted value) have been associated with higher risk for pulmonary complications.[20] Impaired pulmonary function has also been associated with prolonged mechanical ventilation and prolonged hospital stay.[8] The American College of Physician guidelines recommend obtaining pulmonary function tests at least in patients older than 60 years, patients with history of smoking, or patients with signs/symptoms of pulmonary disease. Those with FEV_1 less than 70% could benefit from intense pulmonary rehabilitation to strengthen respiratory muscles before surgery. This rehabilitation may reduce chances of postoperative pulmonary complications.[21,22] Smoking presents a significant challenge in the perioperative management of the patient having postoperative esophagectomy. In addition to the chronically diminished pulmonary function, there can be significant problems with bronchorrhea, sputum retention, atelectasis, and pneumonia.[23]

In our experience, most patients who are current smokers at the time of esophagectomy develop pulmonary complications requiring prolonged mechanical ventilatory support. Patients who are smoking should be counseled regarding smoking cessation at the time of diagnosis.

CARDIOVASCULAR STATUS

The most common postoperative cardiac complication in patients with esophageal cancer is arrhythmia.[17,18] The rates of arrhythmia after esophagectomy are as high as 20% to 30%.[24] The most common rhythm abnormality encountered is atrial fibrillation. The mechanism of atrial fibrillation after esophagectomy remains obscure. This complication can represent a more ominous problem such as esophagogastric anastomotic leak with mediastinitis. The incidence of perioperative myocardial infarction is low (1%–2%).[17,18] However, given that esophagectomy is one of the most physiologically taxing operations, an adequate preoperative cardiac work-up is warranted if risk factors are present such as advanced age, family history, smoking history, hypertension, diabetes, and angina symptoms. Patients presenting with symptoms of congestive heart failure, significant arrhythmia, severe valvular disease, history of myocardial infarction, and anginal symptoms benefit from further cardiac work-up according to the American College of Cardiology (ACC)/American Heart Association (AHA) guidelines.[25,26] The recommendations for performing cardiac stress tests before surgery depend on a history of cardiac events, comorbid conditions, current exercise tolerance, and the planned operative procedure. In addition, staging computed tomography scans can show significant aortic and coronary calcifications, which may also suggest the need for further cardiac evaluation. Stress echocardiography can provide prognostic information on myocardial ischemia and contractile reserve of left ventricle. There is no clear evidence for routine stress testing before surgery for patients undergoing esophagectomy. In some cases, this may require evaluation by a cardiologist for further testing.

Cardiopulmonary exercise testing determines oxygen uptake at increasing levels of exercise, thereby imitating an operative situation. Maximum oxygen uptake (Vo_2-max) can be determined.[27] Forshaw and colleagues[26] evaluated the usefulness of routine preoperative cardiopulmonary exercise testing in 78 consecutive patients having esophagectomy. Vo_2-max of less than 11 ml/kg/min was associated with significant postoperative cardiopulmonary morbidity. However, routine cardiopulmonary exercise testing is a poor predictor of postoperative morbidity. More research is needed to evaluate the optimal method of cardiac stress testing in patients undergoing esophagectomy.

There is currently no clear benefit for routine perioperative β-blockade for prevention of cardiovascular outcomes in patients undergoing noncardiac surgery.[28] However, β-blockers are advised to be continued on patients who are already on them for clinically indicated reasons. Guidelines for the use of perioperative β-blockers have been published by the ACC/AHA. The benefits of perioperative β-blockers depend primarily on the magnitude of the operation, medical comorbidities, and the patient's current use of β-blockers.[29] According to the ACC/AHA guidelines, patients currently taking β-blockers should continue their use at the time of surgery. For those not currently on β-blockers, other medial comorbidities should be considered. An esophagectomy is considered an intermediate-risk surgery. For patients in this category, β-blockers should be considered among patients who are also in the intermediate-risk strata from a medical standpoint. Clinical factors that define this intermediate-risk strata include the presence of diabetes, prior myocardial infarction, compensated heart failure, and renal insufficiency.[25]

Statins have been shown to decrease mortality after noncardiac surgery, probably secondary to their antiinflammatory and plaque-stabilizing effects. A recent meta-analysis evaluating the benefits of perioperative statin use included patients undergoing cardiac and noncardiac surgery.[27] This study included the results of 15 different prospective randomized studies that enrolled a total of 2292 patients. Analysis of the pooled results showed that perioperative statin use decreased the risk of myocardial infarction (relative risk [RR], 0.53; 95% confidence interval [CI] 0.38–0.74), but not the risk of death (RR 0.62; 95% CI 0.34–1.14). Statins also seemed to decrease the overall length of hospital stay. Two studies included in this meta-analysis focused specifically on patients undergoing noncardiac surgery, and they enrolled a combined total of 1030 patients.[30,31] These studies showed that statins reduced the risk of myocardial infarction, and trends toward a reduced risk of mortality did not reach statistical significance. In each of these studies, the duration of statin therapy was approximately 30 days before surgery and 30 days following the operation. Although no study has evaluated patients having esophagectomy and statins, it can be extrapolated that statins may be beneficial and should be restarted soon after esophagectomy.

Most patients with some degree of cardiac dysfunction may be on aspirin along with other medication. Aspirin is generally stopped 7 days before surgery to avoid increased risk of operative bleeding caused by platelet function inhibition, although this practice is not universal among surgeons.

NUTRITIONAL STATUS

Incidence of obesity has steadily increased in the last few decades. Obese patients have increased risk for operative and anesthetic complications. Some studies suggest that obese patients are at greater risk of pulmonary complications and anastomotic leak than nonobese patients.[32] Although surgery in obese patients may be technically challenging, most studies show no increased operative risk and there do not seem to be worse long-term outcomes.[33] Therefore, increased body mass index in itself is not a contraindication for surgery.

Malnutrition is associated with increased risk of postoperative infectious complications.[34] Preoperative nutritional support is of utmost importance. Studies have shown increased surgical morbidity and mortality in patients with hypoalbuminemia as a marker of malnutrition.[34–36] Patients who have obstructing cancers need nutritional support, especially if undergoing neoadjuvant chemotherapy/radiotherapy. A simple and safe technique that adds little to the morbidity and cost of managing patients with esophageal cancer is laparoscopic percutaneous feeding jejunostomy tube placement.[37] Laparoscopy offers the advantage of avoiding inadvertent damage to the gastroepiploic vessels, which are the sole blood supply to the potential gastric conduit at the time of surgery. In addition, laparoscopic approach to jejunostomy feeding tube placement before surgery can also aid in staging the patient's esophageal cancer. Preoperative parental nutritional augmentation has been studied and found to provide no benefit. However, it does increase risk of postoperative infectious complications.[38]

HEPATIC DYSFUNCTION

Other organ dysfunctions can significantly affect postoperative morbidity and mortality of patient with esophageal cancer. Liver cirrhosis has been listed as the 10th most common cause of mortality in the United States.[39] Some patients with esophageal cancer have liver dysfunction. Most surgeons avoid operating on overtly cirrhotic patients. Lu and colleagues[39] performed 16 Ivor Lewis esophagectomies on cirrhotic patients (10 Child A, 4 Child B, 2 Child C). They had an overall 25% mortality with a 100% mortality in Child C cirrhotic patients. Although Child A cirrhotic patients had an overall 10% mortality, this is higher than the current mortality for noncirrhotic patients. Our recommendation is to screen patients with overt signs of liver disease with liver function tests. Cirrhotic patients may need further testing, such as ultrasound-guided percutaneous liver biopsy, to evaluate the degree of disease. Although Child A cirrhotic patients can undergo esophagectomy with acceptable mortality and morbidity, careful consideration is recommended. Early or compensated cirrhotic liver disease may escape detection before surgery despite normal laboratory testing and be discovered at the time of surgery. Intraoperative liver biopsy to determine the degree of fibrosis and surgical judgment should be used cautiously to determine whether to proceed with esophagectomy.

NEOADJUVANT CHEMOTHERAPY/RADIOTHERAPY

Despite advances in perioperative and surgical care, 5-year survival for patients with esophageal cancer is still around 40%.[2,16] Hence there has been great interest in multimodality treatment options to improve the outcomes. Neoadjuvant therapy has been used to enhance locoregional control and improve survival. Some studies have found that neoadjuvant chemotherapy/radiotherapy as a marker of early operative mortality and development of pulmonary complications.[8,9] However, there are other studies in the literature that do not show any increase in postoperative morbidity or mortality.[40,41] Our own experience has not shown any adverse outcome with preoperative neoadjuvant therapy, although occasionally a marked inflammatory response to radiation may make resection more challenging. Timing of surgery after neoadjuvant chemoradiation seems to be an important factor in reducing perioperative complications. Our practice is to wait at least 4 weeks after finishing chemotherapy to allow the patient to recover physiologically before proceeding with surgery. The neoadjuvant radiotherapy presents another set of challenges given the tissue edema that is seen early after radiotherapy and the fibrosis that is seen late after radiotherapy. We consider the safest window after radiation therapy to be approximately 4 to 6 weeks after the last dose. A good general rule is to wait 1 week for every 1000 Gy of radiation administered to the patient. For these reasons as well as others, treatment of esophageal cancer requires a collaborative approach by oncologists, radiation oncologists, and surgeons.

Despite important improvements in the multimodal treatment of upper gastrointestinal tumors in recent years, surgery is still the standard of care and the best way to cure and palliate patients with esophageal cancer. There has also been significant improvement in clinical oncologic staging and in functional preoperative evaluation of patients in the last few decades. This improvement has led to better patient selection and better outcomes. Despite these improvements, esophagectomy is still associated with high operative risk. Diligent perioperative evaluation and risk stratification will lead to better outcomes.

REFERENCES

1. Hulscher JB, van Sandick JW, de Boer AG, et al. Extended transthoracic resection compared with limited transhiatal resection for adenocarcinoma of the esophagus. N Engl J Med 2002;347:1662–9.
2. Siewert JR, Geith M, Wener M, et al. Adenocarcinoma of esophagogastric junction: results of surgical therapy based on anatomic/topographic classification in 1002 consecutive patients. Ann Surg 2000;232:353–61.
3. Van Lanschott JJ, Hulscher JB, Buskens CJ, et al. Hospital volume and hospital mortality for esophagectomy. Cancer 2001;91:1574–8.
4. Wouters MW, Wijnhoven BP, Karim-Kos HE, et al. High volume versus low volume for esophageal resection for cancer: the essential role of case-mix adjustments based on clinical data. Ann Surg Oncol 2008;15:80–7.
5. Sauvanet A, Mariette C, Thomas P, et al. Mortality and morbidity after resection for adenocarcinoma of gastroesophageal junction: predictive factors. J Am Coll Surg 2005;201:253–62.

6. Ferguson MK, Martin TR, Reeder LB. Mortality after esophagectomy: risk factor analysis. World J Surg 1997;21:599–603.
7. Abunasra H, Lewis S, Beggs L, et al. Predictors of operative death after esophagectomy for carcinoma. Br J Surg 2005;92:1029–33.
8. Avenado CE, Flume PA, Silvestri GA, et al. Pulmonary complications after esophagectomy. Ann Thorac Surg 2002;73:922–6.
9. Bailey SH, Bull DA, Harpole DH, et al. Outcomes after esophagectomy: a ten year prospective cohort. Ann Thorac Surg 2003;75:217–22.
10. Jougon JB, Ballester M, Duffy J, et al. Esophagectomy for cancer in the patient aged 70 years and older. Ann Thorac Surg 1997;63:1423–7.
11. Ruol A, Portale G, Castoro C, et al. Management of esophageal cancer in patients aged over 80 years. Eur J Cardiothorac Surg 2007;32:445–8.
12. Poon RT, Law SY, Chu KM, et al. Esophagectomy for carcinoma of the esophagus in the elderly: result of current surgical management. Ann Surg 1998;227:357–64.
13. Cijs TM, Verhoef C, Steyerber EW, et al. Outcome of esophagectomy for cancer in elderly patients. Ann Thorac Surg 2010;90:900–7.
14. Adam DJ, Craig SR, Sang CT, et al. Esophagectomy for the carcinoma in the octogenarian. Ann Thorac Surg 1996;61:190–4.
15. Moskovitz AH, Rizk NP, Venkatraman E, et al. Mortality increases for octogenarians undergoing esophagectomy for esophageal cancer. Ann Thorac Surg 2006;82:2031–6.
16. Internullo E, Moons J, Nafteux P, et al. Outcome after esophagectomy for cancer of the esophagus and GEJ in patients aged over age 75 years. Eur J Cardiothorac Surg 2008;33:1096–104.
17. Whooley BP, Law S, Murthy SC, et al. Analysis of reduced death and complication rates after esophageal resection. Ann Surg 2001;233:338–44.
18. Law S, Wong KH, Kwon KF, et al. Predictive factors for postoperative pulmonary complications and mortality after esophagectomy for cancer. Ann Surg 2004;240:791–800.
19. Ferguson MK, Durkin AE. Preoperative prediction of the risk of pulmonary complications after esophagectomy for cancer. J Thorac Cardiovasc Surg 2002;123:661–9.
20. Kuwano H, Sumiyoshi K, Sonoda K, et al. Relationship between preoperative assessment of organ function and postoperative morbidity in patients with esophageal cancer. Eur J Surg 1998;164:581–6.
21. Nomori H, Kobayashi R, Fuyono G, et al. Preoperative respiratory muscle training. Assessment in thoracic surgery patients with special reference to postoperative pulmonary complications. Chest 1994;105:1782–8.
22. Hulzebos EH, Helders PJ, Favie NJ, et al. Preoperative intensive inspiratory muscle training to prevent postoperative pulmonary complications in high risk patients undergoing CABG surgery: a randomized clinical trial. J Am Med Assoc 2006;296:1851–7.
23. Zingg U, Smithers BM, Gotley DC, et al. Factors associated with postoperative pulmonary morbidity after esophagectomy for cancer. Ann Surg Oncol 2011;18:1460–8.
24. Murthy SC, Law S, Whooley BP, et al. Atrial fibrillation after esophagectomy is a marker for postoperative morbidity and mortality. J Thorac Cardiovasc Surg 2003;126:1162–7.
25. Eagle KA, Berger PB, Calkins H, et al. ACC/AHA guideline update for perioperative cardiovascular evaluation for noncardiac surgery-executive summary. Circulation 2002;105:1257–67.

26. Forshaw MJ, Strauss DC, Davies AR, et al. Is cardiopulmonary exercise testing a useful test before esophagectomy? Ann Thorac Surg 2008;85:294–9.
27. Chopra V, Wesorick DH, Sussman JB, et al. Effect of perioperative statins on death, myocardial infarction, atrial fibrillation and length of stay. Archaeology 2012;147:181–9.
28. Bangalore S, Wetterslev J, Pranesh S, et al. Perioperative beta blockers in patients having non-cardiac surgery: a meta-analysis. Lancet 2008;372:1962–76.
29. Fleisher LA, Beckman JA, Brown KA, et al. ACC/AHA 2006 guidelines update on perioperative cardiovascular evaluation for noncardiac surgery: focused update on perioperative Beta-blocker therapy. J Am Coll Cardiol 2006;47:2343–55.
30. Shouten O, Boersma E, Hoeks SE, et al. Dutch echocardiographic cardiac risk evaluation applying stress echocardiography study group. Fluvastatin and peri-operative events in patients undergoing vascular surgery. N Engl J Med 2009; 361:980–9.
31. Dunkelgrun M, Boersma E, Shouten O, et al. Bisoprolol and fluvastatin for the reduction of perioperative cardiac mortality and myocardial infarction in intermediate-risk patients undergoing noncardiovascular surgery: a randomized controlled trial (DECREASE-IV). Ann Surg 2009;249:921–6.
32. Healy LA, Ryan AM, Gopinath B, et al. Impact of obesity on outcomes in the management of localized adenocarcinoma of the esophagus and esophagogas-tric junction. J Thorac Cardiovasc Surg 2007;134:1284–91.
33. Morgan MA, Lewis WG, Hopper AN, et al. Prognostic significance of body mass indices for patients undergoing esophagectomy for cancer. Dis Esophagus 2007; 20:29–35.
34. Heys SD, Schofield AC, Wahle KW, et al. Nutrition and the surgical patient: triumphs and challenges. Surgeon 2005;3:139–44.
35. Han-Geurts IJ, Hop WC, Tran TC, et al. Nutritional status as a risk factor in esoph-ageal surgery. Dig Surg 2006;23:159–63.
36. Gibbs J, Cull W, Henderson W, et al. Preoperative serum albumin level as a predictor of operative mortality and morbidity: results from the national VA surgical risk study. Archaeology 1999;134:36–42.
37. Jenkinson AD, Lim J, Agrawal N, et al. Laparoscopic feeding jejunostomy in esophagogastric cancer. Surg Endosc 2007;21:299–302.
38. Perioperative total parenteral nutrition in surgical patients. The Veterans Affairs Total Parenteral Nutritional Cooperative Study Group. N Engl J Med 1991;325: 525–32.
39. Lu MS, Liu YH, Wu YC, et al. Is it safe to perform esophagectomy in esophageal cancer patients combined with liver cirrhosis? Interact Cardiovasc Thorac Surg 2005;4:423–5.
40. Merritt RE, Whyte RI, D'Arcy NT, et al. Morbidity and mortality after esophagec-tomy following neoadjuvant chemoradiation. Ann Thorac Surg 2011;92:2034–40.
41. Berger AC, Scott WJ, Freedom G, et al. Morbidity and mortality are not increased after induction chemoradiotherapy followed by esophagectomy in patients with esophageal cancer. Semin Oncol 2005;32:S16–20.

Diagnosis and Management of Barrett's Esophagus

Eric M. Nelsen, MD[a], Robert H. Hawes, MD[b],
Prasad G. Iyer, MD, MS[c],*

KEYWORDS

- Esophageal adenocarcinoma • Screening • Pathogenesis • Management • Ablation

KEY POINTS

- Barrett's esophagus (BE) is the strongest risk factor for and known precursor for esophageal adenocarcinoma (EAC), a lethal malignancy with a rapidly rising incidence.
- Diagnosis requires endoscopic confirmation of columnar metaplasia in the distal esophagus and histologic confirmation of specialized intestinal metaplasia.
- Current recommendations for the management of subjects diagnosed with BE include periodic endoscopic surveillance to detect the development of high-grade dysplasia (HGD) or adenocarcinoma.
- Multimodality endoscopic therapy is effective in the therapy of HGD and early-stage adenocarcinoma with comparable outcomes to esophagectomy in cohort studies.
- Careful endoscopic surveillance to detect recurrent metaplasia or neoplasia after successful endoscopic therapy of BE-related neoplasia is recommended.

INTRODUCTION

BE is characterized by the replacement of squamous epithelium in the esophagus by metaplastic columnar epithelium with goblet cells (specialized intestinal metaplasia).[1] The significance of BE stems from it being the strongest risk factor for EAC, a malignancy with the most rapid increase in incidence (approximately 500%) over the past 3 decades in the Western world and with persistently poor outcomes when diagnosed after the onset of symptoms (survival less than 20% at 5 years).[2]

BE is thought to progress to EAC in a stepwise fashion via increasing grades of dysplasia. The absolute annual risk of progression to EAC remains a subject of debate.

This work was supported by Grant No. RC4DK090413 from the National Institutes of Health, the American College of Gastroenterology, and the Mayo Foundation.
The authors have nothing to disclose.
[a] Department of Internal Medicine, Mayo Clinic, 200 First Street Southwest, Rochester, MN 55905, USA; [b] Center for Interventional Endoscopy, Florida Hospitals, 601 East Rollins Street, Orlando, FL 32803, USA; [c] Barrett's Esophagus Unit, Division of Gastroenterology and Hepatology, Mayo Clinic, 200 First Street Southwest, Rochester, MN 55905, USA
* Corresponding author.
E-mail address: iyer.prasad@mayo.edu

Surg Clin N Am 92 (2012) 1135–1154
http://dx.doi.org/10.1016/j.suc.2012.07.009
0039-6109/12/$ – see front matter © 2012 Elsevier Inc. All rights reserved.

surgical.theclinics.com

Until recently the most accepted rate of progression was 0.5% per year, with a large systemic review of 7780 publications confirming this rate.[3] More recent studies based on large population-based pathology registries have shown the risk to be lower.[4] It is also well known that patients tend to overestimate their risk of progression,[5] which leads to overutilization of surveillance.[6]

Risk factors for progression to EAC in subjects with BE remain unclear, with clinical, demographic and biomarker variables studied with inconsistent results. This has led to recommendations that subjects with BE be placed in surveillance programs based solely on their baseline grade of dysplasia. This approach is riddled with many limitations[7] and is likely not cost effective,[8] particularly for nondysplastic BE. Biomarkers predicting progression to EAC have been identified but have not been validated in large population-based prospective studies, limiting their clinical utility.

The exact effect of BE on life expectancy is not well defined. Data show that EAC remains an uncommon cause of death in patients with BE, with cardiovascular disorders a more common cause of mortality.[9,10] One study reported a 37% increase in mortality; however, 55% of deaths were due to nonesophageal causes.[11] These data highlight the importance not only of managing the risk of EAC but also reducing risks associated with cardiovascular disease in patients with BE. Population-based cohort studies have shown comparable life expectancy (to age-matched and gender-matched general population cohorts) in subjects with BE.[12] This review explores current data and recommendations on the pathogenesis, diagnosis, screening, surveillance, and management of BE.

PATHOGENESIS
Gastroesophageal Reflux

Gastroesophageal reflux disease (GERD) is one of the strongest risk factors for BE, with several studies showing its association with BE.[13,14] Subjects with BE have more severe reflux (greater time with pH less than 4 in the distal esophagus on ambulatory pH monitoring) with reduced lower esophageal sphincter tone and larger hiatal hernias than those with nonerosive and erosive reflux disease. Nonacid reflux has also been implicated in the pathogenesis of BE.[15] Reflux is also more difficult to control in BE subjects, with even high doses of proton pump inhibitors (PPIs) failing to achieve control in a substantial minority of BE subjects.[16,17]

Obesity

The association of BE with elevated body mass index (BMI) has been studied by several investigators with somewhat inconsistent results; one meta-analysis concluded that increased BMI is a risk factor for GERD but not the development of BE.[18] Two epidemiologic studies have reported an association of increased waist circumference and waist-to-hip ratio with a BE diagnosis, independent of BMI.[19,20] Visceral fat area measured by CT has also been shown a risk factor for BE independent of BMI.[21] The distribution of fat as opposed to overall adiposity may play a role in the pathogenesis of BE. Central obesity may also explain the strong male gender and predilection of BE in the white population.

Central obesity leads to increased intrabdominal and intragastric pressure and disruption of the gastroesophageal junction, potentially leading to increased gastroesophageal reflux.[22] The actual correlation between increased waist circumference and increased gastroesophageal reflux, however, is somewhat weak.[23,24] A second mechanism to explain the association of central obesity with BE is the independent or complementary influence of visceral fat (a metabolically active component of abdominal fat) on esophageal inflammation and metaplasia. Adipokines and proinflammatory cytokines produced by visceral fat may contribute to esophageal injury and metaplasia as shown by preliminary studies.[25,26] Whether this effect is independent of reflux-induced injury is unknown. Obesity is also associated with an earlier age of onset of EAC[27] with central obesity also strongly associated with EAC.[28,29]

Familial BE

Genetic influences on the pathogenesis of BE have been hypothesized and explored. A small proportion of subjects with BE (7%) have a documented family history of BE or EAC in first-degree or second-degree relatives.[30] This syndrome has been named, *familial BE*.[31] Multiplex cohorts (those with 3 or more affected family members) may have a younger age of cancer onset compared with duplex families and those without family history. This association was found independent of BMI, regurgitation history, and smoking.[32] Segregation analysis has identified a possible autosomal dominant mechanism as mediating this association.[33]

BE may arise from the transdifferentiation of esophageal squamous cells after exposure to gastroesophageal reflux contents or by the migration (from gastric cardia or bone marrow[34]) and differentiation of pluripotent stem cells under the influence of reflux contents.[35] Evidence for the existence of both pathways has been described by investigators and the exact mechanism of the replacement of squamous epithelium in the esophagus by columnar epithelium remains unknown. Stromal elements, such as bone morphogenic protein 4 and fibroblast growth factors,[36] are also likely involved in BE pathogenesis by stimulating the activation and modulation of pathways, such as the caudal homeobox gene–produced transcription factors (CDX1 and CDX2),[37] Notch, sonic hedgehog, and the Wnt signaling pathways.[38,39]

DIAGNOSIS

BE is currently defined as "the condition in which any extent of metaplastic columnar epithelium that predisposes to cancer development replaces the stratified squamous epithelium that normally lines the distal esophagus."[40] This definition makes the presumption that the end of the tubular esophagus is well defined; this is unfortunately not true because changes with respiration and motility make this a mobile target. Currently, the top of the gastric folds (in a semi-inflated esophagus) is accepted as the marker for the gastroesophageal junction in the West, due to the lack of an alternate validated target.[40,41] Given that interobserver agreement among endoscopists at recognizing a BE segment less than 1 cm long is poor, it is currently accepted that BE is suspected only if at least 1 cm of columnar mucosa is present proximal to the top of the gastric folds (**Fig. 1**).[42] Finally, given the lack of consistent prospective cohort data on the elevated EAC risk with columnar epithelia other than intestinalized metaplasia in the esophagus, in the United States, only specialized columnar metaplasia with goblet cells is accepted as the diagnostic criterion for BE[40,43] in contrast to other European countries. A recent population-based retrospective cohort study found the risk of EAC substantially lower in subjects with columnar metaplasia without goblet cells compared with those with specialized intestinal metaplasia, further reinforcing this criterion.[44] The diagnosis of BE, therefore, requires the endoscopic confirmation of at least 1 cm of columnar mucosa in the distal esophagus with corresponding biopsies showing specialized intestinal metaplasia. The presence of intestinal metaplasia in biopsies from a normally located but irregular gastroesophageal junction identifies an entity called "intestinal metaplasia of the gastroesophageal junction or cardia" and is thought to have a substantially lower EAC risk than BE.[12]

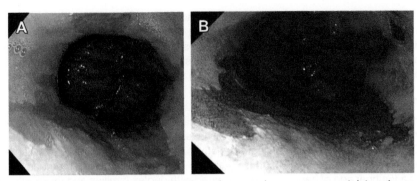

Fig. 1. (*A*) Columnar mucosa seen in distal esophagus: columnar mucosa pink in color, squamous mucosa pale white in color. (*B*) Appearance of columnar mucosa in distal esophagus under NBI highlighting contrast between columnar and squamous mucosa.

The use of chemical agents to highlight esophageal mucosa (chromoendoscopy) has been studied for years with varying results. Methylene blue has had varying results in recognition of BE. A recent meta-analysis of 9 studies showed that there was no increase in detecting intestinal metaplasia compared with standard imaging techniques.[45] Indigo carmine has also been investigated with mixed results; 1 study found it superior in identifying areas with HGD.[46] Currently, chromoendoscopy is not routinely used.[40] Another technique that has been studied is narrow band imaging (NBI). This technique uses narrow band optical filters (which narrow the spectrum of light illuminating the mucosa to shorter wavelength blue and green light) to highlight the vascular and mucosal patterns of the mucosa. This technique also highlights the difference between squamous and columnar epithelium. NBI-directed biopsies found dysplasia in more patients compared with biopsies taken using standard resolution endoscope (57% vs 43%, respectively).[47] Other studies have found its utility lower, with a crossover study looking at chromoendoscopy versus NBI, finding the 2 techniques to have similar rates of detecting HGD and early cancer. Neither technique was found superior to standard white light endoscopy.[48] Other advanced endoscopic imaging techniques, like autofluorescence imaging and confocal laser endomicroscopy, have also been studied extensively, but their success beyond high-resolution white light endoscopy has not been enough to recommend use in routine practice.[40]

SCREENING, EARLY DETECTION
Rationale and Challenges

The basic rationale for screening in BE rests on the concept that EAC arises by a stepwise progression from metaplasia to dysplasia to EAC. Hence, if subjects with BE can be identified (by visualization and sampling of the esophageal mucosa by endoscopic or nonendoscopic methods) they can then be placed into an endoscopic surveillance program, allowing early identification of dysplasia or carcinoma and minimally invasive intervention and improved outcomes. Retrospective cohort studies[49,50] have reported that carcinomas detected in surveillance programs are diagnosed at earlier stages with better outcomes compared with when diagnosed after the onset of symptoms. Modeling studies have found this approach cost effective.[8] Identified risk factors for BE include older age, male gender, white race, obesity (especially central obesity), and family history. BE is known to present later in life. Cohort studies have shown that patients with GERD are more likely to have BE on endoscopy done later in life.[51] This same study found that whites were at higher risk than African Americans or Hispanics for developing BE. This has been shown in several studies, with whites up to 6 times more likely than African Americans to develop BE.[52] Men also seem to have predominance for BE, with a meta-analysis showing the ratio for men to women 2:1.[18]

Challenges to screening are multiple. The lack of a well-defined target population is a significant limitation: the prevalence of BE in those with chronic reflux is between 5% and 10%. Almost 40% to 50% of subjects with BE and EAC, however, do not report frequent or chronic reflux symptoms. Hence, limiting screening to those with chronic reflux symptoms potentially misses a large proportion of cases.[53] Endoscopy is expensive and may lead to complications if used in a large population setting.[54] The sensitivity and specificity of endoscopy in diagnosing BE has been questioned, with several other limitations noted in the management of subjects after a BE diagnosis, particularly in surveillance (sampling error, lack of agreement on diagnostic criteria for dysplasia, and lack of compliance with surveillance recommendations). The survival benefits seen in retrospective studies are also subject to length and lead time biases.[55,56] Prospective studies documenting the beneficial effect of screening and surveillance on EAC-related and overall survival are not available.

Methods

Sedated endoscopy is still the standard of care for screening for BE. Making the diagnosis of BE requires 2 criteria. First endoscopic identification is needed followed by pathologic confirmation of intestinal metaplasia (with goblet cells). Identifying the gastroesophageal junction (end of the tubular esophagus) remains central to the diagnosis of BE. During endoscopy, BE is seen as salmon-colored epithelium that projects into the tubular esophagus (see **Fig. 1**). Endoscopists should report the Prague circumferential and maximum extent of the visualized BE segment to help define the extent of the metaplasia.[57] Biopsies should be taken throughout to confirm the diagnosis of BE. Currently the Seattle protocol calls for 4-quadrant biopsy specimens at intervals of 1 cm to 2 cm throughout the esophagus. Also, areas of irregularities should be separately biopsied because nodularity is associated with higher risk of prevalent malignancy.[58] Once confirmation of BE is made, examination of the extent of dysplasia is needed because it effects the surveillance interval and treatment recommendations. Currently, the American Gastroenterological Association (AGA) recommends confirmation of dysplasia by a second pathologist with expertise in gastrointestinal histopathology,[40] because there remains substantial variability in the confirmation of dysplasia between community and academic pathologists[59] as well as among academic pathologists.[60]

Several new modalities for screening have been investigated. Esophageal capsule is one technique that has been studied; the esophageal capsule has 2 optical domes that have the ability to capture 14 images per second. A recent meta-analysis, however, found the sensitivity and specificity low at 77% and 87%, respectively. This modality is inferior to standard endoscopy and its use in screening is currently not recommended. Esophageal capsule is safe, however, and has a higher rate of patient preference, suggesting that improvements in capsule technology (better imaging and less cost) could make this a suitable tool for screening and surveillance in BE.[61] Another screening technique is unsedated transnasal endoscopy, which has been shown tolerable, safe, and accurate compared with sedated endoscopy.[62] It allows accurate and efficient identification of BE with both visualization and biopsy confirmation. Recent studies have shown this technique acceptable and well tolerated in the general population compared with capsule endoscopy and sedated endoscopy.[63] Another nonendoscopic method for screening studied is the cytosponge, an ingestible esophageal sampling device coupled with an immunohistochemical biomarker, trefoil factor 3. It consists of a gelatin-coated capsule attached to a string, which is swallowed. After 5 minutes, the capsule coating dissolves with the formation of a sponge, which can be then pulled out orally providing cytology specimens of the esophagus. Investigators found it a practical and safe for BE screening. Despite its safety, the sensitivity and specificity of the test were found only 73.3% and 93.8%, respectively, for BE greater than 1 cm in circumferential length.[64] The cost-effectiveness of these nonendoscopic tools remains to be assessed.

Current Recommendations

Recommendations on screening for BE by different gastroenterology societies are listed in **Table 1**. Given the issues discussed previously, recommendations are variable, with modest support for screening in subjects with multiple risk factors,[40] such as male gender, chronic reflux symptoms, age greater than 50 years, white ethnicity, central obesity, and presence of a hiatal hernia. Combining these risk factors together and forming an algorithmic tool to determine who should be screened would be highly beneficial.[40] Screening of the general public is still not recommended,[65] although screening patients with chronic GERD, however, is still a common practice in the United States.

RISK STRATIFICATION
Risk of Progression

The risk of progression in subjects with BE has been the subject of much study. A landmark article estimated the risk of progression at 0.5% per patient year of follow-up. Large meta-analyses[3,66] have confirmed these estimates (**Table 2**). More recently, large population-based studies from Europe (the Netherlands,[67] Northern Ireland,[44] and Denmark[4]) have reported lower estimates of progression, ranging from 0.12% to 0.22% per patient year of follow-up. In better-characterized cohorts

Table 1
Current recommendations regarding screening for BE by gastroenterology societies

AGA[40]	ASGE[115]	ACG[65]	BSG[116]
In patients with multiple risk factors for EAC, screening is recommended (weak recommendation, moderate quality evidence) Screening the general population not recommended (strong recommendation, moderate quality evidence)	Consider in those with chronic GER symptoms or at high risk of BE	Usefulness needs to be established Recommendations should be individualized Greatest yield in white obese males with chronic symptomatic reflux	Not in those with chronic GER Only in those with alarm symptoms associated with GER (dysphagia, recurrent vomiting, weight loss, anemia)

Abbreviations: ACG, American College of Gastroenterology; ASGE, American Society of Gastrointestinal Endoscopy; BSG, British Society of Gastroenterology.

Table 2	
Rates of progression in subjects with BE stratified by grade of dysplasia	
Grade of Dysplasia	**Progression Rate to EAC**
No dysplasia	3.3[117]–5.9[66]/1000/y
LGD	16.9/1000/y[66]
HGD	65.8/1000/y[76]

with defined columnar segments and the confirmation of intestinal metaplasia, however, the incidence of EAC is closer to earlier estimates (0.38% per patient year of follow-up).[44]

Predictors of Progression

Demographic and clinical factors: older age and male gender seem to predict higher risk of progression to HGD and/or EAC in subjects with BE.[3,44] The length of the BE segment may be a risk factor for progression, with 1 recent multicenter cohort study reporting that the risk of progression in nondysplastic BE subjects with a BE segment greater than 6 cm was significantly higher (0.65% per patient year) compared with those with segment lengths shorter than 6 cm (0.09% per patient year).[68] Prior studies and meta-analyses had not found a similar association.[3,69] Increased segment length may also lead to increased risk of progression to EAC in patients without HGD, but currently, a cutoff length at which the risk of HGD/EAC increases is not known.[70] Smoking also seems to increase the risk of developing HGD or EAC in subjects with BE (hazard ratio 2.03; 95% CI, 1.29, 3.17).[71] No association was seen with alcohol consumption in this study. The presence of nodularity in the BE segment also portends a higher likelihood of prevalent advanced neoplasia and higher rate of progression to EAC.[58] Limited data exist on the influence of obesity (overall, as measured by BMI, or central, as measured by anthropometry: waist circumference and waist-to-hip ratio) on progression in subjects with BE.[70]

Medications

Recent observational nonrandomized studies have reported a lower risk of progression to EAC in BE subjects on nonsteroidal anti-inflammatory medications and statins.[72,73] The effect of these 2 classes of medications may be additive.[74]

Grade of dysplasia

Grade of dysplasia is the most widely used marker for risk stratification in subjects with BE despite many limitations: (1) spotty distribution of dysplasia leading to sampling error, (2) significant interobserver variability amongst pathologists, and (3) variation in progression rates in different cohorts. Subjects with low-grade dysplasia (LGD) (**Fig. 2**A) seem to progress at a higher rate than those without dysplasia,[66] although there are reports that contradict this.[75] Patients with HGD (see **Fig. 2**B) progress to EAC at a substantially higher rate of 66 per 1000 patient years.[76]

Biomarkers

Currently, there are several biomarkers that have been studied to help predict the progression of BE, although no panels are ready for clinical use. Biomarkers studied include loss of heterozygosity (LOH) for chromosome p17, aneuploidy/tetraploidy, and methylation-based markers. Patients with aneuploidy or tetraploidy present on biopsy had an increased incidence of 5-year cancer risk than those without, 0%

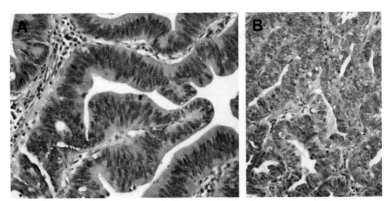

Fig. 2. (*A*) High-power view of LGD (200×) on hematoxylin-eosin stain: nuclei showing strat-ification, without pleomorhphism and maintaining orientation to basement membrane. (*B*) High-power view of HGD (200×) on hematoxylin-eosin stain: nuclei showing hyperchroma-tism, pleiomorphism, loss of polarity to basement membrane.

versus 28% respectively.[77] These investigators used flow cytometry performed on frozen tissue specimens, techniques that are not available at most institutions, thus making it hard to implement testing on large scale. Another marker for neoplastic progression is LOH for the 17p locus. One study concluded that subjects with 17p LOH had increased rates of progression to cancer with a relative risk of 16 compared with those with 2 intact 17p alleles.[78] Unfortunately, this study also required a labor-intensive technique of flow cytometry. This same group looked at using a panel of aneuploidy/tetraploidy, 17p LOH, and 9p LOH, and found a 6-year incidence of cancer of 80% for those with all 3 abnormalities, compared with an incidence of 12% at 10 years for those without any abnormalities.[79] Methylation-based panels have also shown promise in predicting which patients with BE will progress to HGD and/or to EAC. Patients with methylation of p16, RUNX3, and HPP1 were shown to have an increased risk of progression to both HGD and EAC.[80] Although none of these markers has been applied to prospective trials, there may be use for them in the future for risk-stratifying patients with BE. At this time, biomarkers are not used in the current clinical management of BE.

MANAGEMENT
Surveillance

Surveillance guidelines for BE are based currently solely on the degree of dysplasia (**Table 3**). Current guidelines from each gastroenterology society vary, but it is gener-ally accepted that patients found to have no dysplasia should have 2 esophageal examinations with biopsy within 1 year (to decrease the likelihood of missed preva-lent dysplasia) followed by surveillance every 3 to 5 years.[40] Patients with LGD (confirmed by 2 pathologists, at least 1 having expertise in gastrointestinal pathology) should have 2 esophageal examinations within 6 months (to exclude prevalent dysplasia) followed by annual surveillance. A diagnosis of HGD should be confirmed by a pathologist with expertise in gastrointestinal pathology. This should be followed by careful examination with high-resolution white light endoscopy and other imaging techniques, such as NBI to detect visible mucosal abnormalities, which may reflect more advanced neoplasia, such as intramucosal or submucosal adenocarcinoma

Table 3
Summary of current recommendations regarding surveillance of subjects with BE, as determined by grade of dysplasia

	AGA[40]	ASGE[115]	ACG[65]	BSG[116]
No dysplasia	Assess within 1 y and if no dysplasia, repeat in 5 y	Two consecutive examinations within 1 y and follow-up with endoscopy every 3 y	Two examinations with biopsy within 1 y and follow-up with endoscopy every 3 y	Surveillance every 2 y
LGD	Assess in 1 y and re-examine every year if confirmed by 2 pathologists	Follow-up after 6 mo with concentrated biopsies in area of dysplasia, with follow-up every 12 mo thereafter if persistent dysplasia	Treat based on highest grade of dysplasia on 2 examinations within 6 mo and follow-up every year until dysplasia is absent for 2 consecutive endoscopies	Extensive biopsies after acid suppression for 8–12 wk Surveillance every 6 mo if dysplasia persists, every 2–3 y after 2 consecutive examinations showing no dysplasia
HGD	Diagnosis should be confirmed by 2 pathologists Patients should be treated with esophagectomy or endoscopic therapy; follow-up every 3 mo if no therapy	Diagnosis should be confirmed by a pathologist Surgical candidates should have surgery or have endoscopic therapy. If no therapy, surveillance every 3 mo. After 1 y of no malignancy, surveillance can be lengthened	Repeat examination with biopsy within 3 mo with pathology confirmation Follow-up with EMR for any mucosal irregularity then surveillance every 3 mo if no intervention (esophagectomy vs endoscopic ablation)	Confirmation by 2 pathologists, esophagectomy recommended if persistent changes after intensive acid suppression, if not a surgical candidate then endoscopic therapy recommended

Abbreviations: ACG, American College of Gastroenterology; ASGE, American Society of Gastrointestinal Endoscopy; BSG, British Society of Gastroenterology.

(**Fig. 3**). Patients with HGD who do not undergo intensive therapy should be followed with endoscopic surveillance every 3 months.[65] There is some evidence that patients who are followed in surveillance groups have better survival compared with patients who develop EAC outside of surveillance groups. In a recent retrospective study of 2754 subjects, patients who had prior endoscopy 3 to 6 months before diagnosis of EAC had survival median of 11 months compared with 7 months for patients who had never had endoscopy.[50] One of the issues in determining how successful surveillance strategies actually are is the abundance of potential confounders, including lead-time and length-time biases. These confounders were highlighted in a cohort study by Rubenstein and colleagues[56] that showed no survival advantage in patients with prior endoscopy. Randomized data on the influence of surveillance on outcomes in subjects with BE is still awaited. With the advent of better-tolerated and

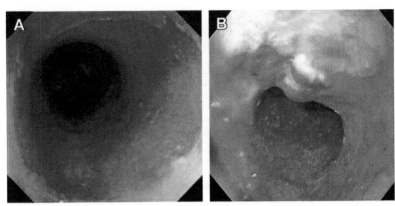

Fig. 3. (*A*) Barrett's segment in subject with HGD without visible abnormalities: flat HGD. (*B*) Barrett's segment in subject with HGD showing visible nodular change on white light imaging: nodular HGD. This should be targeted by endoscopic resection for staging and diagnosis.

safe ablative techniques, surveillance is the least advisable approach, given the possibility of missed advanced neoplasia.

Endoscopic Therapy

The risk of progression for subjects with nondysplastic BE and LGD seem to remain low with long-term studies showing that less than 10% of patients progress to HGD or EAC,[81] with some studies reporting similar rates of progression with both groups[68,75,82] and others reporting higher rates.[83]

Ablation of nondysplastic BE has had varying success. One study reported both endoscopic and histologic reversal in 78% of patients; however, follow-up was only 6 months.[84] Other studies have also showed successful eradication, with one trial comparing argon plasma coagulation group to photodynamic therapy (PDT), finding successful eradication in 97% versus 50%, respectively, in the 2 groups.[85] Once again, longer follow-up of these patients was not done. Some investigators have argued that if eradication led to durable elimination of BE, ablation would be cost effective; however, currently data suggest that surveillance remains essential given the incidence of recurrence of metaplasia and dysplasia after successful ablation, making estimates of cost-effectiveness questionable.[86] Also, treatment is not without complications becuase studies do report stricture formation and bleeding after treatment. Current guidelines do not recommend ablation therapy for nondysplastic BE.[40] Treatment of LGD has been studied with varying success in eradication as well.[87] Although some studies have suggested that subgroups of patients with LGD who are at higher risk of progression can be identified,[88–90] others have not found these factors predictive.[75] In subjects with LGD that has been confirmed by review of an expert pathologist, ablation as a modality of treatment can be discussed as per recent AGA guidelines.[40] The need for continuing surveillance, however, even after successful ablation, given the risk of recurrence should be discussed with patients.

HGD is an accepted indication for endoscopic therapy as an alternative to esophagectomy. Endoscopic mucosal resection (EMR) resects into the submucosa and is used for the evaluation of nodular dysplastic BE and the staging of early carcinoma. It is recommended that any mucosal irregularity, such as nodularity or ulcer, should be assessed with EMR for a more thorough histologic evaluation and exclusion of cancer. Additionally, it is recommended that repeat EGD with biopsies every 1 cm be done within 3 months to exclude coexistent EAC.[65] EMR is helpful in staging of esophageal neoplasia. A study of 25 patients showed it as accurate as esophagectomy in diagnosis of tumor stage for early esophageal neoplasia during preoperative staging.[91] Several studies have shown EMR useful in treatment of HGD and intramucosal cancer.[92,93] Currently, there are no randomized studies comparing it to other modalities of treatment. Ablation of the residual BE segment after focal EMR is recommended to reduce rates of recurrent neoplasia.

There is a plethora of evidence showing that endoscopic treatment is beneficial in treatment of HGD. PDT was shown superior when compared with omeprazole and surveillance in a randomized controlled trial, in terms of reducing the rate of progression to EAC and eliminating HGD.[94] Other studies have also shown success with PDT.[95] Beyond PDT, radiofrequency ablation (RFA) has also shown promise. RFA has the ability to deliver high-energy pulses to the esophageal mucosa creating thermal injury. This energy can be delivered using a circumferential (Halo 360, BARRX, Sunnyvale, California) or focal (Halo 90, BARRX, Sunnyvale, California) device (**Fig. 4**). RFA was shown to achieve eradication of BE in 79% of patients in one study.[96] Additionally it was proved safe and effective in a randomized controlled trial compared with a sham procedure.[87] In this randomized controlled trial, RFA was well tolerated, with only 6% of patients developing strictures; additionally, in those treated with RFA, the rate of progression to EAC was reduced in the RFA arm compared with the sham arm. In addition to endoscopic treatment alone, studies have shown benefit of RFA after EMR: a study of 23 patients achieved eradication in 95% of HGD and 88% of early EAC at 22-month follow-up.[97] The current approach to the management of subjects with BE is summarized in **Fig. 5**.

Recurrence of intestinal metaplasia after successful ablation has been reported. In a 3-year follow-up of the initial Ablation of Intestinal Metaplasia Containing Dysplasia trial,[87] although 3-year rates of remission of intestinal metaplasia and dysplasia were greater than 90%, 10% to 20% of subjects needed retreatment for recurrent intestinal metaplasia and dysplasia, underscoring the importance of continued surveillance after intestinal metaplasia is eliminated.[98] This has also been seen with PDT.[99] Subsquamous BE (columnar mucosa underneath neosquamous mucosa) is an issue that raises concerns given the possibility of undetected progression to HGD/EAC, which has been reported in case studies.[100] Biologic properties of these subsquamous islands may, however, be less sinister than that of exposed columnar tissue. Subsquamous BE may exist before ablation and the rates of subsquamous BE after RFA seem low (0.9%), presuming that postablation biopsies are deep enough to detect

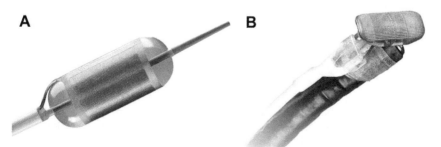

A   **B**

Fig. 4. (*A*) Circumferential ablation device for RFA (Halo 360 ablation catheter, BARRX Medical, Sunnyvale, California). (*B*) Focal ablation device for RFA (Halo 90 ablation catheter, BARRX Medical, Sunnyvale, California).

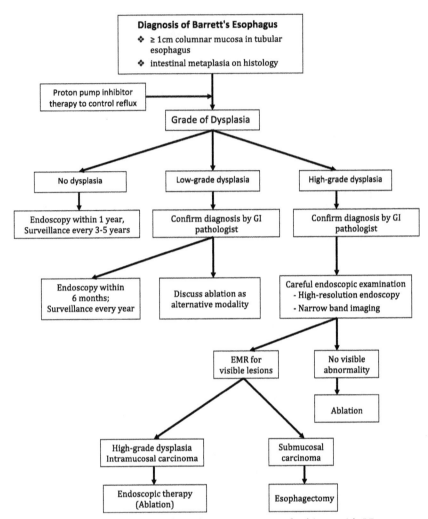

Fig. 5. Summary of current approach to the management of subjects with BE.

subsquamous BE. Some investigators have reported that esophageal biopsies obtained postablation may be superficial with only limited amount of lamina propria present, rendering these biopsies inadequate to exclude subsquamous BE.[101] Despite these concerns, overall, endoscopic therapy has been shown safe and beneficial in the treatment of HGD.

Esophagectomy has long been considered the gold standard for treatment of HGD; however, with the success of endoscopic therapy, this may no longer be certain. One retrospective study comparing survival of early EAC after treatment with PDT in 129 patients versus esophagectomy in 70 patients found similar overall survival in both groups.[102] Similar results have been reported in subjects with HGD treated endoscopically and surgically as well.[102] Esophagectomy carries a high risk for morbidity and mortality, and should be performed at large volume referral centers where many surgeries are done each year.[103] Esophagectomy could be considered for young patients with HGD given the current lack of information on outcomes beyond 5 to 10 years after endoscopic therapy. As long-term data on outcomes after endoscopic therapy continue to accumulate, however, the rationale for esophagectomy may weaken further.

Fundoplication

The potential rationale for fundoplication in the management of subjects with BE rests on 3 areas: symptom control and inducing regression of BE, preventing progression to adenocarcinoma, and reflux control postablation to decrease the odds of recurrent metaplasia and neoplasia. Conclusions in these areas are limited by the lack of randomized data comparing medical and surgical therapy. Case series have reported the regression of metaplasia and dysplasia after the prolonged administration of either PPIs or after fundoplication: however, this is typically seen in subjects with very short segments. More typically, squamous islands appear at biopsy sites after prolonged surveillance and acid reflux control.[104] A comprehensive meta-analysis reached the conclusion that fundoplication did not protect against progression to EAC compared with medical therapy, when data from randomized trials are considered[105] (6.5 cases/1000 patient years in the medical group vs 4.8/1000 patient years in the surgical group) with more recent studies supporting that conclusion.[104] A recent randomized trial comparing laparoscopic antireflux surgery to medical therapy with esomeprazole in subjects with esomeprazole-responsive reflux disease showed similar results.[106] Data on factors predicting recurrence of metaplasia after successful ablation is limited to uncontrolled studies, with some reporting the presence of uncontrolled reflux as a factor predicting recurrent metaplasia and dysplasia.[107,108] No controlled data, however, on the relative advantages of fundoplication versus medical therapy are currently available.

Chemoprevention

The concept of chemoprevention in BE has been investigated by several investigators. The use of PPIs to prevent progression of BE has been studied at length. Most of the evidence is indirect, with laboratory data showing that acid can damage DNA and induce proliferation. There are some nonrandomized observational studies showing that PPIs may reduce the rate of progression in BE and patients who use them have an overall lower incidence of EAC[109,110]; however, it is currently not recommended to use doses of PPIs over the amount needed to prevent symptomatic reflux as a form of chemoprevention. Preventing reflux has driven the concept of antireflux surgery as a means of chemoprevention. Several studies have not found antireflux surgery beneficial in preventing EAC[111,112] and it is not recommended as an antineoplastic measure. Nonsteroidal anti-inflammatory drugs as a form of chemoprevention have shown promise in potentially reducing the risk of developing EAC[113,114]; however, randomized data are awaited. Currently, it is recommended that patients with BE and cardiovascular risk factors be started on low-dose aspirin. Because most patients are on a PPI, the risk of bleeding remains low. Further randomized controlled studies are in progress looking at the benefit of aspirin in BE.

In summary, subjects with BE have a significantly increased risk of progression to EAC. Screening for BE remains challenging due to lack of availability of a suitable tool and lack of a well-defined target population, although progress is being made in this direction. Predictors of progression in BE (in addition to the grade of dysplasia) include increasing age, male gender, and probably longer BE segments: biomarkers to predict progression are in development. Endoscopic therapy for dysplasia in BE has emerged as a first-line approach, with esophagectomy reserved for those who do not respond to endoscopic therapy. The role of obesity in the pathogenesis and progression of subjects with BE remains to be defined.

REFERENCES

1. Sharma P. Clinical practice. Barrett's esophagus. N Engl J Med 2009;361(26): 2548–56.
2. Pohl H, Welch HG. The role of overdiagnosis and reclassification in the marked increase of esophageal adenocarcinoma incidence. J Natl Cancer Inst 2005; 97(2):142–6.
3. Yousef F, Cardwell C, Cantwell MM, et al. The incidence of esophageal cancer and high-grade dysplasia in Barrett's esophagus: a systematic review and meta-analysis. Am J Epidemiol 2008;168(3):237–49.
4. Hvid-Jensen F, Pedersen L, Drewes AM, et al. Incidence of adenocarcinoma among patients with Barrett's esophagus. N Engl J Med 2011;365(15): 1375–83.
5. Shaheen NJ, Green B, Medapalli RK, et al. The perception of cancer risk in patients with prevalent Barrett's esophagus enrolled in an endoscopic surveillance program. Gastroenterology 2005;129(2):429–36.
6. Crockett SD, Lipkus IM, Bright SD, et al. Overutilization of endoscopic surveillance in nondysplastic Barrett's esophagus: a multicenter study. Gastrointest Endosc 2012;75(1):23–31 e22.
7. Spechler SJ. Dysplasia in Barrett's esophagus: limitations of current management strategies. Am J Gastroenterol 2005;100(4):927–35.
8. Inadomi JM, Sampliner R, Lagergren J, et al. Screening and surveillance for Barrett esophagus in high-risk groups: a cost-utility analysis. Ann Intern Med 2003; 138(3):176–86.
9. vanderBurgh A, Dees J, Hop WC, et al. Oesophageal cancer is an uncommon cause of death in patients with Barrett's oesophagus. Gut 1996;39(1): 5–8.
10. Rana PS, Johnston DA. Incidence of adenocarcinoma and mortality in patients with Barrett's oesophagus diagnosed between 1976 and 1986: implications for endoscopic surveillance. Dis Esophagus 2000;13(1):28–31.
11. Solaymani-Dodaran M, Logan RF, West J, et al. Mortality associated with Barrett's esophagus and gastroesophageal reflux disease diagnoses—a population-based cohort study. Am J Gastroenterol 2005;100(12):2616–21.
12. Jung KW, Talley NJ, Romero Y, et al. Epidemiology and natural history of intestinal metaplasia of the gastroesophageal junction and barrett's esophagus: a population-based study. Am J Gastroenterol 2011;106(8):1447–55.
13. Eisen GM, Sandler RS, Murray S, et al. The relationship between gastroesophageal reflux disease and its complications with Barrett's esophagus. Am J Gastroenterol 1997;92(1):27–31.
14. Eloubeidi MA, Provenzale D. Clinical and demographic predictors of Barrett's esophagus among patients with gastroesophageal reflux disease: a multivariable analysis in veterans. J Clin Gastroenterol 2001;33(4):306–9.
15. Song S, Guha S, Liu K, et al. COX-2 induction by unconjugated bile acids involves reactive oxygen species-mediated signalling pathways in Barrett's oesophagus and oesophageal adenocarcinoma. Gut 2007;56(11):1512–21.
16. Katzka DA, Castell DO. Successful elimination of reflux symptoms does not insure adequate control of acid reflux in patients with Barrett's esophagus. Am J Gastroenterol 1994;89(7):989–91.

17. Spechler SJ, Barker PN, Silberg DG. Intragastric acid control in patients who have Barrett's esophagus: comparison of once- and twice-daily regimens of esomeprazole and lansoprazole. Aliment Pharmacol Ther 2009;30(2):138–45.
18. Cook MB, Greenwood DC, Hardie LJ, et al. A systematic review and meta-analysis of the risk of increasing adiposity on Barrett's esophagus. Am J Gastroenterol 2008;103(2):292–300.
19. Edelstein ZR, Farrow DC, Bronner MP, et al. Central adiposity and risk of Barrett's esophagus. Gastroenterology 2007;133(2):403–11.
20. Corley DA, Kubo A, Levin TR, et al. Abdominal obesity and body mass index as risk factors for Barrett's esophagus. Gastroenterology 2007;133(1):34–41 [quiz: 311].
21. El-Serag HB, Kvapil P, Hacken-Bitar J, et al. Abdominal obesity and the risk of Barrett's esophagus. Am J Gastroenterol 2005;100(10):2151–6.
22. Pandolfino JE, El-Serag HB, Zhang Q, et al. Obesity: a challenge to esophagogastric junction integrity. Gastroenterology 2006;130(3):639–49.
23. El-Serag HB, Ergun GA, Pandolfino J, et al. Obesity increases oesophageal acid exposure. Gut 2007;56(6):749–55.
24. El-Serag HB, Tran T, Richardson P, et al. Anthropometric correlates of intragastric pressure. Scand J Gastroenterol 2006;41(8):887–91.
25. Rubenstein JH, Dahlkemper A, Kao JY, et al. A pilot study of the association of low plasma adiponectin and Barrett's esophagus. Am J Gastroenterol 2008; 103(6):1358–64.
26. Rubenstein JH, Kao JY, Madanick RD, et al. Association of adiponectin multimers with Barrett's oesophagus. Gut 2009;58(12):1583–9.
27. Chak A, Falk G, Grady WM, et al. Assessment of familiality, obesity, and other risk factors for early age of cancer diagnosis in adenocarcinomas of the esophagus and gastroesophageal junction. Am J Gastroenterol 2009;104(8):1913–21.
28. Steffen A, Schulze MB, Pischon T, et al. Anthropometry and esophageal cancer risk in the European prospective investigation into cancer and nutrition. Cancer Epidemiol Biomarkers Prev 2009;18(7):2079–89.
29. Corley DA, Kubo A, Zhao W. Abdominal obesity and the risk of esophageal and gastric cardia carcinomas. Cancer Epidemiol Biomarkers Prev 2008;17(2):352–8.
30. Chak A, Lee T, Kinnard MF, et al. Familial aggregation of Barrett's oesophagus, oesophageal adenocarcinoma, and oesophagogastric junctional adenocarcinoma in Caucasian adults. Gut 2002;51(3):323–8.
31. Chak A, Ochs-Balcom H, Falk G, et al. Familiality in Barrett's esophagus, adenocarcinoma of the esophagus, and adenocarcinoma of the gastroesophageal junction. Cancer Epidemiol Biomarkers Prev 2006;15(9):1668–73.
32. Chak A, Chen Y, Vengoechea J, et al. Variation in Age at Cancer Diagnosis in Familial versus Nonfamilial Barrett's Esophagus. Cancer Epidemiol Biomarkers Prev 2012;21(2):376–83.
33. Sun X, Elston R, Barnholtz-Sloan J, et al. A segregation analysis of Barrett's esophagus and associated adenocarcinomas. Cancer Epidemiol Biomarkers Prev 2010;19(3):666–74.
34. Sarosi G, Brown G, Jaiswal K, et al. Bone marrow progenitor cells contribute to esophageal regeneration and metaplasia in a rat model of Barrett's esophagus. Dis Esophagus 2008;21(1):43–50.
35. Souza RF. The role of acid and bile reflux in oesophagitis and Barrett's metaplasia. Biochem Soc Trans 2010;38(2):348–52.
36. Krishnadath KK. Novel findings in the pathogenesis of esophageal columnar metaplasia or Barrett's esophagus. Curr Opin Gastroenterol 2007;23(4):440–5.

37. van Baal JW, Bozikas A, Pronk R, et al. Cytokeratin and CDX-2 expression in Barrett's esophagus. Scand J Gastroenterol 2008;43(2):132–40.
38. Morrow DJ, Avissar NE, Toia L, et al. Pathogenesis of Barrett's esophagus: bile acids inhibit the Notch signaling pathway with induction of CDX2 gene expression in human esophageal cells. Surgery 2009;146(4):714–21 [discussion: 721–12].
39. Peters JH, Avisar N. The molecular pathogenesis of Barrett's esophagus: common signaling pathways in embryogenesis metaplasia and neoplasia. J Gastrointest Surg 2010;14(Suppl 1):S81–7.
40. Spechler SJ, Sharma P, Souza RF, et al. American gastroenterological association technical review on the management of barrett's esophagus. Gastroenterology 2011;140(3):e18–52.
41. McClave SA, Boyce HW Jr, Gottfried MR. Early diagnosis of columnar-lined esophagus: a new endoscopic diagnostic criterion. Gastrointest Endosc 1987;33(6):413–6.
42. Sharma P, McQuaid K, Dent J, et al. A critical review of the diagnosis and management of Barrett's esophagus: the AGA Chicago Workshop. Gastroenterology 2004;127(1):310–30.
43. Liu W, Hahn H, Odze RD, et al. Metaplastic esophageal columnar epithelium without goblet cells shows DNA content abnormalities similar to goblet cell-containing epithelium. Am J Gastroenterol 2009;104(4):816–24.
44. Bhat S, Coleman HG, Yousef F, et al. Risk of malignant progression in Barrett's esophagus patients: results from a large population-based study. J Natl Cancer Inst 2011;103(13):1049–57.
45. Ngamruengphong S, Sharma VK, Das A. Diagnostic yield of methylene blue chromoendoscopy for detecting specialized intestinal metaplasia and dysplasia in Barrett's esophagus: a meta-analysis. Gastrointest Endosc 2009;69(6):1021–8.
46. Sharma P, Weston AP, Topalovski M, et al. Magnification chromoendoscopy for the detection of intestinal metaplasia and dysplasia in Barrett's oesophagus. Gut 2003;52(1):24–7.
47. Wolfsen HC, Crook JE, Krishna M, et al. Prospective, controlled tandem endoscopy study of narrow band imaging for dysplasia detection in Barrett's Esophagus. Gastroenterology 2008;135(1):24–31.
48. Kara MA, Peters FP, Rosmolen WD, et al. High-resolution endoscopy plus chromoendoscopy or narrow-band imaging in Barrett's esophagus: a prospective randomized crossover study. Endoscopy 2005;37(10):929–36.
49. Corley DA, Levin TR, Habel LA, et al. Surveillance and survival in Barrett's adenocarcinomas: a population-based study. Gastroenterology 2002;122(3):633–40.
50. Cooper GS, Kou TD, Chak A. Receipt of previous diagnoses and endoscopy and outcome from esophageal adenocarcinoma: a population-based study with temporal trends. Am J Gastroenterol 2009;104(6):1356–62.
51. Abrams JA, Fields S, Lightdale CJ, et al. Racial and ethnic disparities in the prevalence of Barrett's esophagus among patients who undergo upper endoscopy. Clin Gastroenterol Hepatol 2008;6(1):30–4.
52. Corley DA, Kubo A, Levin TR, et al. Race, ethnicity, sex and temporal differences in Barrett's oesophagus diagnosis: a large community-based study, 1994-2006. Gut 2009;58(2):182–8.
53. Lagergren J, Bergstrom R, Lindgren A, et al. Symptomatic gastroesophageal reflux as a risk factor for esophageal adenocarcinoma. N Engl J Med 1999;340(11):825–31.

54. Dellon ES, Shaheen NJ. Does screening for Barrett's esophagus and adenocarcinoma of the esophagus prolong survival? J Clin Oncol 2005;23(20):4478–82.
55. Rubenstein JH, Inadomi JM. Potential for lead-time and length-time biases in outcomes in esophageal adenocarcinoma. Am J Gastroenterol 2009;104(12): 3106–7 [author reply: 3107–8].
56. Rubenstein JH, Sonnenberg A, Davis J, et al. Effect of a prior endoscopy on outcomes of esophageal adenocarcinoma among United States veterans. Gastrointest Endosc 2008;68(5):849–55.
57. Sharma P, Dent J, Armstrong D, et al. The development and validation of an endoscopic grading system for Barrett's esophagus: the Prague C & M criteria. Gastroenterology 2006;131(5):1392–9.
58. Buttar NS, Wang KK, Sebo TJ, et al. Extent of high-grade dysplasia in Barrett's esophagus correlates with risk of adenocarcinoma. Gastroenterology 2001; 120(7):1630–9.
59. Alikhan M, Rex D, Khan A, et al. Variable pathologic interpretation of columnar lined esophagus by general pathologists in community practice. Gastrointest Endosc 1999;50(1):23–6.
60. Montgomery E, Bronner MP, Goldblum JR, et al. Reproducibility of the diagnosis of dysplasia in Barrett esophagus: a reaffirmation. Hum Pathol 2001;32(4):368–78.
61. Bhardwaj A, Hollenbeak CS, Pooran N, et al. A meta-analysis of the diagnostic accuracy of esophageal capsule endoscopy for Barrett's esophagus in patients with gastroesophageal reflux disease. Am J Gastroenterol 2009;104(6):1533–9.
62. Atkinson M, Chak A. Screening for Barrett's Esophagus. Tech Gastrointest Endosc 2010;12(2):62–6.
63. Chang JY, Talley NJ, Locke GR 3rd, et al. Population screening for Barrett esophagus: a prospective randomized pilot study. Mayo Clin Proc 2011; 86(12):1174–80.
64. Kadri SR, Lao-Sirieix P, O'Donovan M, et al. Acceptability and accuracy of a non-endoscopic screening test for Barrett's oesophagus in primary care: cohort study. BMJ 2010;341:c4372.
65. Wang KK, Sampliner RE. Updated guidelines 2008 for the diagnosis, surveillance and therapy of Barrett's esophagus. Am J Gastroenterol 2008;103(3): 788–97.
66. Wani S, Puli SR, Shaheen NJ, et al. Esophageal adenocarcinoma in Barrett's esophagus after endoscopic ablative therapy: a meta-analysis and systematic review. Am J Gastroenterol 2009;104(2):502–13.
67. de Jonge PJ, van Blankenstein M, Looman CW, et al. Risk of malignant progression in patients with Barrett's oesophagus: a Dutch nationwide cohort study. Gut 2010;59(8):1030–6.
68. Wani S, Falk G, Hall M, et al. Patients with nondysplastic Barrett's esophagus have low risks for developing dysplasia or esophageal adenocarcinoma. Clin Gastroenterol Hepatol 2011;9(3):220–7 [quiz: e226].
69. Rudolph RE, Vaughan TL, Storer BE, et al. Effect of segment length on risk for neoplastic progression in patients with Barrett esophagus. Ann Intern Med 2000;132(8):612–20.
70. Prasad GA, Bansal A, Sharma P, et al. Predictors of progression in Barrett's esophagus: current knowledge and future directions. Am J Gastroenterol 2010;105(7):1490–502.
71. Coleman HG, Bhat S, Johnston BT, et al. Tobacco smoking increases the risk of high-grade dysplasia and cancer among patients with Barrett's esophagus. Gastroenterology 2012;142(2):233–40.

72. Nguyen DM, Richardson P, El-Serag HB. Medications (NSAIDs, statins, proton pump inhibitors) and the risk of esophageal adenocarcinoma in patients with Barrett's esophagus. Gastroenterology 2010;138(7):2260–6.
73. Nguyen DM, El-Serag HB, Henderson L, et al. Medication usage and the risk of neoplasia in patients with Barrett's esophagus. Clin Gastroenterol Hepatol 2009; 7(12):1299–304.
74. Kastelein F, Spaander MC, Biermann K, et al. Nonsteroidal anti-inflammatory drugs and statins have chemopreventative effects in patients with Barrett's esophagus. Gastroenterology 2011;141(6):2000–8 [quiz: e2013–2004].
75. Wani S, Falk GW, Post J, et al. Risk factors for progression of low-grade dysplasia in patients with Barrett's esophagus. Gastroenterology 2011;141(4): 1179–86, 1186 e1171.
76. Rastogi A, Puli S, El-Serag HB, et al. Incidence of esophageal adenocarcinoma in patients with Barrett's esophagus and high-grade dysplasia: a meta-analysis. Gastrointest Endosc 2008;67(3):394–8.
77. Reid BJ, Levine DS, Longton G, et al. Predictors of progression to cancer in Barrett's esophagus: baseline histology and flow cytometry identify low- and high-risk patient subsets. Am J Gastroenterol 2000;95(7):1669–76.
78. Reid BJ, Prevo LJ, Galipeau PC, et al. Predictors of progression in Barrett's esophagus II: baseline 17p (p53) loss of heterozygosity identifies a patient subset at increased risk for neoplastic progression. Am J Gastroenterol 2001; 96(10):2839–48.
79. Galipeau PC, Li X, Blount PL, et al. NSAIDs modulate CDKN2A, TP53, and DNA content risk for progression to esophageal adenocarcinoma. PLoS Med 2007; 4(2):e67.
80. Schulmann K, Sterian A, Berki A, et al. Inactivation of p16, RUNX3, and HPP1 occurs early in Barrett's-associated neoplastic progression and predicts progression risk. Oncogene 2005;24(25):4138–48.
81. Schnell TG, Sontag SJ, Chejfec G, et al. Long-term nonsurgical management of Barrett's esophagus with high-grade dysplasia. Gastroenterology 2001;120(7): 1607–19.
82. Sharma P, Falk GW, Weston AP, et al. Dysplasia and cancer in a large multi-center cohort of patients with Barrett's esophagus. Clin Gastroenterol Hepatol 2006;4(5):566–72.
83. Curvers WL, ten Kate FJ, Krishnadath KK, et al. Low-grade dysplasia in Barrett's esophagus: overdiagnosed and underestimated. Am J Gastroenterol 2010; 105(7):1523–30.
84. Sampliner RE, Faigel D, Fennerty MB, et al. Effective and safe endoscopic reversal of nondysplastic Barrett's esophagus with thermal electrocoagulation combined with high-dose acid inhibition: a multicenter study. Gastrointest Endosc 2001;53(6):554–8.
85. Kelty CJ, Ackroyd R, Brown NJ, et al. Endoscopic ablation of Barrett's oesophagus: a randomized-controlled trial of photodynamic therapy vs. argon plasma coagulation. Aliment Pharmacol Ther 2004;20(11–12):1289–96.
86. Inadomi JM, Somsouk M, Madanick RD, et al. A cost-utility analysis of ablative therapy for Barrett's esophagus. Gastroenterology 2009;136(7):2101–14 e2101–2106.
87. Shaheen NJ, Sharma P, Overholt BF, et al. Radiofrequency ablation in Barrett's esophagus with dysplasia. N Engl J Med 2009;360(22):2277–88.
88. Montgomery E, Goldblum JR, Greenson JK, et al. Dysplasia as a predictive marker for invasive carcinoma in Barrett esophagus: a follow-up study based

on 138 cases from a diagnostic variability study. Hum Pathol 2001;32(4): 379–88.

89. Skacel M, Petras RE, Gramlich TL, et al. The diagnosis of low-grade dysplasia in Barrett's esophagus and its implications for disease progression. Am J Gastroenterol 2000;95(12):3383–7.

90. Skacel M, Petras RE, Rybicki LA, et al. p53 expression in low grade dysplasia in Barrett's esophagus: correlation with interobserver agreement and disease progression. Am J Gastroenterol 2002;97(10):2508–13.

91. Prasad GA, Buttar NS, Wongkeesong LM, et al. Significance of neoplastic involvement of margins obtained by endoscopic mucosal resection in Barrett's esophagus. Am J Gastroenterol 2007;102(11):2380–6.

92. Peters FP, Kara MA, Rosmolen WD, et al. Stepwise radical endoscopic resection is effective for complete removal of Barrett's esophagus with early neoplasia: a prospective study. Am J Gastroenterol 2006;101(7):1449–57.

93. Conio M, Repici A, Cestari R, et al. Endoscopic mucosal resection for high-grade dysplasia and intramucosal carcinoma in Barrett's esophagus: an Italian experience. World J Gastroenterol 2005;11(42):6650–5.

94. Overholt BF, Wang KK, Burdick JS, et al. Five-year efficacy and safety of photo-dynamic therapy with Photofrin in Barrett's high-grade dysplasia. Gastrointest Endosc 2007;66(3):460–8.

95. Pech O, Gossner L, May A, et al. Long-term results of photodynamic therapy with 5-aminolevulinic acid for superficial Barrett's cancer and high-grade intra-epithelial neoplasia. Gastrointest Endosc 2005;62(1):24–30.

96. Sharma VK, Jae Kim H, Das A, et al. Circumferential and focal ablation of Barrett's esophagus containing dysplasia. Am J Gastroenterol 2009;104(2): 310–7.

97. Pouw RE, Wirths K, Eisendrath P, et al. Efficacy of radiofrequency ablation combined with endoscopic resection for Barrett's esophagus with early neo-plasia. Clin Gastroenterol Hepatol 2010;8(1):23–9.

98. Shaheen NJ, Overholt BF, Sampliner RE, et al. Durability of radiofrequency abla-tion in Barrett's esophagus with dysplasia. Gastroenterology 2011;141(2):460–8.

99. Badreddine RJ, Prasad GA, Wang KK, et al. Prevalence and predictors of recur-rent neoplasia after ablation of Barrett's esophagus. Gastrointest Endosc 2010; 71(4):697–703.

100. Gray NA, Odze RD, Spechler SJ. Buried metaplasia after endoscopic ablation of Barrett's esophagus: a systematic review. Am J Gastroenterol 2011;106(11): 1899–908 [quiz: 1909].

101. Gupta N, Mathur SC, Dumot JA, et al. Adequacy of esophageal squamous mucosa specimens obtained during endoscopy: are standard biopsies suffi-cient for postablation surveillance in Barrett's esophagus? Gastrointest Endosc 2012;75(1):11–8.

102. Prasad GA, Wang KK, Buttar NS, et al. Long-term survival following endoscopic and surgical treatment of high-grade dysplasia in Barrett's esophagus. Gastro-enterology 2007;132(4):1226–33.

103. van Lanschot JJ, Hulscher JB, Buskens CJ, et al. Hospital volume and hospital mortality for esophagectomy. Cancer 2001;91(8):1574–8.

104. Wassenaar EB, Oelschlager BK. Effect of medical and surgical treatment of Bar-rett's metaplasia. World J Gastroenterol 2010;16(30):3773–9.

105. Chang EY, Morris CD, Seltman AK, et al. The effect of antireflux surgery on esophageal carcinogenesis in patients with barrett esophagus: a systematic review. Ann Surg 2007;246(1):11–21.

106. Galmiche JP, Hatlebakk J, Attwood S, et al. Laparoscopic antireflux surgery vs esomeprazole treatment for chronic GERD: the LOTUS randomized clinical trial. JAMA 2011;305(19):1969–77.

107. Kahaleh M, Van Laethem JL, Nagy N, et al. Long-term follow-up and factors predictive of recurrence in Barrett's esophagus treated by argon plasma coagulation and acid suppression. Endoscopy 2002;34(12):950–5.

108. Ferraris R, Fracchia M, Foti M, et al. Barrett's oesophagus: long-term follow-up after complete ablation with argon plasma coagulation and the factors that determine its recurrence. Aliment Pharmacol Ther 2007;25(7):835–40.

109. Cooper BT, Chapman W, Neumann CS, et al. Continuous treatment of Barrett's oesophagus patients with proton pump inhibitors up to 13 years: observations on regression and cancer incidence. Aliment Pharmacol Ther 2006;23(6): 727–33.

110. El-Serag HB, Aguirre TV, Davis S, et al. Proton pump inhibitors are associated with reduced incidence of dysplasia in Barrett's esophagus. Am J Gastroenterol 2004;99(10):1877–83.

111. Corey KE, Schmitz SM, Shaheen NJ. Does a surgical antireflux procedure decrease the incidence of esophageal adenocarcinoma in Barrett's esophagus? A meta-analysis. Am J Gastroenterol 2003;98(11):2390–4.

112. Tran T, Spechler SJ, Richardson P, et al. Fundoplication and the risk of esophageal cancer in gastroesophageal reflux disease: a Veterans Affairs cohort study. Am J Gastroenterol 2005;100(5):1002–8.

113. Corley DA, Kerlikowske K, Verma R, et al. Protective association of aspirin/ NSAIDs and esophageal cancer: a systematic review and meta-analysis. Gastroenterology 2003;124(1):47–56.

114. Vaughan TL, Dong LM, Blount PL, et al. Non-steroidal anti-inflammatory drugs and risk of neoplastic progression in Barrett's oesophagus: a prospective study. Lancet Oncol 2005;6(12):945–52.

115. Hirota WK, Zuckerman MJ, Adler DG, et al. ASGE guideline: the role of endoscopy in the surveillance of premalignant conditions of the upper GI tract. Gastrointest Endosc 2006;63(4):570–80.

116. Playford RJ. New British Society of Gastroenterology (BSG) guidelines for the diagnosis and management of Barrett's oesophagus. Gut 2006;55(4):442.

117. Desai TK, Krishnan K, Samala N, et al. The incidence of oesophageal adenocarcinoma in non-dysplastic Barrett's oesophagus: a meta-analysis. Gut 2012; 61(7):970–6.

Management of Stage 1 Esophageal Cancer

Michael Hermansson, MD, PhD, Steven R. DeMeester, MD*

KEYWORDS

- Esophageal cancer • Stage 1 • Vagus-sparing esophagectomy
- Endoscopic resection • Radiofrequency ablation

KEY POINTS

- Barrett surveillance programs and more liberal use of upper endoscopy are leading to the identification of an increasing number of patients with high-grade dysplasia or early stage esophageal adenocarcinoma.
- Endoscopic mucosal resection is currently the only method able to reliably determine the depth of invasion of superficial cancers, and is an important aspect of staging because submucosal invasion imparts a significant risk of lymph node metastases, and therapies that do not include a lymphadenectomy are potentially inadequate.
- A vagal-sparing esophagectomy provides the benefit of complete esophageal resection with elimination of all Barrett segments while minimizing the morbidity associated with traditional esophagectomies that include a vagotomy.
- Currently, a combination of endoscopic resection and ablation is the preferred therapy for most patients with high-grade dysplasia or intramucosal adenocarinoma, and available evidence suggests that survival with endoscopic therapy is equivalent to that after esophagectomy.

SCOPE OF THE PROBLEM

Esophageal cancer is one of the deadliest malignancies in the world. Taken together, there are 418,000 cases of squamous and adenocarcinoma annually throughout the world.[1] Squamous cell is still the predominant form of esophageal cancer in Asia and much of the world, but adenocarcinoma is by far the leading cell type in most Western countries. The two types of esophageal cancer have different etiologies. Squamous cancer occurs as a consequence of tobacco use and alcohol, and although it can develop anywhere in the esophagus, it often occurs proximally. Adenocarcinoma develops secondary to gastroesophageal reflux and Barrett esophagus and occurs most commonly distally or at the gastroesophageal junction.

Department of Surgery, Keck School of Medicine, The University of Southern California, 1510 San Pablo Street, Los Angeles, CA 90033, USA
* Corresponding author.
E-mail address: sdemeester@surgery.usc.edu

Surg Clin N Am 92 (2012) 1155–1167
http://dx.doi.org/10.1016/j.suc.2012.07.014
0039-6109/12/$ – see front matter © 2012 Elsevier Inc. All rights reserved.
surgical.theclinics.com

Once a rare tumor, adenocarcinoma of the esophagus is currently the cancer with the fastest rising incidence in America. Recent data indicate that in the United States since 1975 the rate of increase of adenocarcinoma of the esophagus has outpaced the next closest cancer, melanoma, by nearly three times.[2–4] The current average yearly increase in incidence in the United States exceeds 20%, and among white males the incidence has increased more than 800% since the mid-1970s in some areas of the country.[5–7] This increase has propelled esophageal adenocarcinoma into one of the top 15 cancers in US white males and has led to a complete epidemiologic shift such that in the United States and other industrialized countries adenocarcinoma has replaced squamous cell as the most common esophageal malignancy.[4,5,8]

In addition to the increasing prevalence of the disease, surveillance programs for patients with Barrett esophagus have led to the identification of increasing numbers of patients with high-grade dysplasia or early stage esophageal adenocarcinomas. Similarly, in high-risk Asian populations screening programs are detecting patients with high-grade squamous dysplasia or superficial squamous cell cancer. Although esophagectomy is curative in most of these patients, associated morbidity and mortality remain a hurdle for patient acceptance of the procedure. To minimize morbidity associated with an esophagectomy surgeons have developed minimally invasive techniques and methods to spare the vagus nerves and thereby reduce the incidence of postvagotomy diarrhea or dumping symptoms. In addition, new technologies now allow endoscopic therapy of these lesions with the potential for esophageal preservation. However, neither endoscopic therapy nor vagal-sparing esophagectomy address potentially involved lymph nodes, and are not appropriate in patients that have a significant risk of lymph node metastases. Thus, when planning therapy for a patient with early stage esophageal cancer it is critical to understand the relationship between depth of tumor invasion and the likelihood of lymph node metastases.

STAGING EARLY ESOPHAGEAL CANCER

Staging studies for esophageal cancer include upper endoscopy, endoscopic ultrasound (EUS), endoscopic resection (ER), computed tomography (CT) scans of the chest and abdomen, and positron emission tomography (PET) scan.

Endoscopy

Upper endoscopy provides critical information about the presence and length of a columnar-lined esophagus, and the size and location of any visible lesions. Endoscopic modalities including narrow band imaging and enhanced magnification can facilitate identification of irregular areas in the columnar mucosa of Barrett esophagus, whereas Lugol stain facilitates identification of squamous dysplasia. The endoscopy report should include the distance from the incisor teeth to the upper border of the tumor and the position of the tumor relative to the esophagogastric junction for distal tumors or the cricopharyngeous for proximal tumors. During endoscopic evaluation of the esophagus a critical task is to look for any nodules, ulcers, or irregularities. Such areas are particularly at risk to harbor a cancer. If a random biopsy shows adenocarcinoma but no visible abnormality was seen endoscopically within the columnar mucosa, it has been shown that the cancer is confined to the mucosa in nearly all circumstances.[9] In contrast, if a biopsy showing adenocarcinoma came from a visible lesion, the cancer cannot be assumed to be limited to the mucosa, regardless of the size or appearance of the lesion. Even very small lesions may penetrate into the submucosa, thus the endoscopic appearance of an adenocarcinoma cannot be used to determine the "T" stage. Nonetheless, the risk of submucosal invasion or nodal involvement does increase with increasing tumor length, particularly beyond 2 or 3 cm.[10–12] Further, the Paris classification has related the endoscopic appearance of squamous tumors with the risk of submucosal infiltration. This system includes flat, protruding, and excavating lesions, with flat lesions having the lowest risk and protruding the highest risk.[13]

EUS

Local and regional staging of esophageal cancer is best done with EUS. Standard 7.5- and 12- MHz EUS probes can accurately assess the depth of invasion after the tumor has gone through the submucosa, and also provide information on the presence of abnormal-appearing or enlarged lymph nodes. The addition of fine-needle aspiration improves sensitivity and specificity for nodal EUS staging.[14] However, neither the standard probes nor newer high-resolution 20-MHz probes are able to accurately distinguish intramucosal from submucosal tumor invasion.[15–18] Consequently, in patients with a nodule or superficial lesion staging is best done with an ER to allow pathologic determination of the depth of invasion.[19]

ER

ER, or what initially was called endoscopic mucosal resection, is an endoscopic procedure that allows excision of a disk of esophageal wall down to the muscularis propria. The specimen can then be histologically evaluated and the precise depth of invasion of the lesion determined. Thus, from an ER specimen a pathologist can accurately determine whether a tumor is limited to the mucosa or has penetrated beyond the muscularis mucosa into the submucosa. This distinction is critical because the likelihood of lymph node metastases changes significantly after a tumor breaches the muscularis mucosa and enters the submucosa.[12] Approximately 20% of patients with a tumor invading into the submucosa have lymph node metastases, and a therapy that does not include a lymphadenectomy is not appropriate. The initial technique for ER entailed the use of a cap that was fitted over the end of a standard endoscope. Developed by Dr Inoue from Japan, these caps are available in various sizes and configurations (flat vs angled), and come with a complete kit for the procedure by Olympus.[20] More commonly, the multiband ligator by Cook is now used because it is faster and easier to use, and allows overlapping resections without the cookie-cutter effect that occurs with the Inoue cap technique. To accurately determine margins the specimen should be pinned and fixed for permanent rather than frozen section. In an early series the authors performed an esophagectomy after ER to validate the ER findings, and showed that ER accurately determined the depth of tumor invasion in all cases, and had completely excised the target lesion in 86% of patients.[19] Furthermore, all patients with negative margins on the ER specimen had no evidence of tumor at the ER site on pathologic assessment of the resected specimen. Thus, negative margins are a reliable indicator of complete excision. However, tumor at the cauterized margin of the specimen indicates the potential for residual tumor in the esophagus. A positive lateral margin can be addressed with additional endoscopic therapy, but a positive deep resection margin is an indication for esophagectomy in most cases.

CT and PET-CT

The role of CT and PET-CT in esophageal cancer staging are primarily to evaluate for the presence of distant metastasis because EUS and ER are superior for T and EUS $\pm$ fine-needle aspiration for N staging. The risk of distant metastasis in T1a patients is very small, and therefore these diagnostic modalities are of minimal value in staging superficial esophageal cancers and are not recommended unless ER has shown the tumor to be invasive into the submucosa (T1b).[21] The small size of most early esophageal cancers makes it unlikely that a PET scan will show the primary tumor much less nodal disease even if present.

DEFINITION OF STAGE 1 ESOPHAGEAL CANCER

Under the new American Joint Committee on Cancer (AJCC) seventh edition, stage 1 adenocarcinomas include T1a N0 M0, T1b N0 M0, and T2 N0 M0 G1–2. Stage 1 squamous tumors are T1N0 M0 for all locations and T2–3 N0 M0 if located in the distal esophagus. Grade has been added to the staging system for adenocarcinomas, with high-grade or G3 lesions imposing a higher stage. However, it is uncertain whether there is a clinically significant increase in the risk of lymph node metastases for T1a tumors based solely on tumor grade.[12]

TREATMENT FOR STAGE 1 ESOPHAGEAL CANCER

Treatment for stage 1 esophageal cancer is based on the depth of invasion. Adenocarcinomas or squamous lesions limited to the mucosa (T1a) have a very low risk of lymph node metastases and can be treated endoscopically or by an esophagectomy, including a vagal-sparing esophagectomy. Determining the optimal therapy for these patients requires a thorough understanding of the disease process; the pros, cons, and pitfalls of each therapy; and the expected results.

Endoscopic Therapy for T1a Esophageal Cancer

Important considerations

Endoscopic therapy typically involves a combination of ER and ablation. When considering a new therapy for superficial esophageal cancer there are several things that must be avoided. First, one wants to avoid finding a highly curable lesion in a patient and then treat it ineffectively with the new therapy and lose the patient to the disease process. Second, one wants to avoid creating a whole new set of problems for the patient with the new therapy that they did not have originally. Third, the new therapy should not make it harder to definitely treat the process if the new therapy proves ineffective. Early results suggest that ER and radiofrequency ablation (RFA) for intramucosal adenocarcinoma of the esophagus addresses these concerns better than photodynamic therapy, which was associated with a 30% rate of significant esophageal stricture development, inconsistent eradication of Barrett esophagus, frequent subsquamous or buried Barrett esophagus, and concern that the most genetically abnormal clones of Barrett esophagus were those most likely to persist after therapy.[22–25]

Patient selection

In the authors' opinion there are several considerations that should be used to assist the patient and physician in the decision regarding whether endoscopic therapy or esophagectomy is the best approach in that patient's particular circumstance. These considerations can be divided into tumor factors, esophageal factors, and patient factors. The important tumor factors are that there is only high-grade dysplasia or intramucosal cancer, and that any visible lesion has been completely excised with a negative deep margin. High-risk features for nodal metastases should be absent or considered in the decision to continue with endoscopic therapy. The esophageal factors are more complex, but the first overriding consideration is that the esophagus has to be worth saving. A patient with end-stage reflux manifest by severe regurgitation symptoms, a large nonreducing hiatal hernia, dysphagia, and poor esophageal body function on physiologic testing is a poor candidate for esophageal preservation. Multifocal cancers or widespread squamous high-grade dysplasia are other factors that should encourage esophagectomy. Additionally, high-grade dysplasia that proves refractory to ablation or recurrence of dysplastic Barrett esophagus after initial complete ablation are indications to consider esophagectomy. Finally, there are several patient factors that need to be considered. Patients need to be fully informed of the pros and cons and the risks and benefits of both options for therapy (esophageal preservation vs esophagectomy), and they need to understand that esophageal preservation requires a significant commitment by the patient and the physician. Follow-up endoscopies and biopsies need to be frequent (every 3 months initially) and lifelong because the natural history of endoscopic therapy for these lesions is not yet known. Further, the patient has to be able to live with the uncertainty that a hidden or buried cancer may show up in an advanced stage that may not be curable, and that secondary to recurrence or complications of the endoscopic therapy the patient may at some point require an esophagectomy anyway.

Endoscopic therapies that resect or ablate dysplastic Barrett esophagus or intramucosal cancers are not without complications including a risk for perforation, stricture formation, buried Barrett esophagus beneath the neosquamous epithelium, recurrent or persistent areas of Barrett esophagus, induction of alterations in esophageal body motility, and the potential that ablative therapy could select out the most genetically abnormal or aggressive clones of Barrett esophagus.[23,25,26] Furthermore, endoscopic therapy may complicate a subsequent esophagectomy if resection of the esophagus becomes necessary. Another consideration is that effective control of reflux may be necessary to prevent recurrence of Barrett esophagus, and thus patients that select endoscopic therapy for high-grade dysplasia or intramucosal adenocarcinoma may eventually be recommended to have antireflux surgery. Consequently, the decision to treat intramucosal esophageal cancer with endoscopic therapy cannot be made or taken lightly.

Technique and outcome

ER and ablation should be considered complementary procedures. Although ER can be used to remove all the columnar mucosa, circumferential resections lead to strictures and it is time-consuming to do repeated or long-segment resections. The band ligator technique is currently favored for ER given its ease, safety, and ability to do overlapping resections. There are several techniques for ablation but the most commonly used is RFA. Alternatives include photodynamic therapy and cryoablation, but neither of these techniques has produced results as reliable as those documented with RFA, and complications and poor results have rendered photodynamic therapy essentially obsolete. Ablation with radiofrequency energy is relatively quick, and can be performed circumferentially with a low risk of stricture formation because the depth of injury is limited to the muscularis mucosa. However, RFA should not be done in an area of nodular cancer, because the depth of invasion of the lesion may go beyond the zone of the ablation and leave residual tumor in the esophagus. Instead, any nodules should first be excised using ER.

After ER of any visible lesion, and confirmation of the depth of invasion, the authors' preference is to ablate residual Barrett esophagus or squamous dysplasia with RF energy using the Halo 360-degree or 90-degree device (Covidien, formally BÄRRX Medical, Mansfield, MA). The Halo 360-degree device consists of a high-power RF generator, sizing balloon catheters, and ablation catheters. After sizing the esophageal lumen the ablation catheter is placed by a guidewire. The energy generator provides automated, pressure-regulated air inflation of the ablation catheter and delivers a preset amount of RF energy circumferentially over a 3-cm length of the esophagus. The Halo 90-degree device is a bipolar electrode array that attaches to the end of the endoscope and delivers energy to a targeted area allowing selective, noncircumferential ablation.

At our institution if there are no nodules or ulcers in the Barrett esophagus showing high-grade dysplasia or intramucosal cancer we proceed directly to RFA. However, if any nodule or lesion is present it is first excised using the multiband ligator. If the segment of Barrett esophagus is short we may elect to excise all the Barrett esophagus at that time endoscopically. Alternatively, for longer segments of Barrett esophagus we prefer to allow the mucosa to heal for 8 weeks after ER and then perform the first RFA. An endoscopy with biopsies is performed 8 weeks after RFA to assess for residual intestinal metaplasia. If any is found then another ablation is promptly performed, and this cycle is repeated until all intestinal metaplasia has been successfully eradicated. This is critical because any residual intestinal metaplasia, even without dysplasia, is at risk for progression in these patients. In the authors' experience 18% of patients developed a metachronous tumor while undergoing endoscopic therapy, but none did so after complete ablation of all intestinal metaplasia. After all the intestinal metaplasia has been eradicated the patients enter a surveillance program with endoscopy every 3 months for a year, then every 6 months the second year, then annually.

Currently, little has been published about RFA in patients with early squamous cancer. However, results from two small studies published last year are promising.[27,28] They both included high-grade squamous intraepithelial neoplasia and early squamous cell carcinoma, one study with ER before RFA and the other without previous ER. They both report promising results with 97% complete response after 12 months in one of the studies and 100% complete response after a median of 17 months follow-up in the other study. There was no neoplastic progression in either study but they reported stricture rates of 23% and 14%, respectively, which is higher than reported after RFA for Barrett esophagus.[27,28]

Esophagectomy for T1a Esophageal Cancer

Esophagectomy has been the standard of care for the cure of patients with high-grade dysplasia or intramucosal cancer, and to date no therapy has been proved superior to esophagectomy for the cure of patients with early stage esophageal cancer. Esophagectomy removes the diseased esophagus and essentially eliminates the risk of recurrent mucosal disease in these patients. Furthermore, it is a one-time therapy, with little or no need for subsequent endoscopies or interventions in most patients. Commonly, the esophagus is removed with a transhiatal esophagectomy for high-grade dysplasia or intramucosal cancer, but minimally invasive procedures are becoming more frequent. One drawback to most methods of removing the esophagus is that the vagus nerves are divided during the procedure, and this leads to dumping and post-vagotomy diarrhea in up to 30% of patients.[29] Because patients with high-grade dysplasia or T1a lesions are almost always cured, postesophagectomy quality of life is an important consideration. This prompted the authors to evaluate a technique for vagal preservation with esophagectomy, and early in their experience they confirmed vagal integrity using sham feeds, pancreatic polypeptide measurements, Congo red staining, and nuclear medicine gastric emptying studies.[30] Furthermore, they confirmed that preservation of the pyloric innervation led to a significant reduction in the prevalence of dumping and diarrhea and improved morbidity compared with patients that had a standard esophagectomy with vagotomy.[30,31] The vagal-sparing esophagectomy can be done as an open transabdominal or a laparoscopic approach, requires no mediastinal dissection, and either the stomach or the colon can be used for esophageal replacement, although the authors' preference is the stomach.

Technique of the vagal-sparing esophagectomy

The technique for a vagal-sparing esophagectomy was described in the 1980s by Akiyama and coworkers from Japan.[32] Vagal-sparing procedures are done similar to a transhiatal operation except the esophagus is stripped from the mediastinum and no mediastinal or transhiatal dissection is done. The operation commences in the abdomen, and with a minimum of dissection the hiatus is opened and the anterior and posterior vagal trunks encircled with a vessel-loop. The vagus nerves are retracted gently toward the patient's right, and the gastroesophageal fat pad is dissected beginning on the left of the esophagus and stomach such that it allows the anterior vagus nerve to be brought well over to the right of the esophagus. Failure to do this step leads in most cases to inadvertent injury of the anterior vagus nerve during the subsequent steps of the procedure. After the anterior vagus is safely over to the right of the esophagus a highly selective vagotomy is performed starting just above the crow's foot near the antrum of the stomach. This is necessary if the stomach is to be used as the esophageal replacement, and is beneficial with a colon interposition to reduce gastric acidity and the potential for ulceration in the colon graft. The highly selective vagotomy precisely follows the lesser curve of the stomach up to the point where the distal esophagus is reached and the vagus nerve trunks are completely separated from the esophagus. The authors find that this dissection is facilitated by sequential grasping of the stomach with Babcock clamps along the lesser curve, and by using the Harmonic scalpel for division of the very vascular tissue in this area. Avoidance of a hematoma or bleeding in this area is critical to prevent unintended injury to the distal vagal braches.

At this point the gastroesophageal junction should be completely exposed and the lesser curve above the crow's foot skeletonized. If the stomach is to be used for esophageal replacement then the greater curve is mobilized in the same fashion as for a standard gastric pull-up. However, if the colon is to be used then there is no need to mobilize the greater curve completely. Instead, the omentum is detached from the transverse colon and a window created near the left crus by dividing the most proximal one or two short gastric and posterior pancreaticogastric vessels. This creates a passage from the lesser sac to the hiatus for the colon graft. The colon is mobilized in standard fashion based on the ascending branch of the left colic artery whenever possible.[33] The necessary length of colon is marked out by measuring the distance from the tip of the left ear to the xiphoid anteriorly with an umbilical tape and then marking a similar distance on the colon starting from the point where the left colic vessels tether the graft and going proximally. The colon can then be divided and placed in the pelvis for later use.

Next, attention is directed to the left neck. The esophagus is exposed, and after placing a Penrose drain around the esophagus to facilitate traction blunt dissection is accomplished with a finger to free the upper mediastinal portion of the esophagus. A nasogastric tube is inserted and the esophagus is irrigated with a dilute povidone-iodine solution to reduce mediastinal contamination during the subsequent stripping procedure. The nasogastric tube is then removed.

Next, a gastrotomy is made near the gastroesophageal junction, or alternatively the cardia is divided with a stapler and a small portion of the staple line is opened to provide access to the esophageal lumen. A standard vein stripper is then passed retrograde up the esophagus and brought out the anterior wall of the cervical esophagus as distally as possible. The esophagus is ligated distal to the exit site of the vein stripper in the neck using a heavy suture, and the cervical esophagus divided at the site where the vein stripper comes out. The divided distal end of the esophagus is then suture ligated and tied securely. The authors use several endo-loops to facilitate secure ligation. This is a critical step because if the ligatures slip then the vein stripper merely pulls out, leaving the partially stripped esophagus somewhere in the mediastinum. After changing the vein stripper to the large head the esophagus is inverted on itself by pulling the vein stripper from below. It is useful to leave a long umbilical tape tied to the distal end of the cervical esophagus to provide access to the tract in the posterior mediastinum after the esophagus has been removed. Importantly, in patients with Barrett esophagus and high-grade dysplasia or intramucosal cancer all layers of the esophagus are stripped out so as not to inadvertently leave any Barrett esophagus or tumor behind. However, in patients with benign conditions, such as achalasia, only the mucosa need be stripped out. The esophagus comes out inverted with the mucosa external to the muscular wall similar to taking off a sock inside out. Generally, bleeding is minimal and very little force is required to pull out the esophagus. Resistance should raise concern, and excessive resistance should prompt conversion to a transhiatal procedure.

The next step is to dilate the mediastinal tract to prevent constriction of the graft. The authors sequentially dilate the tract using a 90-mL balloon Foley catheter progressively filled with saline and pulled up through the mediastinum. Typically, two to three passes are made to ensure an adequate tract is created. This is particularly important in patients that have a normal-caliber esophagus at the time of stripping. The graft can then be brought up though the posterior mediastinal tract.

When a gastric pull-up is being used the stomach is tubularized in standard fashion leaving the crow's foot intact. The gastric tube is then pulled up through the posterior mediastinum and an esophagogastric anastomosis constructed in standard fashion. The vascular supply of the gastric tube is typically excellent because the left gastric artery has been preserved and only the branches to the skeletonized lesser curve region were divided. This usually leaves several branches intact to the antrum, and in combination with preserved right gastric and gastroepiploic arteries leads to excellent graft perfusion in most patients. After completing the cervical anastomosis the graft is gently pulled into the abdomen to eliminate redundancy and sutured to the crura to prevent herniation of abdominal organs into the mediastinum. At this point the operation is complete with the exception of passing a nasogastric tube and placing a feeding jejunostomy tube. Because the antral innervation has been preserved no pyloroplasty should be performed.

When a colon graft is used with vagal preservation of the stomach there are several important technical considerations. First, nearly the entire, innervated stomach is left intact and only the cardia immediately below the gastroesophageal junction is excised. A highly selective vagotomy is performed along the lesser curvature to reduce acid secretion and provide protection from the development of cologastric anastomotic ulcers. There is no need to do an extensive mobilization of the greater curvature. Instead, only the proximal most one to two short gastric vessels along with the posterior pancreaticoduodenal vessels are divided so that there is an approximately 10-cm window created near the left crus of the diaphragm. Importantly, the colon graft is passed up posterior to the stomach through this window, into the hiatus, and then up through the posterior mediastinum. The esophagocolo anastomosis is done either with a stapled or hand-sewn technique in an end-to-end fashion. The colon is then pulled firmly back into the abdomen to reduce any redundancy and sutured to the left crus of the diaphragm to prevent twisting of the graft or herniation of abdominal contents into the mediastinum. In particular sutures should be placed between the colon graft and the posterior aspect of the hiatus near the point where the left and right crus meet because herniation can occur underneath the colon graft if these sutures are omitted.

The colon is divided approximately 10 to 15 cm distal to the hiatus taking care not to injure the vascular arcade. A stapled cologastric anastomosis is then done to the proximal posterior fundus using a 75-mm GIA stapler, and a nasogastric tube guided into the stomach. Finally, the colocolostomy is accomplished in standard fashion with care taken to avoid traction on the left colic vessels or the marginal artery supplying the graft. Typically, this requires that the right colon be brought up into the left upper quadrant. Finally, the mesenteric defects are closed and a feeding jejunostomy placed.

When a gastric pull-up is planned the vagal-sparing procedure is readily adapted to a fully laparoscopic approach. The gastric mobilization and the highly selective vagotomy are straightforward laparoscopic procedures. The authors have found that the use of a 4-cm incision in the midline with placement of a handport facilitates stripping the esophagus out (by the handport) and subsequent dilatation of the mediastinal tract. The graft is pulled up attached to a chest tube and the cervical esophagogastric anastomosis accomplished in standard fashion. Similar to an open procedure the gastric tube should be sutured to the left crus to prevent torsion of the graft or herniation of abdominal organs into the posterior mediastinum.

Esophagectomy Versus Endoscopic Therapy in T1a Tumors

Relatively few studies have compared the outcome of esophagectomy versus endoscopic therapy for high-grade dysplasia or intramucosal cancer.[34–36] The authors' group recently published a retrospective review of a 10-year experience using these two strategies in 101 patients.[34] At a median follow-up of 17 months after endoscopic therapy and 34 months after esophagectomy, there was no difference in survival between groups (cancer-related survival was 100% with endotherapy vs 88% with esophagectomy; $P = .54$). There was no procedure-related mortality in either group, but one or more complications occurred in 24 (39%) of 61 patients after esophagectomy compared with none in the 40 patients treated with endotherapy. There was no metachronous cancer development in the esophagus after esophagectomy compared with 18% in the endotherapy group. Furthermore, 26% of patients with only high-grade dysplasia at presentation progressed to cancer during endotherapy before complete eradication of intestinal metaplasia. The median number of treatments to eradicate intestinal metaplasia was three using a combination of ER and RFA in most patients. In the endotherapy group three patients required esophagectomy for persistent or recurrent dysplasia or cancer, all with long-segment Barrett esophagus. After endotherapy patients were maintained on high-dose acid suppression therapy with twice-a-day proton-pump inhibitors or underwent antireflux surgery (n = 8) for control of their reflux disease.

Similar results were recently reported by Pech and coworkers[35] where 76 patients treated endoscopically were matched for tumor stage and age with 38 patients that had an en bloc esophagectomy. The overall recurrence/metachronous cancer rate after endotherapy was 6.6% and complete removal of neoplasia was achieved in 98.7% of patients after a mean of two ERs per patient. There was no significant difference in overall mortality at a median follow-up of 4.1 years after endotherapy and 3.7 years after esophagectomy.[35]

Based on limited published data and relatively short-term follow-up, it seems that endotherapy provides similar survival to esophagectomy with fewer procedure-related complications but at the price of repeated procedures, higher risk for local recurrence or metachronous cancer development, and the need for continued surveillance even with successful therapy. However, most patients and physicians accept these downsides of endotherapy for the benefit of preserving the esophagus and avoiding major surgery. Importantly, not every patient is an appropriate candidate for endotherapy, and esophagectomy, particularly with a vagal-sparing approach, remains a viable treatment option for some of these patients.

Treatment for Submucosal Cancer (T1b)

After a tumor invades into the submucosa the risk of lymph node metastases increases to 20% to 25%. Some studies suggest that the risk is related to the depth of invasion into the submucosa, with the lowest risk for tumors only into the first third or superficial portion of the submucosa. In contrast, the authors were unable to find significant differences in the risk when comparing tumors invasive into the superficial, middle, or deepest thirds of the submucosa.[12] An important and frustrating problem is that currently there is no technique or scan that allows determination of which patients with submucosal tumor invasion have lymph node metastases. Therefore, an esophagectomy with lymph node dissection is recommended in these patients, even though it is recognized that most (~75%) will be node negative after resection and could potentially have been treated successfully endoscopically.

Neoadjuvant therapy is not generally recommended for patients with T1b lesions, particularly given data suggesting that survival may be impaired when neoadjuvant therapy is used in patients with early stage disease.[37] Instead, the preferred approach for most patients with early stage esophageal cancer is primary surgical resection with thoracic and abdominal lymphadenectomy to remove the diseased esophagus and the potentially involved lymph nodes. Options for esophagectomy include transhiatal, transthoracic, and minimally invasive approaches. Long-term survival is reported to be similar for these operations in T1b tumors.[38] However, the subgroup of patients with nodal disease likely benefits from a more extensive lymphadenectomy and as many as 34% of patients with T1b N1 disease has been reported to have metastatic lymph nodes in the mediastinum above the level of dissection performed during a transhiatal resection.[38,39] In a retrospective review of similarly staged patients treated with either a transhiatal or an en bloc resection the authors showed that with extensive nodal disease (≥9) the type of resection did not impact survival because there was nearly universal systemic disease in this group of patients.[40] In contrast, for those with limited nodal disease (one to eight nodes) the type of resection significantly impacted survival in favor of the en bloc resection.[40] Similarly, Omloo and colleagues[39] supported these findings with an analysis of patients that participated in a randomized trial of transhiatal versus transthoracic en bloc esophagectomy in the Netherlands. In those with one to eight involved nodes survival was 64% after en bloc resection and was significantly better than the 23% survival in those that had a transhiatal operation.[39] It remains to be determined whether minimally invasive techniques will allow preservation of the benefits of an en bloc resection with reduction of the morbidity of the procedure.

SUMMARY

Barrett esophagus surveillance programs and more liberal use of upper endoscopy are leading to the identification of an increasing number of patients with high-grade dysplasia or early stage esophageal adenocarcinoma. These patients have several options for therapy, and factors that should be considered include the length of the Barrett esophagus segment, the presence of a nodule or ulcer within the Barrett esophagus, and the age and overall physical condition of the patient. Endoscopic mucosal resection is currently the only method able to reliably determine the depth of invasion of superficial cancers, and is an important aspect of staging because submucosal invasion imparts a significant risk of lymph node metastases, and therapies that do not include a lymphadenectomy are potentially inadequate. A vagal-sparing esophagectomy provides the benefit of complete esophageal resection with elimination of all Barrett esophagus while minimizing the morbidity associated with traditional esophagectomies that include a vagotomy. The ease of the procedure and its applicability to a fully laparoscopic approach are additional factors that should encourage physician and patient acceptance. Currently, a combination of ER and ablation is the preferred therapy for most patients with high-grade dysplasia or intramucosal adenocarinoma, and available evidence suggests that survival with endoscopic therapy is equivalent to that after esophagectomy. However, at this time there is no long-term follow-up confirmation of these findings. Of particular importance will be the incidence of recurrent Barrett esophagus or cancer in the long-term in patients that were initially successfully treated endoscopically.

REFERENCES

1. Ferlay J, Shin HR, Bray F, et al. Estimates of worldwide burden of cancer in 2008: GLOBOCAN 2008. Int J Cancer 2010;15(127):2918–27.
2. Blot WJ, Devesa SS, Kneller RW, et al. Rising incidence of adenocarcinoma of the esophagus and gastric cardia. JAMA 1991;265:1287–9.
3. Kubo A, Corley DA. Marked multi-ethnic variation of esophageal and gastric cardia carcinomas within the United States. Am J Gastroenterol 2004;99:582–8.
4. Pohl H, Welch HG. The role of overdiagnosis and reclassification in the marked increase of esophageal adenocarcinoma incidence. J Natl Cancer Inst 2005; 97:142–6.
5. Devesa SS, Blot WJ, Fraumeni JF. Changing patterns in the incidence of esophageal and gastric carcinoma in the United States. Cancer 1998;83:2049–53.
6. Bollschweiler E, Wolfgarten E, Gutschow C, et al. Demographic variations in the rising incidence of esophageal adenocarcinoma in white males. Cancer 2001;92: 549–55.
7. Kubo A, Corley DA. Marked regional variation in adenocarcinomas of the esophagus and the gastric cardia in the United States. Cancer 2002;95:2096–102.
8. Chen X, Yang CS. Esophageal adenocarcinoma: a review and perspectives on the mechanism of carcinogenesis and chemoprevention. Carcinogenesis 2001; 22:1119–29.
9. Nigro JJ, Hagen JA, DeMeester TR, et al. Occult esophageal adenocarcinoma: extent of disease and implications for effective therapy. Ann Surg 1999;230:433–40.
10. Bolton WD, Hofstetter WL, Francis AM, et al. Impact of tumor length on long-term survival of pT1 esophageal adenocarcinoma. J Thorac Cardiovasc Surg 2009; 138:831–6.
11. Wang BY, Goan YG, Hsu PK, et al. Tumor length as a prognostic factor in esophageal squamous cell carcinoma. Ann Thorac Surg 2011;91:887–93.
12. Leers JM, DeMeester SR, Oezcelik A, et al. The prevalence of lymph node metastases in patients with T1 esophageal adenocarcinoma a retrospective review of esophagectomy specimens. Ann Surg 2011;253:271–8.
13. Endoscopic Classification Review Group. Update on the Paris classification of superficial neoplastic lesions in the digestive tract. Endoscopy 2005;37:570–8.
14. Puli SR, Batapati KR, Bechtold ML, et al. Endoscopic ultrasound: it's accuracy in evaluating mediastinal lymphadenopathy? A meta-analysis and systematic review. World J Gastroenterol 2008;14:3028–37.

15. Buttar N, Wang KK, Lutzke LS, et al. Combined endoscopic mucosal resection (EMR) and photodynamic therapy (PDT) for esophageal neoplasia within Barrett's esophagus. Gastrointest Endosc 2001;54:682–8.
16. Heidemann J, Schilling MK, Schmassmann A, et al. Accuracy of endoscopic ultrasonography in preoperative staging of esophageal carcinoma. Dig Surg 2000;17:219–24.
17. Menzel J, Hoepffner N, Nottberg H, et al. Preoperative staging of esophageal carcinoma: miniprobe sonography versus conventional endoscopic ultrasound in a prospective histopathologically verified study. Endoscopy 1999;31:291–7.
18. Hunerbein M, Ulmer C, Handke T, et al. Endosonography of upper gastrointestinal tract cancer on demand using miniprobes or endoscopic ultrasound. Surg Endosc 2003;17:615–9.
19. Maish MS, DeMeester SR. Endoscopic mucosal resection as a staging technique to determine the depth of invasion of esophageal adenocarcinoma. Ann Thorac Surg 2004;78:1777–82.
20. Tada M, Inoue H, Yabata E, et al. Colonic mucosal resection using a transparent cap-fitted endoscope. Gastrointest Endosc 1996;44:63–5.
21. Little SG, Rice TW, Byble B, et al. Is FDG-PET indicated for superficial esophageal cancer? Eur J Cardiothorac Surg 2007;31:791–6.
22. Overholt BF, Lightdale CJ, Wang KK, et al. Photodynamic therapy with porfimer sodium for ablation of high-grade dysplasia in Barrett's esophagus: international, partially blinded, randomized phase III trial. Gastrointest Endosc 2005;62:488–98.
23. Gray NA, Odze RD, Spechler SJ. Buried metaplasia after endoscopic ablation of Barrett's esophagus: a systematic review. Am J Gastroenterol 2011;106:1899–908.
24. Krishnadath KK, Wang KK, Taniguchi K, et al. Persistent genetic abnormalities in Barrett's esophagus after photodynamic therapy. Gastroenterology 2000;119:624–30.
25. Overholt BF, Panjehpour M, Halberg DL. Photodynamic therapy for Barrett's esophagus with dysplasia and/or early stage carcinoma: long-term results. Gastrointest Endosc 2003;58:183–8.
26. Shaheen NJ, Sharma P, Overholt BF, et al. Radiofrequency ablation in Barrett's esophagus with dysplasia. N Engl J Med 2009;360:2277–88.
27. Bergman JJ, Zhang YM, He S, et al. Outcomes from a prospective trial of endoscopic radiofrequency ablation of early squamous cell neoplasia of the esophagus. Gastrointest Endosc 2011;74:1181–90.
28. van Vilsteren FG, Alvarez Herrero L, Pouw RE, et al. Radiofrequency ablation for the endoscopic eradication of esophageal squamous high grade intraepithelial neoplasia and mucosal squamous cell carcinoma. Endoscopy 2011;43:282–90.
29. Orringer MB, Marshall B, Chang AC, et al. Two thousand transhiatal esophagectomies: changing trends, lessons learned. Ann Surg 2007;246:363–72.
30. Banki F, Mason RJ, DeMeester SR, et al. Vagal-sparing esophagectomy: a more physiologic alternative. Ann Surg 2002;236:324–35.
31. Peyre CG, DeMeester TR. Vagal-sparing esophagectomy. Adv Surg 2008;42:109–16.
32. Akiyama H, Tsurumaru M, Kawamura T, et al. Esophageal stripping with preservation of the vagus nerve. Int Surg 1982;67:125–8.
33. DeMeester SR. Colon interposition following esophagectomy. Dis Esophagus 2001;14:169–72.

34. Zehetner J, DeMeester SR, Hagen JA, et al. Endoscopic resection and ablation versus esophagectomy for high-grade dysplasia and intramucosal adenocarcinoma. J Thorac Cardiovasc Surg 2011;141:39–47.
35. Pech O, Bollschweiler E, Manner H, et al. Comparison between endoscopic and surgical resection of mucosal esophageal adenocarcinoma in Barrett's esophagus at two high-volume centers. Ann Surg 2011;254:67–72.
36. Pacifico RJ, Wang KK, Wongkeesong LM, et al. Combined endoscopic mucosal resection and photodynamic therapy versus esophagectomy for management of early adenocarcinoma in Barrett's esophagus. Clin Gastroenterol Hepatol 2003;1: 252–7.
37. Rice TW, Mason DP, Murthy SC, et al. T2N0M0 esophageal cancer. J Thorac Cardiovasc Surg 2007;133:317–24.
38. Grotenhuis BA, van Heijl M, Zehetner J, et al. Surgical management of submucosal esophageal cancer: extended or regional lymphadenectomy? Ann Surg 2010;252:823–30.
39. Omloo JM, Lagarde SM, Hulscher JB, et al. Extended transthoracic resection compared with limited transhiatal resection for adenocarcinoma of the mid/distal esophagus: five-year survival of a randomized clinical trial. Ann Surg 2007;246: 992–1000.
40. Johansson J, DeMeester TR, Hagen JA, et al. En bloc vs transhiatal esophagectomy for stage T3 N1 adenocarcinoma of the distal esophagus. Arch Surg 2004; 139:627–31.

Management of T2 Esophageal Cancer

Manu Sancheti, MD, Felix Fernandez, MD*

KEYWORDS

- Esophageal cancer • T2 esophageal cancer • Neoadjuvant therapy
- Adjuvant therapy • Esophageal cancer staging • Endoscopic ultrasound

KEY POINTS

- The management of esophageal cancer necessitates a multimodality approach and the constant evolution of treatment algorithm for the best possible outcome.
- T2 esophageal cancer proves to be a diagnostic challenge and a nidus for much debate in terms of its management.
- The outcome of patients with T2 esophageal cancer would benefit by the improvement in staging modalities to more accurately predict true pathologic stage.
- There are limited data to support neoadjuvant therapy for presumed nodal disease versus primary resection followed by adjuvant therapy for proven nodal disease.

INTRODUCTION

The management of esophageal cancer continues to evolve, ranging from surgery alone to various algorithms using neoadjuvant and adjuvant chemotherapy and radiation regimens. Although data are conflicting, patients with nodal disease (ie, N1 disease) or locally advanced disease (ie, T3 tumors) may potentially benefit from neoadjuvant therapy with chemotherapy and radiation followed by surgical resection.[1,2] Surgical therapy is sufficient for superficial cancers without nodal disease (ie, T1N0).[3-5] A small subset of patient with T2 disease (invasion into the muscularis propria) proves to be the most difficult to treat. This difficulty centers around 2 issues. First, the ability to accurately identify T2N0 esophageal cancers with current clinical staging modalities is suspect. Second, the potential benefit of induction therapy for clinical stage T2N0 esophageal cancer remains more controversial than for more advanced stage disease. However, the literature on this subset of patients continues to be limited.

The authors have no disclosures.
Division of Cardiothoracic Surgery, Emory University School of Medicine, Emory University Hospital, 1365A Clifton Road Northeast, Atlanta, GA 30322, USA
* Corresponding author.
E-mail address: felix.fernandez@emoryhealthcare.org

Surg Clin N Am 92 (2012) 1169–1178
http://dx.doi.org/10.1016/j.suc.2012.07.003

It is known that the most important prognostic factor for esophageal cancer is stage and nodal status at diagnosis.[6] Therefore, preoperative clinical staging of the tumor, specifically in relation to nodal status, is vital in the determination of the ideal treatment strategy. The current staging modalities, including endoscopic ultrasonography (EUS), computed tomography (CT), and [18F]fluorodeoxyglucose (FDG) positron emission tomography (PET), or a combination of all, prove to be accurate in the diagnosis of early stage disease and advanced stage disease. That accuracy diminishes in T2N0 disease, leading to understaging a tumor and precluding the patient from receiving neoadjuvant therapy, or overstaging the tumor, leading to unnecessary induction therapy.

This article summarizes the available literature on the management of T2 esophageal cancer. The discussion commences with an explanation of the current T stages and the frequency of nodal metastasis corresponding with depth of invasion. This discussion leads to the various available staging modalities and their performance in accurately staging the disease, specifically in relation to T2 disease. Current treatment strategies for T2N0 disease, albeit controversial, are reviewed.

T Classification

Depth of invasion of esophageal cancer into the esophageal wall correlates with the frequency of lymph node metastases and, therefore, is vital to the determination of the treatment regimen. The depth of invasion is represented by the T classification in the tumor-node-metastasis (TNM) system for esophageal cancer. The current T classification, as set forth by the American Joint Committee on Cancer (AJCC) seventh edition, is as follows[7]:

- T0: no evidence of primary tumor
- Tis: high-grade dysplasia
- T1: invasion of lamina propria, muscularis mucosae, or submucosa
  - T1a: invasion of lamina propria or muscularis mucosae
  - T1b: invasion of submucosa
- T2: invasion of muscularis propria
- T3: invasion of adventitia
- T4: invasion of adjacent structures
  - T4a: resectable tumor invading pleura, pericardium, or diaphragm
  - T4b: unresectable tumor invading other adjacent structures, such as aorta, vertebral body, or trachea

Frequency of Nodal Metastasis According to T Stage

As mentioned earlier, the nodal status of an esophageal malignancy is a critical prognostic factor. For example, a review of almost 3000 patients by Gertler and colleagues[8] showed that survival is markedly affected by increasing nodal positivity, more so than depth of tumor. Preoperative detection of lymph node metastases likely selects a patient for induction therapy. Therefore, in the process of clinically staging a patient, the relation of nodal positivity to the depth of tumor invasion (T stage) is important.

Several case series have reviewed the rate of nodal positivity in esophageal cancer on depth of invasion. The general premise arises that, as the tumor invades more deeply, the incidence of nodal positivity increases, showing that T and N stage are not independent variables. Lu and colleagues[9] reviewed 504 cases and showed a nodal positivity rate ranging from 29.7% to 69.1% as depth of invasion increases. The group with invasion into the muscularis propria (T2) had the 29.7% positivity rate. Rice and colleagues[10] found the rate of lymph node metastases to be 43% for pathologically staged T2 esophageal cancers. In this series, compared with T1 patients, T2 patients were 6 times more likely to have N1 disease. Other series have depicted a range from 22% to 85% as the tumor's depth of invasion increases from T1 to T4.[11] This direct relationship between T stage and nodal positivity is also found in reviewing substages in the T1 group. As the tumor invades more deeply from the lamina propria (T1a) to the deep submucosa (T1b), the nodal positivity rate increases from 0% to 36%.[12]

These reviews show that T2 tumors have a nodal positivity rate in excess of 30%. Because nodal disease confers a worse prognosis, induction therapy is frequently pursued when nodal metastases are detected with clinical staging. Therefore, the question remains for T2 disease: should the clinician more diligently stage the patient given the high risk of nodal positivity or should the clinician more aggressively treat with induction therapy considering that a significant number of patients have positive lymph nodes on pathologic staging?

Performance of Staging Modalities in Esophageal Cancer

The clinical staging of a patient with esophageal cancer is a vital step in the pretreatment evaluation. Clinical stage predicts prognosis and helps select patients for induction therapy. However, current clinical staging modalities continue to be lacking, especially for T2 esophageal cancers. The literature suggests that the depth of invasion of up to 66% of esophageal tumors may be overstaged. In contrast, the nodal positivity of tumors is understaged in up to 55% of cases.[4,13,14] Rice and colleagues[4] showed positive predictive values (PPV) of cT2N0 tumors that were pathologically consistent ranging from 13% to 23%. Likewise, other series have shown a PPV as low as 6%, even when using a combined modality staging system.[14] These data depict the overall inadequacy of current modalities.

The lack of accuracy in clinical staging in T2 disease complicates the clinician's ability to properly treat the patients and has been suggested to adversely affect survival.[4] When reviewing understaged patients (p stage >pT2N0), the error in most instances lies in an inaccuracy in nodal staging. In contrast, in overstaged patients (p stage <pT2N0), the difficulty more often arises in the accurate identification of depth of tumor invasion (T stage).[4]

Understaged patients have worse survival than patients who are pT2N0. These patients may not receive induction therapy and/or extended lymphadenectomy as is usually performed for higher stage tumors. The difference in survival is significant. Up to a 50% decrease in 5-year survival for understaged tumors was shown in one series.[14] This decline is seen in patients who underwent surgery alone and surgery with adjuvant treatment of their esophageal cancer. However, when comparing surgery alone with surgery with adjuvant therapy, the adjuvant therapy did provide a survival benefit.[4]

The current National Comprehensive Cancer Network (NCCN) guidelines suggest that following upper endoscopy and biopsy, the esophageal cancer be staged by using a combination of CT of the chest/abdomen/pelvis, FDG-PET scan, and EUS.[15] This article details the data regarding each modality's specific capabilities in accurately staging esophageal cancer, as well as providing a comparison between them.

CT

After initial diagnosis of esophageal malignancy, CT of the chest, abdomen, and pelvis is usually the next step in the pretreatment evaluation. CT can provide a global view of the tumor, its relationship to surrounding structures, regional/distant lymphadenopathy, and possible metastatic foci. The overall accuracy of CT scan for tumor depth staging ranges from 50% to 80%; whereas the accuracy for nodal involvement ranges from 50% to 70%.[16] A meta-analysis by van Vliet and colleagues[17] similarly showed a pooled sensitivity/specificity for CT of 50%/83% and 52%/91%, for the identification of regional lymph node metastases and distant metastases, respectively. The principal finding of esophageal carcinoma on CT, a thickened esophageal wall, lacks the definition to distinguish between T1, T2, and T3. As a lone modality, CT is not sufficient to clinically stage a patient.

FDG-PET

As a staging modality, FDG-PET provides a means to detect metabolically active tissue that may represent metastatic disease, regional and/or distant. However, its definite role in the algorithm of pretreatment and posttreatment evaluation in esophageal cancer is yet to be fully determined. In reviewing the data regarding FDG-PET, van Vliet and colleagues[17] found a 57%/85% pooled sensitivity/specificity for the identification of regional metastases. These values are minimally improved compared with those of CT scan. However, significant improvement is noted in the identification of distant metastases. This improvement is corroborated by a 2011 review that developed an evidence-based guideline supporting the use of FDG-PET to improve the accuracy of M staging in esophageal tumors.[18] In addition, compared with CT alone, FDG-PET alters the clinical stage of greater than one-third of patients, thus significantly influencing their treatment.[19] These data are opposed by literature stating that routine FDG-PET does not provide additional staging information when performed with another modality, specifically a thorough EUS-guided fine-needle aspiration (FNA).[20] Also, an FDG-PET scan provides little anatomic detail of the esophageal wall. Despite the presence of conflicting data, most clinicians use FDG-PET in clinical staging scenarios, especially with the advent of the fusion FDG-PET/CT scan.

EUS

EUS is a minimally invasive method to measure the depth of invasion of the tumor and the nature of the regional lymph nodes in the clinical staging of esophageal cancer. EUS offers detailed images of the esophageal wall. This definition of the esophageal wall is not offered by CT or FDG-PET. Clinical T2 disease is defined as invasion into, but not through, the fourth ultrasound layer (muscularis propria) on EUS, as shown in **Figs. 1** and **2**. Suspicious lymph nodes based on size, shape, and border can be biopsied via FNA to determine positivity.[4] Large (>1 cm in long axis), round, hypoechoic, nonhomogeneous lymph nodes with indistinct borders are those most likely to be malignant. EUS-guided FNA, can help confirm lymph node metastases with cytology. However, FNA biopsy may not be feasible if the biopsy needle must traverse the tumor to access the lymph node in question. Despite its many advantages, several studies have shown limitations to EUS, especially in the T2 esophageal cancer population.

In the identification of T stage, the overall of accuracy of EUS ranges from 74% to 90%.[14,21] It has been shown to be most inaccurate in the subset of T2 disease. The accuracy of EUS for T2 disease specifically is as low as 31%.[22] Pech and colleagues[21] found that the sensitivity of EUS for T stage drops from 82%–83% in T1 and T3 disease to 43% for T2 disease. In addition, several studies have reported a worse accuracy for early esophageal cancers (T1 and T2N0) compared with locally advanced T3 disease.[4,23–25] As alluded to earlier, the reason for this discrepancy may be the difficulty in differentiating the third ultrasound layer (deep submucosal layer) from the fourth ultrasound layer (muscularis propria).[4] Further, because 2 anatomic boundaries must be assessed to determine T2 disease, the opportunity for error is potentially

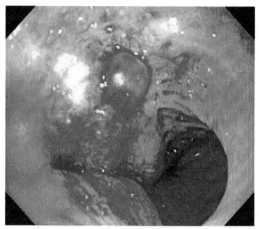

Fig. 1. Endoscopic view of T2 esophageal cancer. (*Courtesy of* Field Willingham, MD, Emory University School of Medicine, Atlanta, GA.)

twice that of T1 or T4 disease. It has been proposed that improvements in EUS technology with increasing megahertz in the probe may provide greater resolution of the layers of the wall of the esophagus. Shimoyama and colleagues[26] showed that a 20-MHz probe on the EUS can accurately differentiate the T1 subtypes in 86% of cases. Using these techniques in the T2 subset may be beneficial. It has also been reported that EUS performed in low-volume centers (<50 procedures/y) has a worse sensitivity than those in high-volume centers (>50 procedures/y).[17]

The performance of EUS in determining nodal status in cT2 disease is equally poor. The overall accuracy and sensitivity of EUS for regional nodal status is approximately

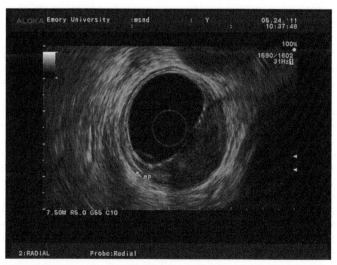

Fig. 2. Esophageal ultrasound view of tumor invading up to the fourth ultrasound layer MP, muscularis propria. (*Courtesy of* Field Willingham, MD, Emory University School of Medicine, Atlanta, GA.)

80% in 1 series by van Vliet and colleagues.[17] However, in the subset of cT2 disease, the rate of finding positive nodes on pathology despite a negative EUS ranges from 38% to 69%.[14,22] Vazquez-Sequerios and colleagues[27] showed that, with the addition of FNA to EUS, the sensitivity and accuracy significantly increase to 93% and 90%, respectively. It has not yet been determined whether this advantage applies to T2 disease specifically. The use of EUS-guided FNA biopsy of periesophageal lymph nodes is strongly encouraged whenever possible and can only augment clinical staging modalities.

Combination of CT, FDG-PET, and EUS

Several studies have compared the performance of the combination of CT, FDG-PET, and EUS as a multimodality staging method for esophageal cancer. Each modality provides a unique asset to determine appropriate clinical stage. FDG-PET and CT (or fusion PET-CT) are useful to determine the surgical resectability of a tumor and the identification of distant disease. The usefulness of EUS comes from its ability to determine depth of invasion and regional nodal status.

Stiles and colleagues[22] indicated that, in their series of cT2 to T3 tumors, the clinical nodal staging was inaccurate in 67% for patients who did not undergo EUS, 63% for patients who did undergo EUS, and 69% for patients who underwent PET and EUS in combination. In a series reported by Crabtree and colleagues[14] of 18 patients with esophageal cancer clinically staged T2N0 with EUS, CT, and PET, only 1 patient (6%) was pT2N0, whereas 9 (50%) were overstaged and 8 (44%) were understaged. This study found that marked/intense uptake on PET scan predicted upstaging of cT1 to T2 esophageal cancer.[14] Therefore, despite their advantages in esophageal cancer staging, the overall performance of these modalities, separate or combined, remain poor for T2 disease.

Treatment of T2N0 Esophageal Cancer

As shown earlier, management of cT2N0 esophageal cancer is controversial, in large part because of difficulties in clinical staging. Because these patients have no evidence of lymph node metastases, they are most often treated with an esophagectomy as primary modality. The survival for cT2N0 ranges from 30% to 58% at 5 years, whereas an appropriately staged pT2N0 tumor more closely mirrors the improved survival of more superficial tumors.[4,14,22] Thus, the inability to accurately clinically stage the patient before initiation of therapy may lead to selection of a less appropriate treatment algorithm and worse survival. The controversy primarily stems around the inaccuracy of nodal staging. If induction therapy is accepted as beneficial for locally advanced esophageal cancer, the central question to be answered is whether neoadjuvant therapy should be administered for all T2 lesions because of the high prevalence of nodal metastases, or whether resection should be pursued initially and adjuvant therapy administered for only node-positive specimens. The current literature, albeit limited, regarding these 2 schools of thought are discussed later.

Neoadjuvant therapy

Multiple studies and meta-analyses justify the benefit of neoadjuvant therapy before surgical resection in esophageal cancer; and its use in current practice is growing.[28–30] However, the use of neoadjuvant therapy in T2N0 disease is yet to be fully supported. Many randomized trials have included T2N0 patients, but numbers are small and/or subset analyses have not been performed.[31–35] The 5-year survival associated with a cT2N0 tumor upstaged pathologically to one with nodal positivity decreased from 90% to 40% in the small subgroup presented by Crabtree and colleagues.[14] As mentioned previously, positive lymph nodes are noted after resection in cT2N0 disease in up to 55% of cases.[4,13,14] With high nodal positivity rates and a reduction in survival for upstaged tumors, the logical pathway is neoadjuvant therapy.

Stiles and colleagues[22] showed that, in their cohort of cT2/3N0 patients, neoadjuvant therapy provided a trend toward improved overall survival from 44.2% to 56.2%, although this was not statistically significant. This study also showed that, in the cT2N0 population, induction therapy did not significantly decrease the rate of nodal metastases.[18]

Kountourakis and colleagues[36] from the MD Anderson Cancer Center retrospectively reviewed their cohort of 49 patients who specifically underwent neoadjuvant therapy followed by esophagectomy for cT2N0 esophageal cancer. The neoadjuvant therapy consisted of fluoropyrimidine/taxane or platinum chemotherapy, followed by 45 to 50 Gy of radiation. At a median follow-up of 28.5 months, a 5-year overall survival of 64.1% and disease-free survival of 58.4% were noted. These rates are improved compared with historical survival rates noted for cT2N0. The study noted that only 10% of this cohort was found to have upstaged tumors pathologically, compared with the 50% to 60% rate previously shown. A lower nodal upstaging rate would be expected, given the administration of induction therapy. Also, complete pathologic response was noted in up to 60% of the specimens and 27% of tumors were downstaged to stage I.[36] These data support the proposed benefit of neoadjuvant therapy in downstaging the tumor and sterilizing regional lymph nodes, thus potentially improving survival.

In contrast, Rice and colleagues[4] showed a decrease in survival with induction therapy for cT2N0 patients. These data from the Cleveland Clinic showed a decrease in 5-year survival from 52% in the surgery alone group to 13% for the group receiving induction therapy plus surgery ($P = .05$). However, the number of patients in the induction therapy subset was small (n = 8) compared with the surgery alone group (n = 53).[4]

Adjuvant therapy

The addition of adjuvant therapy has been associated with an improvement in overall survival, time to recurrence, and recurrence-free survival following resection of locally advanced esophageal cancer.[37,38] However, the routine administration of adjuvant therapy for nodal metastases is also debated by some.[39] Although data are limited, common practice is to administer adjuvant therapy to patients with cT2N0 esophageal cancers that are upstaged following surgery.

The series from Rice and colleagues[4] from the Cleveland Clinic retrospectively reviewed 61 patients over 18 years with cT2N0 esophageal cancer. In examining only the understaged patients (>pT2N0), 10 underwent esophagectomy as lone therapy, whereas 7 underwent surgery followed by adjuvant therapy. Survival for the surgery followed by adjuvant therapy group increased to 43% from 10% for the surgery only group. Although limited by a small patient population, the investigators recommended surgery as primary treatment modality for cT2N0 tumors, followed by adjuvant therapy for upstaged tumors.[4]

Surgical therapy and adequate lymphadenopathy

The primary techniques of esophageal resection include transhiatal esophagectomy, transthoracic esophagectomy, en bloc resection of the esophagus, and minimally invasive esophagectomy. The details of each are beyond the scope of this article, but the primary goal should be to resect the tumor (R0 resection) and perform an adequate lymphadenectomy. The surgeon's choice of procedure should be based on preference, patient/tumor anatomy, and breadth of lymphadenectomy.

According to Rizk and colleagues,[40] in a review of data from the Worldwide Esophageal Cancer Collaboration, survival is improved with a thorough lymphadenectomy based on the clinical T stage of the tumor. For T2 specifically, the study recommends resecting 15 to 22 lymph nodes as optimal therapy.[40] Using this recommendation as a guideline, Stiles and colleagues[22] reviewed 102 patients with cT2/T3 esophageal cancer who underwent resection by mainly the transhiatal and transthoracic en bloc techniques. Transthoracic resection provided a median 29 lymph nodes compared with 18 for a transhiatal approach. Adequate lymphadenectomy was accomplished in 68.6% of transthoracic resection as opposed to 31.3% of transhiatal resections. In addition, an en bloc resection was twice as likely to meet lymphadenectomy criteria compared with less comprehensive resection. Based on these data, the investigators support transthoracic esophageal resection as the ideal technique for the specific subset of cT2/T3 tumors.[22] An association between the number of lymph nodes harvested during esophagectomy and survival has also been previously shown.[41]

SUMMARY

The management of esophageal cancer necessitates a multimodality approach and the constant evolution of treatment algorithm for the best possible outcome. T2 esophageal cancer proves to be a diagnostic challenge and a nidus for much debate in terms of its management. The difficulty stems from the inability of current clinical staging modalities to accurately stage T2 esophageal cancers. This inability, in turn, often leads to selection of an inappropriate treatment strategy. Thus, the outcome of patients with T2 esophageal cancer would, first, be benefited by the improvement in staging modalities to more accurately predict true pathologic stage. Improvement in EUS probes and a wider application of EUS-guided FNA biopsies can potentially augment the accuracy of clinical staging for presumed T2N0 esophageal cancers.

There are limited data to support neoadjuvant therapy for presumed nodal disease versus primary resection followed by adjuvant therapy for proven nodal disease. Given the paucity of data, we adhere to a surgery-first approach for cT2N0 esophageal cancer. This approach allows a decision for adjuvant therapy to be based on the true pathologic stage of the tumor. Although difficult because of the rarity of this subset, a collaborative, randomized study would be the most appropriate next step in answering this challenging question.

REFERENCES

1. Urshel JD, Vasan H, Blewett CJ. A meta-analysis of randomized controlled trials that compared neoadjuvant chemotherapy and surgery to surgery alone for resectable esophageal cancer. Am J Surg 2002;183:274–9.
2. Graham AJ, Shrive FM, Ghali WA, et al. Defining the optimal treatment of locally advanced esophageal cancer: a systematic review and decision analysis. Ann Thorac Surg 2007;83:1257–64.
3. Rice TW, Blackstone EH, Rybicki LA, et al. Refining esophageal cancer staging. J Thorac Cardiovasc Surg 2003;125:1103–13.
4. Rice TW, Mason DP, Murthy SC, et al. T2N0M0 esophageal cancer. J Thorac Cardiovasc Surg 2007;133:317–24.
5. DeMeester SR. Adenocarcinoma of the esophagus and cardia: a review of the disease and its treatment. Ann Surg Oncol 2006;13(1):1312–30.
6. Eloubedi MA, Desmond R, Arguedas MR, et al. Prognostic factors for the survival of patients with esophageal cancer in the U.S.: the importance of tumor length and lymph node status. Cancer 2002;95:1434.

7. Rice TW, Blackstone EH, Rusch VW. 7th edition of the AJCC Cancer Staging Manual: esophagus and esophagogastric junction. Ann Surg Oncol 2010;17(7):1721–4.
8. Gertler R, Stein HJ, Langer R, et al. Long-term outcomes of 2920 patients with cancers of the esophagus and esophagogastric junction: evaluation of the new Union Internationale Contre le Cancer/American Joint Cancer Committee staging system. Ann Surg 2011;253(4):689–98.
9. Lu YK, Li YM, Gu YZ. Cancer of the esophagus and esophagogastric junction: analysis of results of 1025 resections after 5 to 20 years. Ann Thorac Surg 1987;43:176.
10. Rice TW, Zuccaro G, Adelstein DJ, et al. Esophageal carcinoma: depth of invasion is predictive of regional lymph node status. Ann Thorac Surg 1998;65:787–92.
11. Zhang X, Watson DI, Jamieson GG. Lymph node metastases of adenocarcinoma of the esophagus and esophagogastric junction. Chin Med J (Engl) 2007; 120(24):2268–70.
12. Liu L, Hofstetter WL, Rashid A, et al. Significance of the depth of tumor invasion and lymph node metastasis in superficially invasive (T1) esophageal adenocarcinoma. Am J Surg Pathol 2005;29(8):1079–85.
13. Rice TW, Blackstone EH, Adelstein DJ, et al. Role of clinically determined depth of tumor invasion in the treatment of esophageal carcinoma. J Thorac Cardiovasc Surg 2003;125:1091–102.
14. Crabtree TD, Yacoub WN, Puri V, et al. Endoscopic ultrasound for early stage esophageal adenocarcinoma: implications for staging and survival. Ann Thorac Surg 2011;91(5):1509–16.
15. NCCN Clinical Practice Guidelines in Oncology. Esophageal and esophagogastric junction cancers. Fort Washington (PA): National Comprehensive Cancer Network ®; 2011. Available at: www.nccn.org. Accessed December 28, 2011.
16. National Cancer Institute. PDQ® esophageal cancer treatment. Bethesda (MD): National Cancer Institute; 2011. Available at: http://cancer.gov/cancertopics/pdq/treatment/esophageal/HealthProfessional. Accessed December 27, 2011.
17. Van Vliet EP, Heijenbrok-Kal MH, Hunink MG, et al. Staging investigation for oesophageal cancer: a meta-analysis. Br J Cancer 2008;98:547–57.
18. Wong R, Walker-Dilks C, Raifu A. Evidence-based guideline recommendations on the use of positron emission tomography imaging in oesophageal cancer. Clin Oncol (R Coll Radiol) 2012;24(2):86–104.
19. Alam N, Bayam F, Kneale E, et al. The added value of (18F) FDG-PET/CT in staging of oesophageal cancer. Cancer Imaging 2011;11:S116.
20. Keswani RN, Early DS, Edmundowicz SA, et al. Routine positron emission tomography does not alter nodal staging in patients undergoing EUS-guided FNA for esophageal cancer. Gastrointest Endosc 2009;69(7):1210–7.
21. Pech O, Gunter E, Dusemund F, et al. Accuracy of endoscopic ultrasound in preoperative staging of esophageal cancer: results from a referral center for early esophageal cancer. Endoscopy 2010;42(6):456–61.
22. Stiles BM, Mirza F, Coppolino A, et al. Clinical T2-T3N0M0 esophageal cancer: the risk of node positive disease. Ann Thorac Surg 2011;92(2):491–6.
23. Heidemann J, Schilling MK, Schmassmann A, et al. Accuracy of endoscopic ultrasonography in preoperative staging of esophageal carcinoma. Dig Surg 2000;17:219–24.
24. DeWitt J, Kesler K, Brooks JA, et al. Endoscopic ultrasound for esophageal and gastroesophageal junction cancer: impact of increased use of primary neoadjuvant therapy on preoperative locoregional staging accuracy. Dis Esophagus 2005;18:21–7.

25. Kutup A, Link BC, Schurr PG, et al. Quality control of endoscopic ultrasound in preoperative staging of esophageal cancer. Endoscopy 2007;39:715–9.
26. Shimoyama S, Imamura K, Takeshita Y, et al. The useful combination of a higher frequency miniprobe and endoscopic submucosal dissection for the treatment of T1 esophageal cancer. Surg Endosc 2006;20(3):434–8.
27. Vazquez-Sequerios E, Norton ID, Clain JE, et al. Impact of EUS-guided fine-needle aspiration on lymph node staging in patients with esophageal carcinoma. Gastrointest Endosc 2001;53:751–7.
28. Gebski V, Burmeister B, Smithers BM, et al. Survival benefits from neoadjuvant chemoradiotherapy or chemotherapy in oesophageal carcinoma: a meta-analysis. Lancet Oncol 2007;8:226–34.
29. Merkow RP, Bilmoria KY, McCarter MD, et al. Use of multimodality neoadjuvant therapy for esophageal cancer in the United States: assessment of 987 hospitals. Ann Surg Oncol 2012;19(2):357–64.
30. Kelsen DP, Winter KA, Gunderson L, et al. Long-term results of RTOG trial 8911 (USA Intergroup 113): a random assignment trial comparison of chemotherapy followed by surgery compared with surgery alone for esophageal cancer. J Clin Oncol 2007;25(24):3719–25.
31. Bossett JF, Gignoux M, Triboulet JP, et al. Chemoradiotherapy followed by surgery compared with surgery alone in squamous cell cancer of the esophagus. N Engl J Med 1997;337:161–7.
32. Walsh TN, Nonan N, Hoolywood D, et al. A comparison of multimodal therapy and surgery for esophageal adenocarcinoma. N Engl J Med 1996;335:462–7.
33. Nygaard K, Hagen S, Hansen HS, et al. Pre-operative radiotherapy prolongs survival in operable esophageal carcinoma: a randomized, multicenter study of pre-operative radiotherapy and chemotherapy-the second Scandinavian trial in esophageal cancer. World J Surg 1992;16:1104–9.
34. Pennathur A, Luketich JD, Landreneau RJ, et al. Long term results of a phase II trial of neoadjuvant chemotherapy followed by esophagectomy for locally advanced esophageal neoplasm. Ann Thorac Surg 2008;85:1930–6.
35. Le Prise E, Etienne PL, Meunier B, et al. A randomized study of chemotherapy, radiation therapy, and surgery versus surgery for localized squamous cell carcinoma of the esophagus. Cancer 1994;73:1779–84.
36. Kountourakis P, Correa AM, Hofstetter WL, et al. Combined modality therapy of cT2N0M0 esophageal cancer: the University of Texas M.D. Anderson cancer center experience. Cancer 2011;117:925–30.
37. Rice TW, Adelstein DJ, Chidel MA, et al. Benefit of postoperative adjuvant chemoradiotherapy in locoregionally advanced esophageal carcinoma. J Thorac Cardiovasc Surg 2003;126:1590–6.
38. Armanios M, Xu R, Forastiere AA, et al. Adjuvant chemotherapy for resected adenocarcinoma of the esophagus, gastro-esophageal junction, and cardia: phase II trial (E8296) of the Eastern Cooperative Oncology Group. J Clin Oncol 2004;22:4495–9.
39. Power DG, Reynolds JV. Localized adenocarcinoma of the esophagogastric junction-is there a standard of care? Cancer Treat Rev 2010;36(5):400–9.
40. Rizk NP, Ishwaran H, Rice TW, et al. Optimum lymphadenectomy for esophageal cancer. Ann Surg 2010;251:46–50.
41. Peyre CG, Hagen J, DeMeester SR, et al. The number of lymph nodes removed predicts survival in esophageal cancer: an international study on the impact of surgical resection. Ann Surg 2008;248:549–56.

Management of Advanced-Stage Operable Esophageal Cancer

Ankit Bharat, MD, Traves Crabtree, MD*

KEYWORDS

- Esophageal cancer • Neoadjuvant therapy • Surgery

KEY POINTS

- Esophageal cancer is the seventh largest source of cancer-related deaths across the world, with 482,300 new cases annually and 406,800 deaths.
- Although tumor size, length, and site are important, the two most crucial prognostic factors for patients without distant disease are the depth of invasion of the primary tumor and lymphatic metastases.
- Surgical resection, when feasible, provides the best survival advantage.
- Presently there are no prospective randomized trials that compare the different approaches of lymphadenectomy in patients with locally advanced adenocarcinoma.
- Advanced-stage esophageal carcinoma carries a poor prognosis.

INTRODUCTION

Esophageal cancer is the seventh largest source of cancer-related deaths across the world, with 482,300 new cases annually and 406,800 deaths.[1] Incidence rates vary internationally, with the highest rates found in Southern and Eastern Africa and Eastern Asia, and lowest rates observed in Western and Middle Africa and Central America. In the United States, esophageal cancer had an incidence of 16,980 new cases in 2011 with a high mortality of 14,710 deaths.[2]

Esophageal cancer usually occurs as either squamous cell carcinoma in the middle or upper one-third of the esophagus, or as adenocarcinoma in the lower one-third or junction of the esophagus and stomach. Smoking and excessive alcohol consumption account for about 90% of the total cases of squamous cell carcinoma of the esophagus.[3] By contrast, smoking, obesity, and gastroesophageal reflux disease are thought to be the major risk factors for adenocarcinoma. In the past few decades,

Division of Cardiothoracic Surgery, Washington University School of Medicine, Saint Louis, 3108 Queeny Tower, One Barnes-Jewish Hospital Plaza, St Louis, MO 63110-1013, USA
* Corresponding author.
E-mail address: crabtreet@wustl.edu

Surg Clin N Am 92 (2012) 1179–1197
http://dx.doi.org/10.1016/j.suc.2012.07.012
0039-6109/12/$ – see front matter © 2012 Published by Elsevier Inc.

surgical.theclinics.com

there has been a notable increase in esophageal adenocarcinoma in the United States in comparison with squamous cell carcinoma. Overall, the disease is about 3 to 4 times more common in men than in women. However, the incidence is increasing in both genders and is most likely related to lifestyle.[4]

There are no good screening strategies for esophageal cancer. As a result, it is estimated that only about a quarter of all new patients have localized disease. Most patients present with regional or distant metastasis and have a poor prognosis. The 5-year overall survival rate according to the Surveillance, Epidemiology, and End Results (SEER) database is 16.8%, which has improved from past rates of only 5%. The 5-year survival rates for localized, regional, and distant disease are 37.3%, 18.4%, and 3.1%, respectively (http://seer.cancer.gov).

PRESENTATION

The distensible nature of the esophagus leads to a delayed presentation of esophageal cancer unless there is circumferential involvement or considerable penetration into the lumen.[5] Hence, the presenting symptoms are a reflection of the local extent of disease and generally do not occur until late in the disease course. Most patients with esophageal cancer present with dysphagia (74%–83%) and weight loss (58%),[5,6] which are independent indicators of poor prognosis.[6–8] Less common symptoms include gastroesophageal reflux, dyspnea, cough, and odynophagia.[9–11]

DIAGNOSTIC WORKUP

The revised seventh edition of the American Joint Commission on Cancer staging system for esophageal cancer is shown in **Boxes 1** and **2**. Although tumor size, length, and site are important, the two most crucial prognostic factors for patients without distant disease are the depth of invasion of the primary tumor and lymphatic metastases.[6] Careful evaluation of lymph node metastases significantly affects the therapeutic strategy for patients. The diagnostic modalities available for staging esophageal cancer include endoscopic ultrasonography (EUS), computed tomography, and ^{18}F-fluorodeoxyglucose (FDG) positron emission tomography (PET).

The initial diagnostic study is frequently upper endoscopy with biopsy to confirm the diagnosis. An esophagogram may demonstrate a stricture or ulceration.[5,12] A computed tomography (CT) scan may identify distant metastasis and grossly characterize the local extent of the tumor, but PET/CT has become an integral part of esophageal cancer staging. PET/CT improves detection of distant metastasis in more than 10% of cases compared with CT alone, and may prevent the need for more invasive staging strategies such as thoracoscopy and laparoscopy.[13–16]

In patients without distant metastasis, EUS has become essential in defining local invasion and the extent of regional lymph node metastasis. For the assessment of T stage, EUS has a high sensitivity and specificity of 81% to 90% and 94% to 99%, respectively. The accuracy of EUS is better with higher T stage.[17] For assessing lymph node status, EUS sensitivity and specificity is 80% to 85% and 70% to 85%, respectively.[17,18] However, EUS is operator dependent and is unreliable for assessment of lymph nodes deeper than 5 cm. A unique advantage of EUS is the ability to perform fine-needle aspiration (FNA) that is safe and does not require general anesthesia.[19] FNA improves both sensitivity (92%) and specificity (93%) for nodal staging with EUS.[17] EUS is superior to PET/CT for T staging and in identifying locoregional nodes. In a recent study, Walker and colleagues[7] investigated the accuracy of EUS and PET/CT. The accuracy of PET/CT was 91% compared with 100% with EUS for

---

Box 1
TNM nomenclature of esophageal cancer

Primary tumor (T)
Tx   Primary tumor cannot be assessed
T0   No evidence of primary tumor
Tis   High-grade dysplasia
T1a   Tumor invades lamina propria or muscularis mucosae
T1b   Tumor invades submucosa
T2   Tumor invades muscularis propria
T3   Tumor invades adventitia
T4a   Tumor invades resectable adjacent structures (pleura, pericardium, diaphragm)
T4b   Tumor invades unresectable adjacent structures (heart, aorta, and so forth)
Regional lymph Nodes (N)
Nx   Regional lymph nodes cannot be assessed
N0   No regional lymph node metastasis
N1   Metastasis in 1–2 lymph nodes
N2   Metastasis in 3–6 lymph nodes
N3   Metastasis in 7 or more lymph nodes
Distant Metastasis (M)
M0   No distant metastasis
M1   Distant metastasis present
Histologic grade (G)
GX   Grade cannot be assessed—stage as G1
G1   Well differentiated
G2   Moderately differentiated
G3   Poorly differentiated
G4   Undifferentiated—stage as G3 squamous

From Edge SB, Byrd DR, Compton CC, editors. American Joint Committee on Cancer staging system, 7th edition. New York: Springer; 2010; with permission.

T stage. Similarly, for locoregional adenopathy the accuracy of EUS was almost twice that of PET/CT.

Sentinel lymph node sampling has also been evaluated for esophageal cancer staging. However, multidirectional lymphatic flow and an unpredictable pattern of lymph node metastasis make it less appealing for esophageal cancers. It might have some role in patients with Barrett esophagus or early-stage cancer in whom skip lesions are rare,[8,9] but currently it is considered experimental in the context of esophageal cancer.

TREATMENT
Surgical Resection

Surgical resection, when feasible, provides the best survival advantage. However, the type of surgical approach varies based on surgeon and institutional preference. The two most common open approaches used for esophageal resection include the transhiatal esophagectomy (THE) and the transthoracic Ivor Lewis esophagectomy (ILE). The largest randomized trial comparing the 2 surgical approaches included a total of 220 patients with adenocarcinoma who were assigned to THE or ILE with 2-field lymphadenectomy.[10] The transhiatal group had shorter duration of surgery, less blood loss, and less overall morbidity. By contrast, significantly more lymph nodes were resected in the ILE group. Nevertheless, there was no significant difference in perioperative mortality. In addition, the R0 resection rate was similar for both groups. There was no statistically significant difference between the 2 groups in terms of survival. However, in a subgroup analysis, a survival advantage was demonstrated in patients

Box 2					
TNM Staging of esophageal cancer					
Stage	**T**	**N**	**M**	**Grade**	**Location**
Squamous Cell Carcinoma					
0	Tis	N0	M0	1, X	Any
Ia	T1	N0	M0	1, X	Any
Ib	T1	N0	M0	2–3	Any
	T2–3	N0	M0	1, X	Lower, X
IIa	T2–3	N0	M0	1, X	Upper, Middle
	T2–3	N0	M0	2–3	Lower, X
IIb	T2–3	N0	M0	Any	Upper, Middle
	T1–2	N1	M0	Any	Any
IIIa	T1–2	N2	M0	Any	Any
	T3	N1	M0	Any	Any
	T4a	N0	M0	Any	Any
IIIb	T3	N2	M0	Any	Any
IIIc	T4a	N1-2	M0	Any	Any
	T4b	Any	M0	Any	Any
	Any	N3	M0	Any	Any
IV	Any	Any	M1	Any	Any
Adenocarcinoma					
0	Tis	N0	M0	1, X	Any
Ia	T1	N0	M0	1, X	Any
Ib	T1	N0	M0	2–3	Any
	T2–3	N0	M0	1, X	Lower, X
IIa	T2–3	N0	M0	1, X	Upper, Middle
	T2–3	N0	M0	2–3	Lower, X
IIb	T2–3	N0	M0	2–3	Upper, Middle
	T1–2	N1	M0	Any	Any
IIIa	T1–2	N2	M0	Any	Any
	T3	N1	M0	Any	Any
	T4a	N0	M0	Any	Any
IIIb	T3	N2	M0	Any	Any
IIIc	T4a	N1-2	M0	Any	Any
	T4b	Any	M0	Any	Any
	Any	N3	M0	Any	Any
IV	Any	Any	M1	Any	Any

From Edge SB, Byrd DR, Compton CC, editors. American Joint Committee on Cancer staging system, 7th edition. New York: Springer; 2010; with permission.

with 1 to 8 positive lymph nodes among those undergoing the transthoracic approach (64% vs 23%, $P = .02$). Also, there was a trend toward a better 5-year overall survival with ILE in the intent-to-treat population (39% vs 29%, $P<.05$).[11] However, when patients with preoperatively unresectable/incurable disease were excluded and the data were analyzed per protocol specification, there was no longer a trend seen in 5-year survival rates between the two approaches. Other trials, including meta-analyses, have confirmed a lack of survival difference between the two techniques and thus the choice of operation is dependent on the surgeon's comfort level with each approach.[12–14] Others advocate the use of a 3-incision or 3-hole technique that allows for a 3-field lymphadenectomy. This approach is discussed later in the context of nodal dissection with esophagectomy.

Because of concerns about the morbidities associated with esophagectomy, minimally invasive approaches have been attempted. In one of the largest series from

Luketich's group,[15] 222 patients underwent minimally invasive esophagectomies using thoracoscopic and laparoscopic approaches. A completion rate of over 90% was achieved with an overall operative mortality of 1.4% and comparable long-term outcomes with open esophagectomies. Although a randomized controlled trial has been not performed, it appears that under experienced hands, a minimally invasive approach may result in outcomes similar to those of open techniques in a select group of patients.

Lymphadenectomy

The lymphatic drainage of the esophagus is highly complex, with abundant lymph-capillary networks throughout the mucosa. Embryologically, the esophagus develops simultaneously from the mesenchyme of the head and neck and of the body, merging at the level of tracheal bifurcation. Lymphatic spread is influenced by this development. Tumors above the level of the carina tend to drain cranially into the thoracic duct and supraclavicular lymph nodes. Below the carina, tumors drain into the cysterna chyli and lymph nodes of the inferior mediastinum, and along the left gastric artery to the celiac trunk. Lymphatic stasis because of tumor spread can lead to flow reversal, resulting in unpredictable spread. In addition, the unique network of intramural lymphatic vessels that drain into local lymph nodes has the potential for skip lesions.[16–18]

Several terms have been used to describe the extent of lymphadenectomy during esophagectomy. Three-field lymphadenectomy (**Fig. 1**) includes resection of nodal

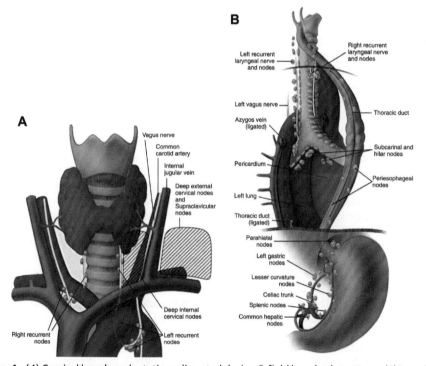

Fig. 1. (A) Cervical lymph node stations dissected during 3-field lymphadenectomy. (B) Lymph nodes dissected during right thoracotomy and laparotomy with 3-field lymphadenectomy. (From Altorki NK, Lerut T. Three-field lymph node dissection for cancer of the esophagus. In: Patterson GA, Cooper JD, Deslauriers J, et al, editors. Pearson's thoracic and esophageal surgery. 3rd edition. Philadelphia: Churchill Livingstone; 2008. p. 608; with permission.)

tissue in the abdomen (abdominal lymphadenectomy), mediastinum (mediastinal lymphadenectomy), and neck (cervical lymphadenectomy). It encompasses all nodal tissue in abdominal compartments from 1 through 12 (equivalent to a D2 lymphadenectomy), periesophageal nodal tissue in the chest, including thoracic duct, subcarinal space, aortopulmonary window, and main stem bronchial nodes, as well as lymph nodes along both recurrent laryngeal nerves.

Mediastinal lymphadenectomy can be classified as standard, extended, and total. Standard mediastinal lymphadenectomy refers to a complete clearance of lymph nodes from the lower posterior mediastinum. Extension along the ride side of trachea is termed extended lymphadenectomy, whereas a total mediastinal lymphadenectomy includes everything in extended lymphadenectomy plus dissection of the left paratracheal area, left recurrent laryngeal nerve, and subaortic lymph nodes.[19,20]

Cervical lymphadenectomy includes removal of the following three groups of nodes: the deep internal, external, and lateral nodes bilaterally. The deep internal nodes are medial to the internal jugular vein, closely related to the recurrent laryngeal nerve, and include the paraesophageal and paratracheal lymph nodes in the neck. The deep external nodes are grouped around the internal jugular vein and include the supraclavicular glands inferiorly. The deep lateral nodes are situated along the spinal accessory nerve in the lower part of the neck.[21]

Two-field lymphadenectomy includes the same abdominal and thoracic compartments as the 3-field dissection, without cervical nodes. Peritumoral lymphadenectomy, by contrast, includes dissection of the nodes in direct proximity to the tumor, the esophagus, and the upper stomach.[22]

At present there are no prospective randomized trials that compare the different approaches of lymphadenectomy in patients with locally advanced adenocarcinoma. One randomized controlled trial has compared 2-field and 3-field lymphadenectomy in squamous cell carcinoma. With 30 patients randomized to each arm, 5-year survival rates were 48% with 2-field and 66% with 3-field lymphadenectomy (not significant).[23] Other studies have reported similar survival between 2-field and 3-field lymphadenectomy, although the 3-field approach has been associated with higher operative morbidity including higher recurrent laryngeal nerve paralysis and pulmonary complications.[24–26] Neoadjuvant chemoradiation is now routinely used for locally advanced esophageal carcinoma with N1 disease,[27–29] and some argue that it may further diminish the role of 3-field lymphadenectomy. Hence, ILE with 2-field lymphadenectomy or THE with abdominal D2 lymphadenectomy as well as excision of infracarinal posterior mediastinal lymph nodes are both considered viable treatment options.[30]

Three-field lymphadenectomy has been recommended by some for carcinomas located above the tracheal bifurcation, because of the higher incidence of nodal involvement in the upper thorax and neck.[18] The basis for 3-hole esophagectomy is inclusion of cervical lymphadenectomy (3-field lymphadenectomy) as part of the esophagectomy. Prior studies have shown that cervical lymph nodes could harbor tumor metastasis in up to 30% to 40% of patients in whom curative resection had been performed.[31] Therefore, extended lymphadenectomy with 3-hole esophagectomy may have an impact on tumor staging, although its role on survival is unclear.

In a study by Altorki and colleagues,[31] 36% of esophagectomy patients had clinically unsuspected cervicothoracic disease irrespective of the location (lower third 33%, middle third 59%). The investigators reported overall and disease-free 5-year survivals of 50% and 46%, respectively, in 80 patients treated with 3-field lymphadenectomy. However, those with metastasis to the cervical lymph nodes had overall 3- and 5-year survival of 33% and 25%, respectively. In Japanese centers 3-field lymphadenectomy is routinely performed. In a Japanese series of squamous cancers of the lower thoracic esophagus, the 5-year survival rates were 5.6% after 2-field dissection compared with 30% following 3-field dissection, with 42% of the lymph nodes located in the upper and middle mediastinum.[32] However, as already discussed, other studies have reported no difference and therefore the role of neck lymphadenectomy is debatable, especially in tumors located in the middle or lower third of the esophagus that are more commonly seen in the Western world.[33–36]

NEOADJUVANT THERAPY

The main prognostic variables following surgery are lymph node metastasis and margin involvement.[37] Some studies have shown that only 25% to 40% of patients have a resectable tumor at the time of diagnosis and only 70% of these tumors are amenable to R0 resection.[38,39] For early-stage esophageal cancer (T1N0, T2N0), surgery is the first-line therapy and provides 5-year survival rates of 50% to 80%.[40,41] If lymph node metastases are found in the pathologic specimen or if R0 resection is not obtained, adjuvant therapy may be considered, although it is unclear whether this provides a significant survival benefit.[42–44]

For clinical T3 or T4 tumors, or N1 disease, surgery alone provides poor results, with 3-year survival in the 10% to 25% range.[28,45] Therefore, in such cases neoadjuvant therapy is often recommended. The goal of neoadjuvant therapy is to increase R0 resection rate by decreasing the size of the tumor, treat micrometastases, decrease local and distant metastases, and thereby improve overall survival.

Radiation Therapy

Radiation therapy as a single modality in the neoadjuvant setting has failed to demonstrate survival benefit. Five phase III randomized clinical trials comparing preoperative radiation with surgery alone (**Table 1**) have not demonstrated an increase in resectability or overall survival with preoperative radiation alone.[46–50] Although Nygaard and colleagues[48] suggested a benefit in 3-year overall survival, this was achieved after pooling patients who had received neoadjuvant chemoradiotherapy as well. At best, a meta-analysis including data from 1147 patients who almost exclusively had

Table 1
Phase III randomized trials of neoadjuvant radiotherapy (NRT) versus surgery (S) alone

Authors,[Ref] Year	N	RT Treatment	Histology	5-Year OS NRT (%)	5-Year OS S (%)	P
Launois et al,[47] 1981	134	4000 rad Cobalt 8 d preop	SCC	10	12	NS
Gignoux et al,[46] 1987	208	N/A	SCC	11	10	NS
Wang et al,[50] 1989	206	400 cGy 2–4 wk preop	SCC	35	30	NS
Arnott et al,[49] 1992	176	20 Gy in 10 treatments over 2 wk	AC/SCC	9	17	NS
Nygaard et al,[48] 1992	89	35 Gy preop	SCC	21[a]	9[a]	NS

Abbreviations: AC, adenocarcinoma; N/A, no data available; NS, not significant; OS, overall survival; SCC, squamous cell carcinoma.
[a] 3-year survival.

squamous cell carcinoma revealed a statistically insignificant trend toward improved 5-year survival (odds ratio [OR] 0.89, 95% confidence interval [CI] 0.78–1.01; $P = .062$).[51] Based on available data, radiation is not typically recommended as a single-line neoadjuvant therapy.

Chemotherapy

The randomized trials that have compared neoadjuvant chemotherapy with surgery alone are listed in **Table 2**. In the largest study of both adenocarcinoma (53.6%) and squamous cell carcinoma (46.4%), 204 patients underwent preoperative chemotherapy using 5-fluorouracil (5-FU) and cisplatin, while 227 were treated with surgery alone.[52] Median survival was 16.1 months for surgery alone versus 14.9 months for neoadjuvant chemotherapy ($P = .53$). R1 resections were more common in the surgery group alone (15% vs 4%).[52] In another large study published by the Medical Research Council,[53] 802 patients were included of whom 66% had adenocarcinoma. A significant survival benefit was seen in the neoadjuvant therapy group (median survival 16.8 months vs 13.4 months, 5-year survival 23% vs 17%; $P<.05$). The survival benefit was seen in the adenocarcinoma group but not with squamous cancer (**Table 3**). There was also improvement in the R0 resection rates (60% vs 54%; $P<.001$). The main differences in the 2 studies were the smaller sample size in the former study[52] as well as higher chemotherapy dose causing a greater incidence of toxicities. Surgical resection was only possible in 75% of patients in this study because of the high incidence of chemotherapy-related toxicities, compared with 95% in the latter. A recent meta-analysis that included 9 clinical trials suggested that neoadjuvant chemotherapy is beneficial in adenocarcinoma (hazard ratio [HR] 0.78; $P = .014$) but not in squamous cell carcinoma (HR 0.88; $P = .12$).[54]

Chemoradiation

Although historically there has been limited experience with neoadjuvant chemoradiation, there is an increasing amount of data evaluating neoadjuvant chemoradiation for

Table 2
Randomized trials of neoadjuvant chemotherapy versus surgery alone

Authors,[Ref] Year	Treatment	n	Histology	3-Year OS (%)	P
Schlag,[95] 1992	C F	22	SCC	a	NS
	Surgery	24			
Nygaard et al,[48] 1992	B C	44	SCC	3	NS
	Surgery	41		9	
Maipang et al,[96] 1994	B V C	24	SCC	31	NS
	Surgery	22		36	
Law et al,[97] 1997	C F	74	SCC	40	NS
	Surgery	73		13	
Kelsen et al,[52] 1998	C F	213	AC/SCC	19	NS
	Surgery	227		20	
Ancona et al,[98] 2001	C F	47	SCC	34	NS
	Surgery	47		22	
MRC,[53] 2002	C F	400	AC/SCC	43	<.01
	Surgery	402		34	

Abbreviations: AC, adenocarcinoma; B, bleomycin; C, cisplatin; F, fluorouracil; MRC, Medical Research Council; NS, not significant; OS, overall survival; SCC, squamous cell carcinoma; V, vinblastine.
[a] Median survival 10 months in both groups.

Table 3
Randomized trials of neoadjuvant chemoradiotherapy versus surgery alone that include adenocarcinoma

Authors,[Ref] Year	Treatment	n	5-Year Survival (%)	Histology	P
Urba et al,[57] 2001	C F V + 45 Gy	50	30[a]	AC/SCC	NS
	Surgery	50	16		
Tepper et al,[58] 2008	C F + 50.4 Gy	30	39	AC/SCC	<.01
	Surgery	26	16		
Burmeister et al,[56] 2005	C F + 35 Gy	128	17	AC/SCC	NS
	Surgery	128	13		
Walsh et al,[55] 1996	C F + 40 Gy	58	32[a]	ACC	<.05
	Surgery	55	6		

Abbreviations: AC, adenocarcinoma; C, cisplatin; F, fluorouracil; NS, not significant; SCC, squamous cell carcinoma; V, vinblastine.
[a] 3-year survival.

the treatment of esophageal cancer. In a study of 103 patients with adenocarcinoma, neoadjuvant chemoradiation improved 3-year survival (32% vs 6%, $P = .01$) and median survival (16 months vs 11 months with surgery alone).[55] This study was criticized for incomplete preoperative staging and lack of intent-to-treat analysis. Furthermore, the patients in the surgery-alone group had a surprisingly low survival (6% at 3 years) compared with existing standards. In another study with 128 patients in each arm, patients undergoing neoadjuvant chemoradiation were more likely to undergo R0 resection versus surgery alone (80% vs 59%).[56] However, disease-free (17 months vs 13 months) and overall survival (22 months vs 19.3 months) were similar. Urba and colleagues[57] demonstrated a trend toward better survival with chemoradiation in a cohort of 100 patients (30% vs 16%; $P = .15$), while Tepper and colleagues[58] reported an improvement in 5-year survival, with chemoradiation at 39% (95% CI 21%–57%) versus surgery alone at 16% (95% CI 5%–33%).

Meta-analyses have reported an overall survival advantage with neoadjuvant chemoradiation for both adenocarcinoma and squamous cell carcinoma. An early study by Urshel and Vasan[59] included 9 randomized controlled trials with 1116 patients, and reported a 3-year survival benefit that favored neoadjuvant chemoradiotherapy (OR 0.66; $P = .016$). The survival benefit was even more pronounced when chemotherapy and radiotherapy were given concurrently (OR 0.45; $P = .005$). Furthermore, patients who received neoadjuvant chemoradiation were more likely to have an R0 resection (OR 0.53; $P = .007$), with 21% demonstrating complete pathologic response. The more recent meta-analysis published by Gebski and colleagues[54] evaluated 1209 patients in 10 trials and found a survival benefit with neoadjuvant chemoradiotherapy compared with surgery alone, with a 19% decreased risk of death, corresponding to a 13% absolute difference in survival at 2 years.

Neoadjuvant Chemoradiation Versus Chemotherapy Alone

There remains controversy, however, regarding the relative efficacy of chemotherapy versus chemoradiation in the neoadjuvant setting. The only randomized trial comparing chemotherapy alone with chemotherapy with radiation was closed prematurely because of problems with patient recruitment. With a limited cohort, these results demonstrated that chemoradiation was associated with a better pathologic response and lymph node downstaging. There was a trend toward better 3-year survival with chemoradiation (47.4% vs 27.7%; $P = .07$). However, a nonsignificant increase in postoperative mortality was found with chemoradiation (10.2% vs 3.8%; $P = .26$).[60] Advocates of chemoradiation argue that overall survival is improved and that perioperative mortality can be limited in experienced hands, whereas chemotherapy advocates believe that the relative survival advantage is negligible if present at all, and highlight the risk of increased postoperative morbidity and mortality associated with radiation. At present there is an active Canadian trial (NCT 01404156) recruiting patients to compare neoadjuvant chemotherapy with concurrent chemoradiation using carboplatin and paclitaxel. The estimated primary completion date is February 2013.

Chemoradiation Alone Without Surgery

An additional area of controversy involves the relative efficacy of induction chemoradiation followed by surgery versus chemoradiation alone. Stahl and colleagues[61] reported on patients with locally advanced (T3–4 N0–1) squamous cell carcinoma with good performance status. In the surgery arm, induction therapy consisted of chemotherapy (5-FU, leucovorin, etoposide, and cisplatin) followed by concurrent chemoradiotherapy with cisplatin and etoposide (days 2–8) and 40 Gy of radiation before ILE. In the chemoradiation and no-surgery arm, the radiation dose was increased to 65 Gy after the same induction therapy. The surgery arm demonstrated better progression-free survival (2-year 64.3% vs 40.7%; $P = .003$) but the overall survival at 2 years was equivalent between both treatment groups (surgery: 39.9% and chemoradiation: 35.4%, log-rank test of equivalence; $P = .007$). However, the treatment-related mortality was 12.8% in the surgery group compared with 3.5% ($P = .03$) in the chemoradiation-therapy arm, which would be considered excessive using the current standards.

The FFCD 9102 trial included 259 patients with operable T3-4 N0-1 esophageal carcinoma predominantly populated by patients with squamous cell carcinoma (89.2%).[62] Patients underwent induction chemoradiation with 2 sessions of 5-FU and cisplatin in addition to 46 Gy of radiation versus definitive chemoradiotherapy without surgery. Surgery was associated with higher mortality rates (9.3% vs 0.8%; $P = .002$). No statistically significant difference was found in the median (17.7 months vs 19.3 months) or 2-year survival (34% vs 40%; $P = .44$). Variability in treatment regimens and heterogeneity of tumors in these studies preclude definitive consensus on the relative efficacy of these modalities.

Studies have suggested that the complete clinical response rate to chemoradiation is generally lower in adenocarcinoma compared with squamous cell carcinoma (45.6% vs 70.2%; $P = .013$).[63] Others have confirmed that chemoradiation alone can provide a complete clinical response in 50% to 65% of cases with a median survival of 17 to 26 months and 2-year survival of 30% to 40%.[64] It is speculated that the complete clinical response correlates with higher complete pathologic response seen in patients with squamous cell carcinoma. Hence, the higher percentage of complete response in patients with locally advanced squamous cell carcinoma might be responsible for diminishing the relative benefits of surgery. Unfortunately, current nonsurgical staging modalities are unreliable in identifying patients with complete response after induction therapy, as is outlined next.

ASSESSMENT OF THE RESPONSE OF NEOADJUVANT THERAPY

The modalities available to assess the clinical response of induction therapy include CT, EUS, and FDG PET/CT. Unfortunately, as mentioned previously, the accuracy of these modalities is low following induction therapy. Westerterp and colleagues[65] reported on the relative accuracy of these imaging modalities by constructing summary receiver-operating characteristic curves. The accuracy for these modalities was 54% for CT, 86% for EUS, and 85% for FDG PET. Hence, the accuracy of CT was lower than that of FDG PET ($P<.006$) and EUS ($P<.003$), whereas the accuracy of FDG PET and EUS were similar ($P = .84$). It is estimated that the sensitivity of PET and EUS range from 20% to 100% and 42% to 100% while the specificity ranges from 36% to 100% and 27% to 100%, respectively. Furthermore, there was no difference in the accuracy between early FDG PET and FDG PET after completion of neoadjuvant therapy.[66]

Overall, EUS has demonstrated poor accuracy following neoadjuvant therapy. Post-chemotherapy EUS accurately predicted pathologic stage in only 30% of resected patients. The accuracy of EUS in determining the T stage was 80% with the accuracy for N stage being 35%, in contrast to an accuracy of 85% for EUS predicting patho-logic stage in patients undergoing primary surgical resection.[67] Thus, EUS currently is unreliable in accurately characterizing the clinical response to induction therapy.

For PET, the reported sensitivity, specificity, positive predictive value, and negative predictive value for primary tumor response assessment were reported as 27.3% to 93.3%, 41.7% to 95.2%, 70.8% to 93.3%, and 71.4% to 93.5%, respectively, and for N restaging 16.0% to 67.5%, 85.7% to 100%, 33% to 100%, and 91.7% to 93.3%, respectively.[68] At present, FDG uptake by PET can correlate with tumor response but cannot distinguish patients who achieve complete pathologic response. As such, no modality can presently predict complete pathologic response after induction therapy. The active clinical trial NCT 01333033 is prospectively evaluating the efficacy of PET scanning after combination chemotherapy, and should be completed by April 2013.

T4 TUMORS

Overall, T4 tumors of the esophagus have a very poor prognosis. The reported inci-dence of T4 lesions is 12% to 34%.[69–72] Current diagnostic modalities such as CT, PET, and EUS have been historically inaccurate. These diagnostic modalities correctly diagnosed tumor invasion (T4) in only 51% of patients with a false-positive rate of 40%.[73] This inaccuracy is compounded by the use of induction therapy in patients with presumed T4 tumors, given the greater difficulty in distinguishing between inflam-mation and tumor invasion after induction therapy.

Based on available data, esophagectomy alone, even with resection of involved neighboring organs, does not improve outcomes in comparison with nonsurgical therapy.[74–76] At present, either definitive chemoradiation or chemoradiation followed by surgery remain the 2 treatment options for presumed clinical T4 tumors.[77–85] Given the poor accuracy of current nonsurgical staging modalities in terms of differentiating T3 versus T4 lesions, multimodality strategies may offer the best survival advantage in this setting. When there is clear preoperative evidence of local tumor invasion into adjacent organs the role of surgery remains limited, but can be offered to patients with T4a tumors.

Definitive Chemoradiation

In lieu of surgical intervention, definitive chemoradiation is often used in these patients. The combination of 5-FU and cisplatin is considered the most effective chemothera-peutic regimen, generally given with a concurrent external radiation dose of 50 to 66 Gy.

Tumor response and recurrence

The complete response rate varies from 17% to 39% with an overall response rate of up to 88%. The overall 1-, 3-, and 5-year survival rates after definitive chemoradiation were 26% to 45%, 0% to 23%, and 0% to 14%, respectively. Patients with complete clinical response have a much better prognosis than those without.[79,86] Seto and colleagues[79] reported 1-, 3-, and 5-year survival rates of patients showing a clinical response was 83%, 33%, and 33% compared with only 23%, 0%, and 0% in those without a clinical response. Itoh and colleagues[86] reported that 4 of 6 (67%) patients with adequate clinical response also revealed good local control after definitive chemoradiation.

Chemoradiation Followed by Surgery

Several studies have evaluated the outcomes of patients undergoing chemoradiation followed by surgery for T4 tumors. The primary chemotherapy is the combination of 5-FU and cisplatin. Concurrent radiation is typically used at a dose of 30 to 60 Gy, which is lower than that used for definitive chemoradiation. Typically the chemoradiation is administered 4 to 6 weeks before surgery.[82,83,85]

Tumor response and recurrence

For T4 tumors, it is estimated that 20% to 83% will achieve clinical response to chemoradiation.[80,83,84] However, only 8% to 29% will develop a complete pathologic response. Following chemoradiation, the curative R0 resection rate for T4 tumors varies from 32% to 44%. The most commonly resected en bloc structures include respiratory tract, lung, and pericardium.[80,83,84] Median perioperative morbidity and mortality rates are 62% and 6%, respectively. The most common complications include recurrent nerve palsy, tracheal ischemia, empyema, and anastomotic leaks.[80,83–85] The reported 1-, 3-, and 5-year survival rates are 24% to 73%, 5% to 45%, and 0% to 38%, respectively.

As with all esophageal cancer, the best chance for improved long-term survival is R0 resection.[73,87] This approach necessitates the resection of adjacent organs, which carries the risk of considerable morbidity and mortality. The impact of neoadjuvant therapy and tumor downstaging followed by surgery is evolving, and may show promise with future studies of tumor-specific therapies.[83,88] Even among patients undergoing an R0 resection, long-term survival may vary depending on what organs are involved. A worse prognosis was seen in patients with tumors infiltrating the respiratory tract in comparison with tumors infiltrating the aorta alone or other organs. Patients with respiratory tract invasion also seem to show a poorer response to chemoradiation. Although data are limited, it appears that chemoradiation followed by surgery may offer a short-term survival advantage compared with definitive chemoradiation alone (57% vs 39.5% at 1 year),[79,80] although this has not translated into a significant long-term survival benefit.

As discussed earlier, determining the relative response to induction therapy may help define prognosis and guide subsequent treatment decisions. It is intriguing that nonresponders to chemoradiation in the chemoradiation-surgery group have improved survival in comparison with nonresponders in the definitive chemoradiation group (median 1-, 3-, and 5-year overall survival 58%, 30%, and 20% vs 24.5%, 3.5%, and 0%).[79] In patients with complete pathologic response following chemoradiation, surgery may not add any benefit. Fujita and colleagues[80] compared chemoradiation with chemoradiation plus surgery in patients who achieved complete pathologic response following induction therapy, and showed similar 5-year survival (23% in both groups). By contrast, in patients who did not have a significant response after chemoradiation (nonresponders), those who underwent surgery after chemoradiation showed longer survival than those without surgery (1- and 2-year survival rates 64% and 33% vs 20% and 20%, respectively). It is postulated that among patients who show a complete response to chemoradiation, the long-term prognosis is determined by distant metastasis, and surgical resection might not add an additional survival benefit, although currently there are no nonsurgical staging modalities that reliably identify complete responders, making this issue even more complicated. Alternatively, these data suggest that surgical resection, when feasible, might add survival benefit in patients with T4 tumors who do not respond to chemoradiation. These issues are important ones that require additional clinical data to define the role of surgery in patients with locally advanced esophageal cancer.

ADJUVANT THERAPY FOLLOWING RESECTION
Chemotherapy

The data regarding adjuvant therapy in patients undergoing esophagectomy with a curative intent remains controversial. The Japanese JCOG9204[42] trial published in 2003 evaluated surgery plus chemotherapy versus surgery alone for localized squamous cell carcinoma. The study included 242 patients who were randomly assigned to surgery alone (122) or surgery plus chemotherapy (120). The 5-year disease-free survival was 45% with surgery alone and 55% with surgery plus chemotherapy ($P =$ .03). Despite this, there was no difference in overall 5-year survival rate of 52% (surgery alone) and 61% (surgery with chemotherapy) ($P =$ .13). However, the investigators did report benefit in 5-year survival in patients with N1 disease with adjuvant chemotherapy (38% vs 52%; $P =$ .04). A prior study by the same group, however, failed to report any survival benefit.[43] A prospective nonrandomized trial showed a slight benefit in 3-year disease-free survival with adjuvant chemotherapy (47.6% vs 35.6% with surgery alone; $P =$ .04) but no difference in 5-year overall survival (50.7% in the adjuvant chemotherapy group and 43.7% in the surgery alone group; $P =$ .2).[89] It is noteworthy that these studies did not have neoadjuvant therapy as part of their protocol. There is currently no study that evaluates the role of adjuvant chemotherapy in residual tumor or pathologic N1 disease in patients who have undergone neoadjuvant therapy.

Radiotherapy

In a retrospective review of the SEER database including 1046 patients, Schreiber and colleagues[90] compared patients with T3-4N0 and T1-4N1 tumors who underwent either surgery alone or postoperative radiation. In this study adjuvant radiation was found to be the most important predictor of improved survival (HR 0.70, 95% CI 0.59–0.83; $P<$.001). However, this was a retrospective study containing unmatched controls.

A randomized French trial[91] published in 1991 including 221 patients revealed no difference in overall survival in patients with or without node-positive disease. Similarly, another randomized study from Hong Kong[92] in 1993 included 130 patients. The overall median survival of patients after postoperative radiotherapy was 8.7 months, which was shorter than the 15.2 months for the control groups ($P =$ .02). A Chinese study[93] published in 2003 included 495 patients and randomized them into surgery alone versus surgery followed by radiotherapy. There was no difference in 5-year overall survival (31.7% in surgery alone vs 41.3% in surgery plus radiotherapy; $P =$ .4). However, the 5-year survival rates were reported to be better in patients with stage III patients who underwent radiotherapy (13.1% vs 35.1%, $P =$ .002). Again, none of these patients received neoadjuvant therapy, even those with stage III tumors. Hence, the role of adjuvant radiotherapy in the present era remains unclear owing to the lack of clinical trials.

Chemoradiation

The use of adjuvant chemoradiation is also controversial in patients with esophageal cancer, and clinical trial data are limited on this issue. However, there are limited data that suggest a survival advantage in patients with tumors of the gastroesophageal junction.[94] In the INT 0116 trial of 556 patients with resected adenocarcinoma of stomach and gastroesophageal junction, patients randomized to adjuvant chemoradiotherapy received 4 cycles of adjuvant leucovorin-modulated fluorouracil, with the second cycle concurrent with radiotherapy (45 Gy), following surgical resection. The median overall survival was 27 months versus 36 months (HR 1.35; $P = .005$), favoring adjuvant chemoradiation. Compliance and toxicity remain a concern regarding administration of a toxic regimen of chemoradiation after esophagectomy. The search for better-tolerated regimens has led to an active Canadian trial (NCT 00400114) examining sunitinib malate (Sutent), which allegedly is well tolerated in patients who have undergone surgical resection following induction therapy.

SUMMARY

Advanced-staged esophageal carcinoma carries a poor prognosis. There has been a significant increase in adenocarcinoma relative to squamous cell carcinoma. Numerous initial trials that defined the current treatment strategies included squamous cell carcinomas, which was much more common at that time. Several clinical trials are under way to investigate newer strategies in for the treatment of both adenocarcinoma and squamous cell carcinoma. At present, a multimodal approach offers the best chance of survival.

REFERENCES

1. Jemal A, Bray F, Center MM, et al. Global cancer statistics. CA Cancer J Clin 2011;61:69–90.
2. Siegel R, Ward E, Brawley O, et al. Cancer statistics, 2011: the impact of eliminating socioeconomic and racial disparities on premature cancer deaths. CA Cancer J Clin 2011;61(4):212–36.
3. Engel LS, Chow WH, Vaughan TL, et al. Population attributable risks of esophageal and gastric cancers. J Natl Cancer Inst 2003;95:1404–13.
4. Brown LM, Devesa SS, Chow WH. Incidence of adenocarcinoma of the esophagus among white Americans by sex, stage, and age. J Natl Cancer Inst 2008; 100:1184–7.
5. Daly JM, Fry WA, Little AG, et al. Esophageal cancer: results of an American College of Surgeons Patient Care Evaluation Study. J Am Coll Surg 2000;190: 562–72 [discussion: 572–3].
6. Rice TW, Rusch VW, Ishwaran H, et al. Cancer of the esophagus and esophagogastric junction: data-driven staging for the seventh edition of the American Joint Committee on Cancer/International Union Against Cancer Cancer Staging Manuals. Cancer 2010;116(16):3763–73.
7. Walker AJ, Spier BJ, Perlman SB, et al. Integrated PET/CT fusion imaging and endoscopic ultrasound in the pre-operative staging and evaluation of esophageal cancer. Mol Imaging Biol 2011;13(1):166–71.
8. Feith M, Stein HJ, Siewert JR. Pattern of lymphatic spread of Barrett's cancer. World J Surg 2003;27:1052–7.
9. Stein HJ, Feith M, Siewert JR. Individualized surgical strategies for cancer of the esophagogastric junction. Ann Chir Gynaecol 2000;89:191–8.

10. Hulscher JB, van Sandick JW, de Boer AG, et al. Extended transthoracic resection compared with limited transhiatal resection for adenocarcinoma of the esophagus. N Engl J Med 2002;347:1662–9.
11. Omloo JM, Lagarde SM, Hulscher JB, et al. Extended transthoracic resection compared with limited transhiatal resection for adenocarcinoma of the mid/distal esophagus: five-year survival of a randomized clinical trial. Ann Surg 2007;246: 992–1000 [discussion: 1000–1].
12. Chu KM, Law SY, Fok M, et al. A prospective randomized comparison of transhiatal and transthoracic resection for lower-third esophageal carcinoma. Am J Surg 1997;174:320–4.
13. Goldminc M, Maddern G, Le Prise E, et al. Oesophagectomy by a transhiatal approach or thoracotomy: a prospective randomized trial. Br J Surg 1993;80: 367–70.
14. Pennathur A, Zhang J, Chen H, et al. The "best operation" for esophageal cancer? Ann Thorac Surg 2010;89:S2163–7.
15. Luketich JD, Alvelo-Rivera M, Buenaventura PO, et al. Minimally invasive esophagectomy: outcomes in 222 patients. Ann Surg 2003;238:486–94 [discussion: 494–5].
16. Hosch SB, Stoecklein NH, Pichlmeier U, et al. Esophageal cancer: the mode of lymphatic tumor cell spread and its prognostic significance. J Clin Oncol 2001; 19:1970–5.
17. Rice TW. Superficial oesophageal carcinoma: is there a need for three-field lymphadenectomy? Lancet 1999;354:792–4.
18. Lerut T, Nafteux P, Moons J, et al. Three-field lymphadenectomy for carcinoma of the esophagus and gastroesophageal junction in 174 R0 resections: impact on staging, disease-free survival, and outcome: a plea for adaptation of TNM classification in upper-half esophageal carcinoma. Ann Surg 2004;240:962–72 [discussion: 972–4].
19. Siewert JR, Stein HJ, Bottcher K. Lymphadenectomy in tumors of the upper gastrointestinal tract. Chirurg 1996;67(9):877–88 [in German].
20. Siewert JR, Stein HJ. Lymph-node dissection in squamous cell esophageal cancer—who benefits? Langenbecks Arch Surg 1999;384(2):141–8.
21. Hennessy TP. Lymph node dissection. World J Surg 1994;18(3):367–72.
22. Jamieson GG, Lamb PJ, Thompson SK. The role of lymphadenectomy in esophageal cancer. Ann Surg 2009;250(2):206–9.
23. Nishihira T, Hirayama K, Mori S. A prospective randomized trial of extended cervical and superior mediastinal lymphadenectomy for carcinoma of the thoracic esophagus. Am J Surg 1998;175(1):47–51.
24. Cense HA, van Eijck CH, Tilanus HW. New insights in the lymphatic spread of oesophageal cancer and its implications for the extent of surgical resection. Best practice & research. Clin Gastroenterol 2006;20(5):893–906.
25. Fang WT, Chen WH. Current trends in extended lymph node dissection for esophageal carcinoma. Asian Cardiovasc Thorac Ann 2009;17(2):208–13.
26. Tabira Y, Okuma T, Sakaguchi T, et al. Three-field dissection or two-field dissection?—A proposal of new algorithm for lymphadenectomy. Hepatogastroenterology 2004;51:1015–20.
27. Fiorica F, Di Bona D, Schepis F, et al. Preoperative chemoradiotherapy for oesophageal cancer: a systematic review and meta-analysis. Gut 2004;53:925–30.
28. Malthaner RA, Wong RK, Rumble RB, et al. Neoadjuvant or adjuvant therapy for resectable esophageal cancer: a systematic review and meta-analysis. BMC Med 2004;2:35.

29. Greer SE, Goodney PP, Sutton JE, et al. Neoadjuvant chemoradiotherapy for esophageal carcinoma: a meta-analysis. Surgery 2005;137:172–7.
30. Orringer MB, Marshall B, Chang AC, et al. Two thousand transhiatal esophagectomies: changing trends, lessons learned. Ann Surg 2007;246:363–72 [discussion: 372–4].
31. Altorki N, Kent M, Ferrara C, et al. Three-field lymph node dissection for squamous cell and adenocarcinoma of the esophagus. Ann Surg 2002;236:177–83.
32. Igaki H, Tachimori Y, Kato H. Improved survival for patients with upper and/or middle mediastinal lymph node metastasis of squamous cell carcinoma of the lower thoracic esophagus treated with 3-field dissection. Ann Surg 2004; 239(4):483–90.
33. Schuhmacher C, Novotny A, Ott K, et al. Lymphadenectomy with tumors of the upper gastrointestinal tract. Chirurg 2007;78(3):203–6, 208–12, 214–6. [in German].
34. Doki Y, Ishikawa O, Takachi K, et al. Association of the primary tumor location with the site of tumor recurrence after curative resection of thoracic esophageal carcinoma. World J Surg 2005;29:700–7.
35. Law S, Wong J. Current management of esophageal cancer. J Gastrointest Surg 2005;9(2):291–310.
36. Hsu CP, Hsu NY, Shai SE, et al. Pre-tracheal lymph node metastasis in squamous cell carcinoma of the thoracic esophagus. Eur J Surg Oncol 2005;31:749–54.
37. Slim K, Blay JY, Brouquet A, et al. Digestive oncology: surgical practices. J Chir (Paris) 2009;146(Suppl 2):S11–80 [in French].
38. Enzinger PC, Mayer RJ. Esophageal cancer. N Engl J Med 2003;349(23): 2241–52.
39. Tytgat GN, Bartelink H, Bernards R, et al. Cancer of the esophagus and gastric cardia: recent advances. Dis Esophagus 2004;17:10–26.
40. Collard JM, Otte JB, Fiasse R, et al. Skeletonizing en bloc esophagectomy for cancer. Ann Surg 2001;234:25–32.
41. Mariette C, Piessen G, Balon JM, et al. Surgery alone in the curative treatment of localised oesophageal carcinoma. Eur J Surg Oncol 2004;30:869–76.
42. Ando N, Iizuka T, Ide H, et al. Surgery plus chemotherapy compared with surgery alone for localized squamous cell carcinoma of the thoracic esophagus: a Japan Clinical Oncology Group Study—JCOG9204. J Clin Oncol 2003;21:4592–6.
43. Ando N, Iizuka T, Kakegawa T, et al. A randomized trial of surgery with and without chemotherapy for localized squamous carcinoma of the thoracic esophagus: the Japan Clinical Oncology Group Study. J Thorac Cardiovasc Surg 1997; 114:205–9.
44. Rice TW, Adelstein DJ, Chidel MA, et al. Benefit of postoperative adjuvant chemoradiotherapy in locoregionally advanced esophageal carcinoma. J Thorac Cardiovasc Surg 2003;126:1590–6.
45. Law S. Optimal surgical approach for esophagectomy: the debate still goes on? Ann Thorac Cardiovasc Surg 2009;15(5):277–9.
46. Gignoux M, Roussel A, Paillot B, et al. The value of preoperative radiotherapy in esophageal cancer: results of a study of the E.O.R.T.C. World J Surg 1987;11: 426–32.
47. Launois B, Delarue D, Campion JP, et al. Preoperative radiotherapy for carcinoma of the esophagus. Surg Gynecol Obstet 1981;153:690–2.
48. Nygaard K, Hagen S, Hansen HS, et al. Pre-operative radiotherapy prolongs survival in operable esophageal carcinoma: a randomized, multicenter study of pre-operative radiotherapy and chemotherapy. The second Scandinavian trial in esophageal cancer. World J Surg 1992;16:1104–9 [discussion: 1110].

49. Arnott SJ, Duncan W, Kerr GR, et al. Low dose preoperative radiotherapy for carcinoma of the oesophagus: results of a randomized clinical trial. Radiother Oncol 1992;24:108–13.
50. Wang M, Gu XZ, Yin WB, et al. Randomized clinical trial on the combination of preoperative irradiation and surgery in the treatment of esophageal carcinoma: report on 206 patients. Int J Radiat Oncol Biol Phys 1989;16:325–7.
51. Arnott SJ, Duncan W, Gignoux M, et al. Preoperative radiotherapy for esophageal carcinoma. Cochrane Database Syst Rev 2005;(4):CD001799.
52. Kelsen DP, Ginsberg R, Pajak TF, et al. Chemotherapy followed by surgery compared with surgery alone for localized esophageal cancer. N Engl J Med 1998;339:1979–84.
53. Surgical resection with or without preoperative chemotherapy in oesophageal cancer: a randomised controlled trial. Lancet 2002;359(9319):1727–33.
54. Gebski V, Burmeister B, Smithers BM, et al. Survival benefits from neoadjuvant chemoradiotherapy or chemotherapy in oesophageal carcinoma: a meta-analysis. Lancet Oncol 2007;8:226–34.
55. Walsh TN, Noonan N, Hollywood D, et al. A comparison of multimodal therapy and surgery for esophageal adenocarcinoma. N Engl J Med 1996;335:462–7.
56. Burmeister BH, Smithers BM, Gebski V, et al. Surgery alone versus chemoradiotherapy followed by surgery for resectable cancer of the oesophagus: a randomised controlled phase III trial. Lancet Oncol 2005;6:659–68.
57. Urba SG, Orringer BM, Turrisi A, et al. Randomized trial of preoperative chemoradiation versus surgery alone in patients with locoregional esophageal carcinoma. J Clin Oncol 2001;19:305–13.
58. Tepper J, Krasna MJ, Niedzwiecki D, et al. Phase III trial of trimodality therapy with cisplatin, fluorouracil, radiotherapy, and surgery compared with surgery alone for esophageal cancer: CALGB 9781. J Clin Oncol 2008;26:1086–92.
59. Urschel JD, Vasan H. A meta-analysis of randomized controlled trials that compared neoadjuvant chemoradiation and surgery to surgery alone for resectable esophageal cancer. Am J Surg 2003;185(6):538–43.
60. Stahl M, Walz MK, Stuschke M, et al. Phase III comparison of preoperative chemotherapy compared with chemoradiotherapy in patients with locally advanced adenocarcinoma of the esophagogastric junction. J Clin Oncol 2009;27:851–6.
61. Stahl M, Stuschke M, Lehmann N, et al. Chemoradiation with and without surgery in patients with locally advanced squamous cell carcinoma of the esophagus. J Clin Oncol 2005;23:2310–7.
62. Bedenne L, Michel P, Bouche O, et al. Chemoradiation followed by surgery compared with chemoradiation alone in squamous cancer of the esophagus: FFCD 9102. J Clin Oncol 2007;25:1160–8.
63. Tougeron D, Di Fiore F, Hamidou H, et al. Response to definitive chemoradiotherapy and survival in patients with an oesophageal adenocarcinoma versus squamous cell carcinoma: a matched-pair analysis. Oncology 2007;73:328–34.
64. Di Fiore F, Lecleire S, Rigal O, et al. Predictive factors of survival in patients treated with definitive chemoradiotherapy for squamous cell esophageal carcinoma. World J Gastroenterol 2006;12:4185–90.
65. Westerterp M, van Westreenen HL, Reitsma JB, et al. Esophageal cancer: CT, endoscopic US, and FDG PET for assessment of response to neoadjuvant therapy–systematic review. Radiology 2005;236:841–51.
66. Ngamruengphong S, Sharma VK, Nguyen B, et al. Assessment of response to neoadjuvant therapy in esophageal cancer: an updated systematic review of

diagnostic accuracy of endoscopic ultrasonography and fluorodeoxyglucose positron emission tomography. Dis Esophagus 2010;23:216–31.

67. Machlenkin S, Melzer E, Idelevich E, et al. Endoscopic ultrasound: doubtful accuracy for restaging esophageal cancer after preoperative chemotherapy. Isr Med Assoc J 2009;11:166–9.

68. Rebollo Aguirre AC, Ramos-Font C, Villegas Portero R, et al. 18F-fluorodeoxiglucose positron emission tomography for the evaluation of neoadjuvant therapy response in esophageal cancer: systematic review of the literature. Ann Surg 2009;250:247–54.

69. Junginger T, Dutkowski P. Selective approach to the treatment of oesophageal cancer. Br J Surg 1996;83(10):1473–7.

70. Lerut TE, de Leyn P, Coosemans W, et al. Advanced esophageal carcinoma. World J Surg 1994;18:379–87.

71. Holscher AH, Bollschweiler E, Bumm R, et al. Prognostic factors of resected adenocarcinoma of the esophagus. Surgery 1995;118:845–55.

72. Fok M, Law SY, Wong J. Operable esophageal carcinoma: current results from Hong Kong. World J Surg 1994;18(3):355–60.

73. Matsubara T, Ueda M, Kokudo N, et al. Role of esophagectomy in treatment of esophageal carcinoma with clinical evidence of adjacent organ invasion. World J Surg 2001;25:279–84.

74. Shimada HS, Okazumi S, Matsubara H, et al. Impact of the number and extent of positive lymph nodes in 200 patients with thoracic esophageal squamous cell carcinoma after three-field lymph node dissection. World J Surg 2006;30: 1441–9.

75. Shimada H, Kitabayashi H, Nabeya Y, et al. Treatment response and prognosis of patients after recurrence of esophageal cancer. Surgery 2003;133:24–31.

76. Ichiyoshi Y, Kawahara H, Taga S, et al. Indications and operative techniques for combined aortoesophageal resection. Jpn J Thorac Cardiovasc Surg 1999;47: 318–24.

77. Ancona E, Ruol A, Castoro C, et al. First-line chemotherapy improves the resection rate and long-term survival of locally advanced (T4, any N, M0) squamous cell carcinoma of the thoracic esophagus: final report on 163 consecutive patients with 5-year follow-up. Ann Surg 1997;226:714–23.

78. John MJ, Flam MS, Mowry PA, et al. Radiotherapy alone and chemoradiation for nonmetastatic esophageal carcinoma. A critical review of chemoradiation. Cancer 1989;63:2397–403.

79. Seto Y, Chin K, Gomi K, et al. Treatment of thoracic esophageal carcinoma invading adjacent structures. Cancer Sci 2007;98:937–42.

80. Fujita H, Sueyoshi S, Tanaka T, et al. Esophagectomy: is it necessary after chemoradiotherapy for a locally advanced T4 esophageal cancer? Prospective nonrandomized trial comparing chemoradiotherapy with surgery versus without surgery. World J Surg 2005;29:25–30 [discussion: 30–1].

81. de Manzoni G, Pedrazzani C, Pasini F, et al. Chemoradiotherapy followed by surgery for squamous cell carcinoma of the thoracic esophagus with clinical evidence of adjacent organ invasion. J Surg Oncol 2007;95:261–6.

82. Miyoshi N, Yano M, Takachi K, et al. Myelotoxicity of preoperative chemoradiotherapy is a significant determinant of poor prognosis in patients with T4 esophageal cancer. J Surg Oncol 2009;99:302–6.

83. Noguchi T, Moriyama H, Wada S, et al. Resection surgery with neoadjuvant chemoradiotherapy improves outcomes of patients with T4 esophageal carcinoma. Dis Esophagus 2003;16(2):94–8.

84. Ikeda K, Ishida K, Sato N, et al. Chemoradiotherapy followed by surgery for thoracic esophageal cancer potentially or actually involving adjacent organs. Dis Esophagus 2001;14:197–201.
85. Yano M, Tsujinaka T, Shiozaki H, et al. Concurrent chemotherapy (5-fluorouracil and cisplatin) and radiation therapy followed by surgery for T4 squamous cell carcinoma of the esophagus. J Surg Oncol 1999;70:25–32.
86. Itoh Y, Fuwa N, Matsumoto A, et al. Outcomes of radiotherapy for inoperable locally advanced (T4) esophageal cancer-retrospective analysis. Radiat Med 2001;19:231–5.
87. Tachibana M, Dhar DK, Kinugasa S, et al. Surgical treatment for locally advanced (T4) squamous cell carcinoma of the thoracic esophagus. Dysphagia 2002;17: 255–61.
88. Fujita H, Sueyoshi S, Tanaka T, et al. Prospective non-randomized trial comparing esophagectomy-followed-by-chemoradiotherapy versus chemoradiotherapy-followed-by-esophagectomy for T4 esophageal cancers. J Surg Oncol 2005; 90:209–19.
89. Lee J, Lee KE, Im YM, et al. Adjuvant chemotherapy with 5-fluorouracil and cisplatin in lymph node-positive thoracic esophageal squamous cell carcinoma. Ann Thorac Surg 2005;80:1170–5.
90. Schreiber, D, Rineer J, Vongtama D, et al. Impact of postoperative radiation after esophagectomy for esophageal cancer. Journal of thoracic oncology: official publication of the International Association for the Study of Lung Cancer 2010; 5(2):244–50.
91. Teniere P, Hay JM, Fingerhut A, et al. Postoperative radiation therapy does not increase survival after curative resection for squamous cell carcinoma of the middle and lower esophagus as shown by a multicenter controlled trial. French University Association for Surgical Research. Surg Gynecol Obstet 1991;173: 123–30.
92. Fok M, Sham JS, Choy D, et al. Postoperative radiotherapy for carcinoma of the esophagus: a prospective, randomized controlled study. Surgery 1993;113: 138–47.
93. Xiao ZF, Yang ZY, Liang J, et al. Value of radiotherapy after radical surgery for esophageal carcinoma: a report of 495 patients. Ann Thorac Surg 2003;75:331–6.
94. Macdonald JS, Smalley SR, Benedetti J, et al. Chemoradiotherapy after surgery compared with surgery alone for adenocarcinoma of the stomach or gastro-esophageal junction. N Engl J Med 2001;345:725–30.
95. Schlag PM. Randomized trial of preoperative chemotherapy for squamous cell cancer of the esophagus. The Chirurgische Arbeitsgemeinschaft Fuer Onkologie der Deutschen Gesellschaft Fuer Chirurgie Study Group. Arch Surg 1992; 127(12):1446–50.
96. Maipang T, Vasinanukorn P, Petpichetchian C, et al. Induction chemotherapy in the treatment of patients with carcinoma of the esophagus. J Surg Oncol 1994; 56(3):191–7.
97. Law S, Fok M, Chow S, et al. Preoperative chemotherapy versus surgical therapy alone for squamous cell carcinoma of the esophagus: a prospective randomized trial. J Thorac Cardiovasc Surg 1997;114(2):210–7.
98. Ancona E, Ruol A, Santi S, et al. Only pathologic complete response to neoadjuvant chemotherapy improves significantly the long term survival of patients with resectable esophageal squamous cell carcinoma: final report of a randomized, controlled trial of preoperative chemotherapy versus surgery alone. Cancer 2001;91(11):2165–74.

Management of Gastroesophageal Junction Tumors

Matthew P. Fox, MD[a], Victor van Berkel, MD, PhD[b],*

KEYWORDS

- Gastroesophageal junction tumors • Esophagectomy • Lymphadenectomy
- Chemoradiotherapy

KEY POINTS

- The incidence of adenocarcinomas of the esophagogastric junction is rising dramatically.
- While the overall prognosis for these tumors remains poor, surgery and multimodality therapy can be curative.
- Endoscopic therapy or limited resection is indicated for tumors confined to the mucosa.
- Tumors penetrating into the submucosa have a high likelihood of lymph node involvement and require radical resection.
- For Siewert 1 tumors, transthoracic en bloc esophagectomy with 2-field lymph node dissection is the procedure of choice. Transhiatal (THE) esophagectomy should be considered in patients with compromised pulmonary function.
- For type 2 and 3 tumors, either esophagectomy with proximal gastrectomy or THE extended total gastrectomy with D2 lymphadenectomy may be performed provided adequate margins are obtained.
- All patients with T3 or greater tumors or nodal involvement should be considered for chemoradiotherapy, preferably in the neoadjuvant setting.
- Platinum-based chemotherapy is indicated for palliation of stage 4 disease.

INTRODUCTION

Over the past few decades, the incidence of adenocarcinoma of the esophagogastric junction (AEG) has risen dramatically in western countries.[1,2] The mechanism of this change is unclear. Despite endoscopic screening and advances in multimodality therapy, the prognosis of these tumors remains poor, with an overall 5-year survival

[a] Department of Surgery, School of Medicine, University of Louisville, 201 Abraham Flexner Way, Suite 1200, Louisville, KY 40202, USA; [b] Division of Cardiothoracic Surgery, Department of Surgery, School of Medicine, University of Louisville, 201 Abraham Flexner Way, Suite 1200, Louisville, KY 40202, USA
* Corresponding author.
E-mail address: victor.vanberkel@louisville.edu

Surg Clin N Am 92 (2012) 1199–1212
http://dx.doi.org/10.1016/j.suc.2012.07.011
0039-6109/12/$ – see front matter © 2012 Elsevier Inc. All rights reserved.

rate of approximately 20%.[3] This article will discuss the current pathologic classification, epidemiology, staging, and standard treatment of these tumors.

SIEWERT CLASSIFICATION

Because of their location, a great deal of controversy has been present regarding whether AEGs represent gastric or esophageal cancer. Siewert attempted to rectify this problem in 1996 with a standardized system classifying these tumors based on topographic anatomic criteria.[4,5] By definition, all of these tumors must invade the esophagogastric junction (EGJ). Type 1 tumors were defined as those with an epicenter 1 to 5 cm above the EGJ. Type 2 tumors were defined as having a center 1 cm above to 2 cm below the EGJ. Finally, type 3 tumors were defined as being centered 2 to 5 cm below the EGJ (**Fig. 1**). Therefore, type 1 tumors represent distal esophageal adenocarcinoma. Type 2 tumors are true adenocarcinomas of the cardia, and type 3tumors are subcardial gastric cancers. It is worth noting that precise endoscopic localization of the EGJ can be difficult,[6] leading to possible misclassification of tumors preoperatively. This classification system was adopted at the Second International Gastric Cancer Congress in 1997 and has since been used extensively without modification.

EPIDEMIOLOGY AND ETIOLOGY OF ADENOCARCINOMA OF THE EGJ

The relation between Barrett's esophagus and adenocarcinoma of esophagus is well established.[7,8] Given their esophageal epicenter, it is no surprise that type 1 AEGs have the strongest association with Barrett's esophagus, with approximately 80% of resected specimens showing intestinal metaplasia.[9] Conversely, Barrett's metaplasia was present in only 5.6% and 0.8% of patients with type 2 and 3 tumors, respectively. Asian case series have shown a weaker association between Barrett and type 1 AEGs.[10] Furthermore, in different populations, the ratio of type 1 to type 2 and 3 tumors is different; eastern counties have a relative preponderance for type 2 and 3 carcinomas compared with the United States and Europe.[11,12]

This differential distribution in tumor location is likely due to the rise in esophageal adenocarcinoma (EAC) in the West. In the United States, the relative incidence of

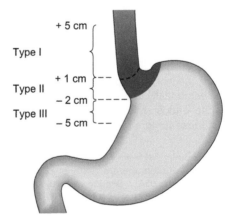

Fig. 1. Classification of adenocarcinoma of the esophagogastric junction according to the localization of the center of the tumor by Siewert and colleagues (1987). (*From* Hölscher AH. Adenocarcinoma of the cardia. In: Patterson GA, Cooper JD, Deslauriers J, et al, editors. Pearson's thoracic and esophageal surgery. 3rd edition. Philadelphia: Churchill Livingstone; 2008. p. 493; with permission.)

EAC increased by 400% in white men and 300% in white women over 26 years.[13] In the same study, African American men had a 100% relative increase in EAC, while incidence of squamous carcinoma (SCC) of the esophagus remained unchanged. In a review of the surveillance, epidemiology, and end result (SEER) database from 1992 to 1998, Kubo and Corely showed the incident rate of esophageal adenocarcinomas increased, while the rate of cardial carcinomas remained steady across time.[14] Other studies have shown a slight increase in type 2 and type 3 cancers.[15] When combined with data showing the steep decline of distal gastric cancers in the West, there is clear epidemiologic evidence that AEGs represent a heterogeneous set of tumors with etiologies that are partially related to, but are distinct from, EAC, distal gastric cancer, and esophageal SCC.

DIAGNOSIS AND STAGING

Before the advent of the American Joint Committee on Cancer (AJCC) 7th edition staging manual, AEGs could be staged using either the esophageal or gastric adenocarcinoma systems, potentially leading to discordant staging that could adversely affect therapy. The 7th edition attempts to harmonize esophageal and gastric cancer staging, and all AEGs are staged according to the esophageal system.[16]

A typical staging workup for esophageal cancer includes combined computed tomography (CT)/positron emission tomography (PET) scans of the chest, abdomen, and pelvis along with endoscopic ultrasound. For esophageal cancers, the sensitivity and specificity of both these methods are well documented, and they provide complimentary information. In a study of esophageal cancers undergoing esophagectomy with neoadjuvant therapy, esophageal ultrasound (EUS) was able to distinguish between early (T1-2, N0) and advanced disease (T3-4, N1) in 83% of patients.[17] EUS may also potentially be useful in identifying mucosal carcinomas that may be candidates for endoscopic therapy.[18] Its assessment of T and N stage is likely more accurate than PET, which has been shown to accurately determine T stage in only 40% of cases,[19] and has a sensitivity of only 50% for detecting regional nodal disease.[20,21] Additionally, EUS may assist traditional upper endoscopic techniques in defining the Siewert classification.[22] EUS has been shown to be accurate for gastric cancers[23] and AEGs.[24] Limitations with EUS include invasiveness, reproducibility,[25–27] and most importantly, an inability to identify distant metastases.

PET is therefore a useful adjunct. In a recent retrospective review of 83 patients with esophageal cancer undergoing pretherapy PET/CT and EUS, PET was found to provide additional staging information that altered treatment in 10% of patients.[28] Another retrospective review of 130 patients undergoing CT, EUS, and PET/CT showed PET excluded surgery from 25% of patients deemed resectable by CT and EUS alone.[29] These results are similar to a prospective study of 74 patients in whom PET upstaged 20% of patients deemed resectable by CT/EUS.[30]

While PET's usefulness in EAC and type 1 AEGs is well documented, its place in the staging of gastric cancer and type 2/3 AEGs is less clear. In a review of 52 patients with type 1 and type 2 tumors, Ott and colleagues[31] showed all of the type 1 tumors were PET-avid, whereas only 75% of type 2 tumors were. This coincides with a study in distal gastric cancer, which produced a PET detection rate of 60%. When the authors stratified patients by histology, tumors with intestinal histology showed a higher PET detection rate (83%) compared with nonintestinal type tumors (41%).[32] This literature illustrates the differing biology of esophageal and gastric adenocarcinoma and further supports the hypothesis that type 2 AEGs are a heterogeneous mix of esophageal and gastric cancers.

As the sensitivity of PET for detecting metastases in type 2 and type 3 AEGs is reduced, staging laparoscopy may play a role in the pretreatment assessment. This technique has been validated in gastric cancer[33] as well as distal esophageal and gastro-esophageal junction (GEJ) adenocarcinoma.[34] However, in the largest series of the patients advocating the use of routine staging laparoscopy, EUS was performed in only 10% of patients.[35] To the authors' knowledge, no study has ever directly compared PET with staging laparoscopy for AEGs.

SURGICAL TREATMENT

Multiple studies have shown that R0 resection remains among the most significant predictors of long-term survival in patients with an AEG.[36–38] Consequently, the therapeutic goals should be complete surgical resection of the tumor and any associated intestinal metaplasia with adequate lymphadenectomy. If doubt exists over the ability to achieve an R0 resection, neoadjuvant therapy should be considered.[39,40] As with any operation, the functional and physiologic status of the patient should be considered and optimized before proceeding. Some controversy remains over the required extent of resection and lymphadenectomy, along with the correct operative approach. These issues will be discussed in depth for each Siewert classification.

Siewert 1 Tumors

Given the increase in screening of patients with Barrett's esophagus, many of these patients are presenting with early stage tumors.[41] Consequently, there has been renewed interest in limited resections, which may offer shorter recovery times, less morbidity, and better quality of life compared with radical esophagectomy.[42] Options include endoscopic mucosal resection,[43] local resection such as the Merendino procedure,[42,44] and vagal-sparing esophagectomy.[45] The technical aspects of these procedures are beyond the scope of this article; however, consideration must be given to length of the tumor and any associated high-grade dysplasia. Both must be completely resected or ablated, with negative margins. Oncologic outcomes for tumors confined to the mucosa after any of these procedures and radical esophagectomy are similar,[45,46] although large-scale trials are still needed.

Once the tumor has infiltrated the submucosa, the rate of lymph node metastases increases drastically with the 10% to 67% of patients having nodal involvement, depending on the depth of invasion.[47,48] Consequently, the operation of choice remains radical esophagectomy with proximal gastrectomy and reconstruction with a gastric tube. The necessary extent of lymphadenectomy and decision to perform a transthoracic (TTE) or transhiatal (THE) resection remain controversial. For type 1 AEGs, the rate of metastases to the lower mediastinum and abdomen is approximately 60% and 74%, respectively.[49] One study advocating a 3-field lymphadenectomy showed cervical nodal metastases in 17.6% of type 1 AEGs.[50] However, given the rarity of upper mediastinal recurrences, it is questionable whether an extensive superior lymphadenectomy is needed.[51] Due to the propensity for paracardial, lesser curvature, and celiac axis metastases, a complete lymph node dissection should be performed in these locations.

The question of whether to perform a TTE or THE resection is also controversial. Five randomized controlled trials have been performed comparing THE with TTE.[52–56] The largest trial randomized 220 patients with adenocarcinoma of the distal esophagus or gastric cardia to either TTE with an extended en bloc lymphadenectomy via a right thoracic approach or THE.[56] The TTE group also underwent mandatory dissection of the celiac, common hepatic artery, and splenic hilar nodes. The THE group only had a celiac node dissection performed if there was clinical suspicion of involvement. Reconstruction with a gastric tube and cervical anastomosis was performed in both groups. Postoperative morbidity was higher in the TTE group, including pulmonary complications (57% vs 27%, $P<.001$), chylous leakage (10% vs 2%, $P=.02$), longer median ventilator time (2 days vs 1 day, $P<.001$), intensive care unit (ICU) stay (6 days vs 2 days, $P<.001$), and hospital stay (19 days vs 15 days, $P<.001$). However, there was no difference in in-hospital mortality (4% vs 2%, $P = .45$).

With regard to oncologic outcomes, the rate of R0 resection in this study was not different (71% vs 72%, $P = .28$), but the mean number of lymph nodes harvested was higher with TTE(31 vs 16, $P<.001$). More importantly, there was a statistically nonsignificant trend toward better long-term survival in the TTE group (median survival 2 years vs 1.8 years $P = .38$, estimated 5-year survival of 39% vs 29%).[56] A follow-up study with more complete data published in 2007 showed a similar 5-year survival between the 2 groups (36% vs 34%, $P = .71$). However, in the Siewert type 1 tumors, there was again a strong trend toward better overall 5-year survival in the TTE group (51% vs 37%, $P = .33$), and particularly in the subgroup of patients with 1 to 8 positive nodes (64% vs 23%, $P = .02$).[57] Although cofounded by the differences in abdominal node dissection, these results strongly suggest that an oncologic survival benefit is present for en bloc TTE esophageal resection for type 1 tumors. While there may be some increased risk of pulmonary complications, anastomotic complications are reduced by the use of an intrathoracic anastomosis, and intrathoracic leaks are no longer associated with high mortality.[58]

Minimally invasive esophagectomy, while beyond the scope of this article, is likely a valid alternative to traditional open THE or TTE. Preliminary data suggest oncologic outcomes and lymph node harvests are similar to that of TTE when a thoracoscopic dissection of the esophagus is performed.[59,60] Randomized trials are ongoing to ascertain its optimal role.[61]

Siewert 2 and 3 Tumors

There are few randomized trials comparing surgical approaches to type 2 and type 3 tumors. Generally, type 3 tumors have been treated as a true gastric cancer, while type 2 tumors have been treated as both gastric and esophageal cancer. Lymphatics from both sites generally drain to the paracardial and lesser curvature nodes first. Isolated mediastinal metastases are found in less than 12% of cases. Nodal recurrences are most frequent in the para-aortic nodes.[62,63] Patients with positive mediastinal nodes have an extremely poor prognosis.[64]

As both esophagectomy and gastrectomy harvest the most frequently involved lymph node stations, both are oncologically sound provided adequate margins are obtained. A retrospective review of 505 patients undergoing either of these procedures suggested 3.8 cm as the proximal margin length most predictive of cure.[65] In this study, there was no difference between gastrectomy and esophagectomy in operative mortality, R1 resection lymph node harvest, or overall survival when controlling for stage. Similar results have been obtained in other retrospective studies.[37,66]

A single phase 3 randomized trial (Japan Clinical Oncology Group 9502) randomized 167 patients with Siewert 2 and 3 tumors to extended total gastrectomy with D2 lymphadenectomy via the THE route or the same procedure along with lower mediastinal lymphadenectomy via a left thoracoabdominal (LTA) approach. Complications (49% vs 34%, $P = .006$) and in-hospital mortality (4% vs 0%, $P = .06$) were higher in the LTA group. Five-year survival was lower in the LTA group (37.9% vs 52.3%). Results were similar in the type 2 and type 3 tumor subgroups.[67]

While a mediastinal lymph node dissection in these patients has not been proven to be beneficial, extended abdominal lymph node dissection (D2 lymphadenectomy, **Fig. 2**) appears to confer an oncologic benefit. The original Dutch Gastric Cancer Trial randomized patients with gastric adenocarcinoma to D1 or D2 lymphadenectomy along with total or distal gastrectomy. As part of their dissection, the D2 patients received a distal pancreatectomy and splenectomy. Their overall complication rate (43% vs 25%, $P<.001$) and in-hospital mortality rate (10 vs 4%, $P = .004$) were higher.[68] However, after 15-year follow-up, gastric cancer-related death was lower in the D2 group (37% vs 48%, $P = .01$). Other studies have shown that pancreatectomy and splenectomy are not necessary for D2 lymphadenectomy,[69] and D2 lymphadenectomy may be accomplished with low morbidity, 17.9%, and mortality, 2.2%.[70]

Given the overall similarity in outcomes between esophagectomy and gastrectomy in these patients, the authors feel either procedure is valid provided adequate negative margins are obtained. If gastrectomy is performed, a D2 lymph node dissection should be considered. If esophagectomy is performed, a THE approach may be beneficial given the low likelihood of mediastinal lymph node involvement.

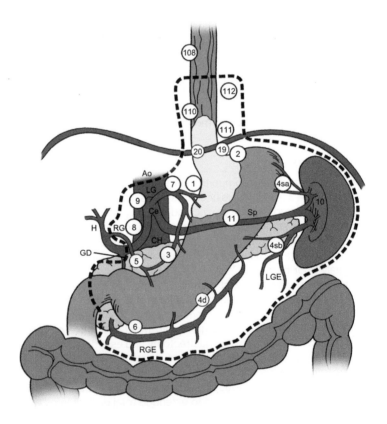

Fig. 2. Abdominal lymphatic stations to achieve a D2 lymphadenectomy. (*From* Peracchia A, Rosati R. Total gastrectomy and Roux-en-Y reconstruction. In: Patterson GA, Cooper JD, Deslauriers J, et al, editors. Pearson's thoracic and esophageal surgery. 3rd edition. Philadelphia: Churchill Livingstone; 2008. p. 615; with permission.)

As with esophagectomy, the role of minimally invasive surgery for total gastrectomy is unclear. Presently, a few case series from Asian centers and a meta-analysis exist showing similar oncologic results between laparoscopic and open operations with reduced postoperative pain and length of stay.[71] Further prospective trials are required to elicit laparoscopic surgery's true role for type 2 and type 3 AEGs.

MULTIMODALITY THERAPY

While complete surgical resection remains the largest influence outcome in patients with AEGs, only 11% to 21% of patients will present with potentially resectable disease and have the physiologic capacity to tolerate surgery.[72] Additionally, 70% of patients have systemic recurrences,[73] and increasingly radical surgery has not produced better results. Consequently, there has been much interest in perioperative chemotherapy and/or radiotherapy for esophageal, gastric and EGJ tumors.

Adjuvant Therapy

The SWOG 9008/INT 0116 trial randomized 556 patients with resected stage 1B–4 gastric or EGJ cancer to surgery with postoperative adjuvant chemoradiotherapy or to surgery alone. Adjuvant therapy consisted of 425 mg of fluorouracil per square meter of body surface area per day, plus 20 mg of leucovorin per square meter per day, for 5 days, followed by 4500 cGy of radiation at 180 cGy per day, given 5 days per week for 5 weeks, with modified doses of fluorouracil and leucovorin on the first 4 and the last 3 days of radiotherapy. One month after the completion of radiotherapy, 2 5-day cycles of fluorouracil (425 mg/m^2/d) plus leucovorin (20 mg/m^2/d) were given 1 month apart.[74] The median overall survival was 36 months in the multimodality group compared with 27 months in the surgery only cohort ($P<.005$). While this trial illustrated the usefulness of adjuvant therapy in gastric cancer, only 21% of tumors were located in the cardia. Furthermore, 90% of patients underwent a D0 or D1 lymph node dissection, which is limited compared with the currently accepted D2 dissection. The ongoing CALGB-80101 trial is comparing this regimen to chemoradiation with epirubicin, cisplatin, and 5-FU.

Adjuvant chemotherapy alone in gastric cancer was studied in the Japanese SCTS-GC trial. One thousand fifty-nine patients with stage 1 or 3 gastric cancer who had undergone curative gastrectomy with D2 lymphadenectomy were randomized to oral S-1, a fluoropyramidine, for 1 year, or surgery alone.[75] The 3-year overall survival rate in the adjuvant therapy group was 80.5% compared with 70.1%. Unfortunately, the proportion of AEGs composing the study cohort was not reported. Although the results of this trial can be extended to AEGs in Asian countries, which are predominantly type 2/3 and similar to gastric cancer, it is questionable whether they apply to western patients who are more likely to have type 1 tumors and undergo less extensive lymphadenectomy. Furthermore, the metabolism of S-1 in Asian and western patients is different, although a recent global phase 3 study comparing cisplatin/S-1 to cisplatin/5-FU in patients with metastatic gastroesophageal junction or gastric cancer showed this can be accounted for, suggesting this regimen may be effective in western patients with Siewert 2 or 3 tumors.[76]

Neoadjuvant Therapy

In the INT-0116 study, only 64% of patients were able to complete the treatment. These results were similar to adjuvant therapy trials showing difficulty with treatment tolerance. Therefore, most recent trials have focused upon neoadjuvant therapy.

The Medical Research Council Adjuvant Gastric Infusional Chemotherapy (MAGIC Trial) compared 3 cycles of epirubicin, cisplatin, and 5-FU before and after surgery to surgery alone in patients with resectable gastric, GEJ, and lower esophageal adenocarcinoma.[77] Importantly, this study protocol did not include the use of neoadjuvant radiation therapy. Five-year survival was significantly improved in the multimodality group (36% vs 23%, $P = .009$). Although only 14.5% of patients had lower esophageal tumors, and 11.5% had GEJ tumors, there was no significant interaction between tumor location and survival. These results were confirmed by a multicenter French phase 3 that randomized patients with distal esophageal, EGJ, or stomach adenocarcinoma to perioperative cisplatin/5-FU or surgery alone.[78] The perioperative chemotherapy group had improved overall and disease-free survival as well as an increased rate of R-0 resection. Importantly, 64% of the patients had AEGs.

Definitive Chemoradiotherapy

Given the efficacy of neoadjuvant chemoradiotherapy, there has been interest in the use of definitive chemoradiotherapy (dCRT) for esophageal cancer.[79] Most trials comparing dCRT to esophagectomy were comprised primarily of patients with SCC. Furthermore, the literature suggests that in adenocarcinoma the rate of complete pathologic response is less than squamous carcinoma,[80] and survival is significantly worse after dCRT compared with surgery.[81] Consequently, the authors believe that surgery is indicated for all resectable AEG patients who are a reasonable operative risk.

PALLIATIVE THERAPY FOR ADVANCED DISEASE

Approximately one-third of AEG patients present with stage 4 disease.[15] While surgical, endoscopic, or radiotherapeutic treatment may be needed on a case-by-case basis for local palliation and symptom control, systematic chemotherapy remains the mainstay of treatment for these patients. Multiple trials and meta-analyses have shown improved survival and quality of life with palliative chemotherapy in gastric cancer.[82–85] Only 2 randomized trials have shown such benefits in esophageal adenocarcinoma.[86,87] After initially being developed for SCC, cisplatin/5-FU has been considered the standard treatment regimen for metastatic esophageal and gastric adenocarcinoma with a response rate of 34%.[88] Various phase 2 trials have shown improved response rates with the addition of anthracycline agents (doxorubicin or epirubicin)[86,87,89–91] or taxanes (docetaxel or paclitaxel).[92,93]

Other trials have focused on limiting the toxic effects of chemotherapeutic agents. The randomized epirubacin, cisplatin, and fluorouracil [ECF] for advanced and locally advanced esophagogastric cancer 2 (REAL-2) trial demonstrated survival noninferiority when cisplatin and 5-FU in the ECF regimen were replaced with oxaliplatin and oral capecitabine.[94] The recent fluorouracil in advanced gastric or gastroesophageal adenocarcinoma (FLAG) trial showed survival noninferiority of cisplatin/S-1 compared with cisplatin/5-FU along with an improved safety profile.[76]

There has been substantial investigation into targeted biologic agents in the treatment of metastatic gastroesophageal cancer. Approximately 10% of AEGs in the United States overexpress HER2. Trastuzumab, a monoclonal HER-2 antibody, has been widely used in the treatment of breast cancer. The trastuzumab for gastric adenocarcinoma (ToGA) trial randomized patients with stomach or EGJ HER2-positive adenocarcinoma to chemotherapy with and without trastuzumab. Response rate (47% vs 35%) and median overall survival (13.8 months and 11.1 months) were significantly better in the treatment group.[95,96] The utility of other agents, such as cetuximab, gefitinib, and erlotinib, are currently under investigation.

SUMMARY

The incidence of adenocarcinomas of the EGJ is rising dramatically. Although the overall prognosis for these tumors remains poor, surgery and multimodality therapy can be curative. For tumors confined to the mucosa, endoscopic therapy or limited resection is indicated. Tumors penetrating into the submucosa have a high likelihood of lymph node involvement and require radical resection. TTE en bloc esophagectomy with 2-field lymph node dissection is the procedure of choice for patients with Siewert 1 tumors. In patients with compromised pulmonary function, THE esophagectomy should be considered. All patients with T3 or greater tumors or nodal involvement should be considered for chemoradiotherapy, preferably in the neoadjuvant setting. For palliation of stage 4 disease, platinum-based chemotherapy is indicated.

If adequate margins can be obtained, either esophagectomy with proximal gastrectomy or THE extended total gastrectomy with D2 lymphadenectomy may be performed for type 2 and type 3 tumors.

REFERENCES

1. Devesa S, Blot W, Fraumeni J. Changing patterns in the incidence of esophageal and gastric carcinoma in the United States. Cancer 1998;83:2049–53.
2. Pera M, Manterola C, Vidal O, et al. Epidemiology of esophageal adenocarcinoma. J Surg Oncol 2005;92:151–9.
3. Whitson BA, Groth SS, Li Z, et al. Survival of patients with distal esophageal and gastric cardia tumors: a population-based analysis of gastroesophageal junction carcinomas. J Thorac Cardiovasc Surg 2010;139:43–8.
4. Siewert JR, Stein H. Adenocarcinoma of the gastroesophageal junction: classification, pathology and extent of resection. Dis Esophagus 1996;9:173–82.
5. Siewert JR, Stein H. Classification of carcinoma of the oesphagogastric junction. Br J Surg 1998;85:1457–9.
6. Ishimura N, Amano Y, Kinoshita Y. Endoscopic definition of esophagogastric junction for diagnosis of Barrett's esophagus: importance of systematic education and training. Dig Endosc 2009;21:213–8.
7. Hameeteman W, Tytgat GN, Houthoff HJ, et al. Barrett's esophagus: development of dysplasia and adenocarcinoma. Gastroenterology 1989;96:1249–56.
8. Bresalier RS. Barrett's esophagus and esophageal adenocarcinoma. Ann Rev Med 2009;60:221–31.
9. Siewert JR, Feith M, Stein HJ. Biologic and clinical variations of adenocarcinoma at the esophago–gastric junction: relevance of a topographic–anatomic subclassification. J Surg Oncol 2005;90:139–46.
10. Bai JG, Lv Y, Dang CX. Adenocarcinoma of the esophagogastric junction in China according to Siewert's classification. Jpn J Clin Oncol 2006;36:364–7.
11. Hasegawa S, Yoshikawa T, Cho H, et al. Is adenocarcinoma of the esophagogastric junction different between Japan and western countries? The incidence and clinicopathological features at a Japanese high-volume cancer center. World J Surg 2009;33:95–103.
12. Fang WL, Wu CW, Chen JH, et al. Esophagogastric junction adenocarcinoma according to Siewert classification in Taiwan. Ann Surg Oncol 2009;16:3237–44.
13. Brown LM, Devesa SS. Epidemiologic trends in esophageal and gastric cancer in the United States. Surg Oncol Clin N Am 2002;11:235–56.
14. Kubo A, Corley DA. Marked multi-ethnic variation of esophageal and gastric cardia carcinomas within the United States. Am J Gastroenterol 2004;99:582–8.

15. Pohl H, Welch HG. The role of overdiagnosis and reclassification in the marked increase of esophageal adenocarcinoma incidence. J Natl Cancer Inst 2005;97: 142–6.

16. Rice TW, Blackstone EH, Rusch VW. 7th edition of the AJCC Cancer Staging Manual: esophagus and esophagogastric junction. Ann Surg Oncol 2010;17: 1721–4.

17. Barbour AP, Rizk NP, Gerdes H, et al. Endoscopic ultrasound predicts outcomes for patients with adenocarcinoma of the gastroesophageal junction. J Am Coll Surg 2007;205:593–601.

18. Rampado S, Bocus P, Battaglia G, et al. Endoscopic ultrasound: accuracy in staging superficial carcinomas of the esophagus. Ann Thorac Surg 2008;85: 251–6.

19. Lowe VJ, Booya F, Fletcher JG, et al. Comparison of positron emission tomography, computed tomography, and endoscopic ultrasound in the initial staging of patients with esophageal cancer. Mol Imaging Biol 2005;7:422–30.

20. van Westreenen HL, Westerterp M, Bossuyt PM, et al. Systematic review of the staging performance of 18F-fluorodeoxyglucose positron emission tomography in esophageal cancer. J Clin Oncol 2004;22:3805–12.

21. Sandha GS, Severin D, Postema E, et al. Is positron emission tomography useful in locoregional staging of esophageal cancer? Results of a multidisciplinary initiative comparing CT, positron emission tomography, and EUS. Gastrointest Endosc 2008;67:402–9.

22. Pedrazzani C, Bernini M, Giacopuzzi S, et al. Evaluation of Siewert classification in gastro–esophageal junction adenocarcinoma: what is the role of endoscopic ultrasonography? J Surg Oncol 2005;91:226–31.

23. Ang TL, Ng TM, Fock KM, et al. Accuracy of endoscopic ultrasound staging of gastric cancer in routine clinical practice in Singapore. Chin J Dig Dis 2006;7: 191–6.

24. Blackshaw G, Lewis WG, Hopper AN, et al. Prospective comparison of endosonography, computed tomography, and histopathological stage of junctional oesophagogastric cancer. Clin Radiol 2008;63:1092–8.

25. Meining A, Rosch T, Wolf A, et al. High interobserver variability in endosonographic staging of upper gastrointestinal cancers. Z Gastroenterol 2003;41:391–4.

26. Burtin P, Napoleon B, Palazzo L, et al. Interobserver agreement in endoscopic ultrasonography staging of esophageal and cardia cancer. Gastrointest Endosc 1996;43:20–4.

27. Catalano MF, Sivak MV Jr, Bedford RA, et al. Observer variation and reproducibility of endoscopic ultrasonography. Gastrointest Endosc 1995;41:115–20.

28. Thurau K, Palmes D, Franzius C, et al. Impact of PET-CT on primary staging and response control on multimodal treatment of esophageal cancer. World J Surg 2011;35:608–16.

29. Gananadha S, Hazebroek EJ, Leibman S, et al. The utility of FDG-PET in the preoperative staging of esophageal cancer. Dis Esophagus 2008;21:389–94.

30. Heeren PA, Jager PL, Bongaerts F, et al. Detection of distant metastases in esophageal cancer with (18)F-FDG PET. J Nucl Med 2004;45:980–7.

31. Ott K, Weber WA, Fink U, et al. Fluorodeoxyglucose-positron emission tomography in adenocarcinomas of the distal esophagus and cardia. World J Surg 2003;27:1035–9.

32. Stahl A, Ott K, Weber WA, et al. FDG PET imaging of locally advanced gastric carcinomas: correlation with endoscopic and histopathological findings. Eur J Nucl Med Mol Imaging 2003;30:288–95.

33. Mahadevan D, Sudirman A, Kandasami P, et al. Laparoscopic staging in gastric cancer: an essential step in its management. J Minim Access Surg 2010;6: 111–3.
34. de Graaf GW, Ayantunde AA, Parsons SL, et al. The role of staging laparoscopy in oesophagogastric cancers. Eur J Surg Oncol 2007;33:988–92.
35. Krasna MJ, Reed CE, Nedzwiecki D, et al. CALGB 9380: a prospective trial of the feasibility of thoracoscopy/laparoscopy in staging esophageal cancer. Ann Thorac Surg 2001;71:1073–9.
36. Ott K, Bader FG, Lordick F, et al. Surgical factors influence the outcome after Ivor-Lewis esophagectomy with intrathoracic anastomosis for adenocarcinoma of the esophagogastric junction: a consecutive series of 240 patients at an experienced center. Ann Surg Oncol 2009;16:1017–25.
37. Johansson J, Djerf P, Oberg S, et al. Two different surgical approaches in the treatment of adenocarcinoma at the gastroesophageal junction. World J Surg 2008;32:1013–20.
38. Lerut T, Coosemans W, Decker G, et al. Surgical techniques. J Surg Oncol 2005; 92:218–29.
39. Stiles BM, Mirza F, Coppolino A, et al. Clinical T2-T3N0M0 esophageal cancer: the risk of node positive disease. Ann Thorac Surg 2011;92:491–6.
40. Matuschek C, Bolke E, Peiper M, et al. The role of neoadjuvant and adjuvant treatment for adenocarcinoma of the upper gastrointestinal tract. Eur J Med Res 2011; 16:265–74.
41. Wong T, Tian J, Nagar AB. Barrett's surveillance identifies patients with early esophageal adenocarcinoma. Am J Med 2010;123:462–7.
42. Stein HJ, Feith M, Mueller J, et al. Limited resection for early adenocarcinoma in Barrett's esophagus. Ann Surg 2000;232:733–42.
43. Ell C, May A, Pech O, et al. Curative endoscopic resection of early esophageal adenocarcinomas (Barrett's cancer). Gastrointest Endosc 2007;65:3–10.
44. Merendino KA, Dillard DH. The concept of sphincter substitution by an interposed jejunal segment for anatomic and physiologic abnormalities at the esophagogastric junction; with special reference to reflux esophagitis, cardiospasm and esophageal varices. Ann Surg 1955;142:486–506.
45. Peyre CG, DeMeester SR, Rizzetto C, et al. Vagal-sparing esophagectomy: the ideal operation for intramucosal adenocarcinoma and Barrett with high-grade dysplasia. Ann Surg 2007;246:665–71.
46. Hölscher AH, Vallböhmer D, Schröder W, et al. Limited surgery for "early" cancer of the esophagus. Eur Surg 2007;39:273–80.
47. Westerterp M, Koppert LB, Buskens CJ, et al. Outcome of surgical treatment for early adenocarcinoma of the esophagus or gastro-esophageal junction. Virchows Arch 2005;446:497–504.
48. Liu L, Hofstetter WL, Rashid A, et al. Significance of the depth of tumor invasion and lymph node metastasis in superficially invasive (T1) esophageal adenocarcinoma. Am J Surg Pathol 2005;29:1079–85.
49. Dresner SM, Lamb PJ, Bennett MK, et al. The pattern of metastatic lymph node dissemination from adenocarcinoma of the esophagogastric junction. Surgery 2001;129:103–9.
50. Lerut T, Nafteux P, Moons J, et al. Three-field lymphadenectomy for carcinoma of the esophagus and gastroesophageal junction in 174 R0 resections: impact on staging, disease-free survival, and outcome. Ann Surg 2004;240:962–74.
51. Hulscher JB, van Sandick JW, Tijssen JG, et al. The recurrence pattern of esophageal carcinoma after transhiatal resection. J Am Coll Surg 2000;191:143–8.

52. Jacobi CA, Zieren HU, Muller JM, et al. Surgical therapy of esophageal carcinoma: the influence of surgical approach and esophageal resection on cardiopulmonary function. Eur J Cardiothorac Surg 1997;11:32–7.
53. Areja D, Subhan A, Mirza MR, et al. Transhiatal versus Ivor-Lewis procedure for the treatment of carcinoma esophagus. Pak J Surg 2006;22:126–9.
54. Chu KM, Law SY, Fok M, et al. A prospective randomized comparison of transhiatal and transthoracic resection for lower-third esophageal carcinoma. Am J Surg 1997;174:320–4.
55. Goldminc M, Maddern G, Le Prise E, et al. Oesophagectomy by a transhiatal approach or thoracotomy: a prospective randomized trial. Br J Surg 1993;80: 367–70.
56. Hulscher JB, Van Sandick JW, de Boer A, et al. Extended transthoracic resection compared with limited transhiatal resection for adenocarcinoma of the esophagus. N Engl J Med 2002;347:1662–9.
57. Omloo JM, Lagarde SM, Hulscher JB, et al. Extended transthoracic resection compared with limited transhiatal resection for adenocarcinoma of the mid/distal esophagus: five-year survival of a randomized clinical trial. Ann Surg 2007;246: 992–1000.
58. Escofet X, Manjunath A, Twine C, et al. Prevalence and outcome of esophagogastric anastomotic leak after esophagectomy in a UK regional cancer network. Dis Esophagus 2010;23:112–6.
59. Dantoc MM, Cox MR, Eslick GD. Does minimally invasive esophagectomy (MIE) provide for comparable oncologic outcomes to open techniques? A systematic review. J Gastrointest Surg 2012;16:486–94.
60. Gao Y, Wang Y, Chen L, et al. Comparison of open three-field and minimally-invasive esophagectomy for esophageal cancer. Interact Cardiovasc Thorac Surg 2011;12:366–9.
61. Biere SS, Maas KW, Bonavina L, et al. Traditional invasive vs. minimally invasive esophagectomy: a multi-center, randomized trial (TIME-trial). BMC Surg 2011; 11:2.
62. Yamashita H, Katai H, Morita S, et al. Optimal extent of lymph node dissection for Siewert type II esophagogastric junction carcinoma. Ann Surg 2011;254: 274–80.
63. Wayman J, Bennett MK, Raimes SA, et al. The pattern of recurrence of adenocarcinoma of the oesophago–gastric junction. Br J Cancer 2002;86:1223–9.
64. Wakatsuki K, Takayama T, Ueno M, et al. Characteristics of gastric cancer with esophageal invasion and aspects of surgical treatment. World J Surg 2009;33: 1446–53.
65. Barbour AP, Rizk NP, Gonen M, et al. Adenocarcinoma of the gastroesophageal junction: influence of esophageal resection margin and operative approach on outcome. Ann Surg 2007;246:1–8.
66. Schumacher G, Schmidt SC, Schlechtweg N, et al. Surgical results of patients after esophageal resection or extended gastrectomy for cancer of the esophagogastric junction. Dis Esophagus 2009;22:422–6.
67. Sasako M, Sano T, Yamamoto S, et al. Left thoracoabdominal approach versus abdominal–transhiatal approach for gastric cancer of the cardia or subcardia: a randomised controlled trial. Lancet Oncol 2006;7:644–51.
68. Bonenkamp JJ, Hermans J, Sasako M, et al. Extended lymph-node dissection for gastric cancer. N Engl J Med 1999;340:908–14.
69. Kunisaki C, Makino H, Suwa H, et al. Impact of splenectomy in patients with gastric adenocarcinoma of the cardia. J Gastrointest Surg 2007;11:1039–44.

70. Degiuli M, Sasako M, Ponti A. Morbidity and mortality in the Italian Gastric Cancer Study Group randomized clinical trial of D1 versus D2 resection for gastric cancer. Br J Surg 2010;97:643–9.
71. Wei HB, Wei B, Qi CL, et al. Laparoscopic versus open gastrectomy with D2 lymph node dissection for gastric cancer: a meta-analysis. Surg Laparosc Endosc Percutan Tech 2011;21:383–90.
72. Verhoef C, van de Weyer R, Schaapveld M, et al. Better survival in patients with esophageal cancer after surgical treatment in university hospitals: a plea for performance by surgical oncologists. Ann Surg Oncol 2007;14:1678–87.
73. Abate E, DeMeester SR, Zehetner J, et al. Recurrence after esophagectomy for adenocarcinoma: defining optimal follow-up intervals and testing. J Am Coll Surg 2010;210:428–35.
74. Macdonald JS, Smalley SR, Benedetti J, et al. Chemoradiotherapy after surgery compared with surgery alone for adenocarcinoma of the stomach or gastroesophagael junction. N Engl J Med 2001;345:725–30.
75. Sakuramoto S, Sasako M, Yamaguchi T, et al. Adjuvant chemotherapy for gastric cancer with S-1, an oral fluoropyrimidine. N Engl J Med 2007;357:1810–20.
76. Ajani JA, Rodriguez W, Bodoky G, et al. Multicenter phase III comparison of cisplatin/S-1 with cisplatin/infusional fluorouracil in advanced gastric or gastroesophageal adenocarcinoma study: the FLAGS trial. J Clin Oncol 2010;28:1547–53.
77. Cunnignham D, Allum WH, Stenning SP, et al. Perioperative chemotherapy versus surgery alone for resectable gastroesophageal cancer. N Engl J Med 2006;355:11–20.
78. Ychou M, Boige V, Pignon JP, et al. Perioperative chemotherapy compared with surgery alone for resectable gastroesophageal adenocarcinoma: an FNCLCC and FFCD multicenter phase III trial. J Clin Oncol 2011;29:1715–21.
79. Morgan MA, Lewis WG, Casbard A, et al. Stage-for-stage comparison of definitive chemoradiotherapy, surgery alone and neoadjuvant chemotherapy for oesophageal carcinoma. Br J Surg 2009;96:1300–7.
80. Tougeron D, Di Fiore F, Hamidou H, et al. Response to definitive chemoradiotherapy and survival in patients with an oesophageal adenocarcinoma versus squamous cell carcinoma: a matched-pair analysis. Oncology 2007;73:328–34.
81. Tougeron D, Scotte M, Hamidou H, et al. Definitive chemoradiotherapy in patients with esophageal adenocarcinoma: an alternative to surgery? J Surg Oncol 2012;105:761–6.
82. Glimelius B, Ekstrom K, Hoffman K, et al. Randomized comparison between chemotherapy plus best supportive care with best supportive care in advanced gastric cancer. Ann Oncol 1997;8:163–8.
83. Wagner AD, Unverzagt S, Grothe W, et al. Chemotherapy for advanced gastric cancer. Cochrane Database Syst Rev 2010;(3):CD004064.
84. Thuss-Patience PC, Kretzschmar A, Bichev D, et al. Survival advantage for irinotecan versus best supportive care as second-line chemotherapy in gastric cancer—a randomised phase III study of the Arbeitsgemeinschaft Internistische Onkologie (AIO). Eur J Cancer 2011;47:2306–14.
85. Wagner AD, Grothe W, Haerting J, et al. Chemotherapy in advanced gastric cancer: a systematic review and meta-analysis based on aggregate data. J Clin Oncol 2006;24:2903–9.
86. Ross P, Nicolson M, Cunningham D, et al. Prospective randomized trial comparing mitomycin, cisplatin, and protracted venous-infusion fluorouracil (PVI 5-FU) with epirubicin, cisplatin, and PVI 5-FU in advanced esophagogastric cancer. J Clin Oncol 2002;20:1996–2004.

87. Webb A, Cunningham D, Scarffe JH, et al. Randomized trial comparing epirubicin, cisplatin, and fluorouracil versus fluorouracil, doxorubicin, and methotrexate in advanced esophagogastric cancer. J Clin Oncol 1997;15:261–7.

88. Ohtsu A. Randomized phase III trial of fluorouracil alone versus fluorouracil plus cisplatin versus uracil and tegafur plus mitomycin in patients with unresectable, advanced gastric cancer: The Japan Clinical Oncology Group Study (JCOG9205). J Clin Oncol 2003;21:54–9.

89. Lee JJ, Kim SY, Shin IS, et al. Randomized phase III trial of cisplatin, epirubicin, leucovorin, 5-fluorouracil (PELF) combination versus 5-fluorouracil alone as adjuvant chemotherapy in curative resected stage III gastric cancer. Cancer Res Treat 2004;36:140–5.

90. Zaniboni A, Barni S, Labianca R, et al. Epirubicin, cisplatin, and continuous infusion 5-fluorouracil is an active and safe regimen for patients with advanced gastric cancer. An Italian Group for the Study of Digestive Tract Cancer (GISCAD) report. Cancer 1995;76:1694–9.

91. Highley MS, Parnis FX, Trotter GA, et al. Combination chemotherapy with epirubicin, cisplatin and 5-fluorouracil for the palliation of advanced gastric and oesophageal adenocarcinoma. Br J Surg 1994;81:1763–5.

92. Roth AD, Fazio N, Stupp R, et al. Docetaxel, cisplatin, and fluorouracil; docetaxel and cisplatin; and epirubicin, cisplatin, and fluorouracil as systemic treatment for advanced gastric carcinoma: a randomized phase II trial of the Swiss Group for Clinical Cancer Research. J Clin Oncol 2007;25:3217–23.

93. Thuss-Patience PC, Kretzschmar A, Repp M, et al. Docetaxel and continuous-infusion fluorouracil versus epirubicin, cisplatin, and fluorouracil for advanced gastric adenocarcinoma: a randomized phase II study. J Clin Oncol 2005;23: 494–501.

94. Cunningham D, Starling N, Rao S, et al. Capecitabine and oxaliplatin for advanced esophagogastric cancer. N Engl J Med 2008;358:36–46.

95. Bang YJ, Van Cutsem E, Feyereislova A, et al. Trastuzumab in combination with chemotherapy versus chemotherapy alone for treatment of HER2-positive advanced gastric or gastro-oesophageal junction cancer (ToGA): a phase 3, open-label, randomised controlled trial. Lancet 2010;376:687–97.

96. Pearson FG, Patterson GA. Pearson's thoracic & esophageal surgery. 3rd edition. Philadelphia: Churchill Livingstone/Elsevier; 2008.

Definitive Chemoradiotherapy for Esophageal Carcinoma

S. Lewis Cooper, MD[a], J. Kyle Russo, MD[a], Steve Chin, MD[b,c],*

KEYWORDS

- Radiotherapy • Esophagus • Esophageal • Carcinoma • Definitive
- Chemoradiotherapy

KEY POINTS

- The management of esophageal cancer is complex and should be managed in a multidisciplinary setting including thoracic surgery, medical oncology, radiation oncology, diagnostic radiology, pathology, gastroenterology, and nutrition.
- Superficial esophageal cancer (cT1N0) is best managed by endoscopic therapy (endoscopic mucosal dissection or endoscopic mucosal resection) or esophagectomy, but definitive radiotherapy may benefit a small population of patients with squamous cell carcinoma and who are not candidates for other therapies.
- Locally advanced esophageal cancer is best treated with neoadjuvant chemoradiotherapy (CRT) followed by esophagectomy, but areas of future research include identifying patients who may not benefit from esophagectomy after CRT.
- Patients who have unresectable disease, are not operative candidates, or refuse surgery should receive definitive CRT and can be expected to have a 2-year survival of 40% to 55%.
- Patients with a radiographic complete response on positron emission tomography can have a 2-year survival as high as 70%.

INTRODUCTION

Although some modest survival gains in esophageal carcinoma have been made over the past 4 decades, survival remains poor. Globally, esophageal cancer is the sixth leading cause of cancer mortality, with an estimated 406,800 deaths and 482,300 new cases in 2008.[1] Esophageal cancer will affect about 17,460 people in the United States in 2012 and an estimated 15,070 people will die of the disease.[2] The 5-year survival has improved from 5% in 1977 to 19% in 2007. Gains have been made in

The authors have nothing to disclose.
[a] Department of Radiation Oncology, Medical University of South Carolina, Charleston, SC, USA; [b] Neuropsycho-Oncology, Department Psychiatry and Behavioral Sciences, Medical University of South Carolina, Charleston, SC, USA; [c] Division of Hematology and Oncology, Medical University of South Carolina, Charleston, SC, USA
* Corresponding author. 96 Jonathan Lucas Street-903 CSB, Charleston, SC 29425.
E-mail address: chin@musc.edu

Surg Clin N Am 92 (2012) 1213–1248
http://dx.doi.org/10.1016/j.suc.2012.07.013   surgical.theclinics.com
0039-6109/12/$ – see front matter Published by Elsevier Inc.

the 22% of patients presenting with localized disease (5-year survival 49.3%) and 32% of patients presenting with regional disease (5-year survival 20.6%); 5-year survival remains 2.8% in the 32% of patients presenting with distant disease.[2] Men have a 3 to 4 times higher incidence of esophageal cancer than women.[1] Squamous cell carcinoma (SCC) and adenocarcinoma (AC) are the 2 most common histologies of esophageal cancer, but other histologies include small cell carcinoma, lymphoma, and sarcomas. The incidence of SCC and AC varies geographically based on the risk factors most prevalent in a given population. Overall, the incidence of esophageal cancer is increasing in the United States as a result of increased rates of AC.[1,3,4] A list of acronyms is given in **Box 1**.

TREATMENT

The management of esophageal cancer is complex and should be managed in a multi-disciplinary setting, including thoracic surgery, medical oncology, radiation oncology,

Box 1	
List of acronyms	
AC	Adenocarcinoma
AJCC	American Joint Cancer Committee on Cancer
BED	Biological equivalent course
BT	Brachytherapy
CBCT	Cone beam computed tomography
cCR	Clinical complete response
CF	Conventional fractionation
CRT	Chemoradiotherapy
CTV	Clinical target volume
CT	Computed tomography
EUS	Endoscopic ultrasonography
EMD	Endoscopic mucosal dissection
EMR	Endoscopic mucosal resection
GEJ	Gastroesophageal junction
GTV	Gross tumor volume
ICT	Induction chemotherapy
IHC	Immunohistochemistry
IMRT	Intensity modulated radiation therapy
INT	Intergroup
ITV	Internal target volume
LD	Limited disease
MAPK	Mitogen-activated protein kinase
pCR	Pathologic complete response
PET	Positron emission tomography
PET-CR	PET complete response
PLE	Pharyngolaryngoesophagectomy
PTV	Planning target volume
RP	Radiation pneumonitis
RT	Radiation therapy
RTOG	Radiation Therapy Oncology Group
SCC	Squamous cell carcinoma
SCEC	Small cell esophageal carcinoma
SCLC	Small cell lung cancer
SIB	Simultaneous integrated boost
SUV	Standardized uptake value
TE	Tracheoesophageal
UES	Upper esophageal sphincter

diagnostic radiology, pathology, gastroenterology, and nutrition. Careful staging and evaluation are critical to determine the optimal treatment options for each patient. Superficial esophageal cancers are generally managed with endoscopic therapies or with esophagectomy, but some centers have experience with definitive radiation therapy (RT). Locally advanced esophageal cancers are generally treated with neoadjuvant chemoradiotherapy (CRT) followed by esophagectomy for operable candidates and by definitive CRT for nonoperative candidates or those who refuse surgery. Patients who have invasion of the aorta, trachea, heart, great vessels, or the presence of a tracheoesophageal (TE) fistula (T4b) are inoperable, and patients with involvement of the pleura, pericardium, or diaphragm are potentially resectable (T4a).[5] Cervical esophagus primaries and small cell carcinoma are preferentially treated with definitive CRT. Because of the challenges associated with treating esophageal cancer, treatment should be performed at centers with significant experience.[6,7]

Radiotherapy

Early results with RT alone for esophageal cancer were disappointing, with poor survival and high rates of local failure; however, RT alone may still play an important role in a small subset of patients (**Table 1**).[8–22] Initially, RT alone was given to patients who were nonoperative candidates or refused surgery, although RT was presented as an equal alternative to surgery in some cases because of high operative mortality of 11% to 23%.[8] Imprecision in staging and targeting led to the treatment of large treatment volumes as well as the possibility that gross disease was not in the treatment portals. The first large retrospective series to compare the results of RT with surgery yielded a 5-year survival of 5% and 26%, respectively.[8] Another large review of more than 8000 patients who received RT alone also reported a 5-year survival of 6%.[9] Patterns of failure were not reported in many early studies because the tools to evaluate this end point were not available, but it became clear that the poor survival of patients treated with RT alone was predominantly caused by local failure. One study found that 78% of patients treated with RT alone died of persistent local and regional tumor.[10] Another study evaluated more than 1000 patients with esophageal cancer treated with RT alone who survived greater than 5 years and found that 40% of deaths were caused by local failure.[12]

Because of poor local control, efforts were made to increase the biological effective dose given to the tumor by using regimens with altered fractionation or hypofractionation, or by giving smaller-volume boost doses.[15–22] One series giving 3 Gy per fraction produced a 5-year overall survival of 21%, but local control was not reported.[17] Four studies looking at different fractionation regimens in patients with SCC of the esophagus yielded a 5-year survival with RT alone between 31.5% and 36.9%.[15,16,22] Two studies randomized 85 and 98 patients with SCC of the esophagus to 64 to 68.4 Gy at 1.8 to 2 Gy per fraction (conventional fractionation [CF]) to 40 to 41.4 Gy at 1.8 to 2 Gy per fraction with a 24 to 27 Gy in 16 to 18 fractions boost given twice daily (late course accelerated fractionation [LCAF]). One trial found a significant improvement in 5-year survival from 15% to 34% and improved local control with LCAF, but the other trial did not find a 3-year survival or local control benefit to LCAF.[18,19] Another randomized study compared surgery with LCAF radiotherapy in 269 patients. The surgery arm had significantly lower 5-year local failure rates of 27.8% versus 57.3%, but the 5-year overall survival and progression-free survival were the same.[22]

One of the reasons for the poor local control seen in early series of patients treated with RT alone may have been inadequate staging techniques and the inability to target sites of disease. A review of 101 patients treated with RT alone to 50 to 52.5 Gy in 15 to 16 fractions found that the use of diagnostic computed tomography (CT) scan for

Table 1
Selected results of definitive radiation alone in the treatment of esophageal cancer

Study, Publication Year	Patient Number (Accrual Dates)	Dose	Local Control	Survival	Toxicity	Notes
Historical series						
Appelqvist et al,[8] 1979	50 (1965–74)	Mean dose 60.3 Gy at 1.6–2.2 Gy/fx, 84% SC	NR	5-y OS 5%	8% TE fistula	Tumors <5 cm
Earlam and Cuhna-Melo,[9] 1980	8489 (1954–79)	Variable	NR	5-y OS 6%	Not reported	Review of 49 articles of RT alone
Mantravadi et al,[10] 1982	173 (1960–79)	55 Gy median dose (30–75 Gy) at 1.8–2 Gy/fx	78% of those who did not have surgery died of LRF	5.8-mo median OS RT alone 11-mo median OS for preoperative RT	15% TE fistula: all with recurrence	17% had surgery
Newaishy et al,[11] 1982	444 (1956–74)	50–55 Gy/20fx	NR	5-y OS 9%	43.7% stricture, 9% fatal fistula, 5.4% hemorrhage	Tumors <10 cm All SCC
Yang et al,[12] 1983	1136 (1958–74)	ESD 27–93 rad 87%–50–80 rad	40% died of local recurrence	Only patients surviving >5 y included	NR	45% <5 cm 37% upper one-third
De-Ren,[13] 1989	869 (NR)	^{60}Co, 50–79 Gy at 1.5–2 Gy/fx	27.3% progression 58.2% recurrence	5-y OS 8.1% 5-y OS 25% for <5 cm lesion	Fatal toxicity: 6.3% hemorrhage, 1.9% perforation, 0.8% fistula	54% had lost pathologic data, remainder SCC
Okawa et al,[14] 1989	311 (1968–83)	60–70 Gy at 2 Gy/fx	NR	5-y OS 9.0% 5-y OS 17.7% for <5 cm lesion	NR	
Petrovich et al,[15] 1991	241 (1963–86)	57%: mean 55 Gy 19%: mean 50 Gy + 40 Gy BT boost	39% of patients died of LRF	5-y OS 2% RT 5-y OS 11% c BT boost	22% esophagitis 1% TE fistula 1% severe stenosis	76% received RT alone 19% received neoadjuvant RT

Study	N (dates)	Dose/fractionation	LRF	Survival	Toxicity	Comments
Kikuchi,[16] 1993	60 (1985–91)	62–64 Gy/40fx twice a day concomitant boost	42.8% 5-y LRF	5-y CSS 31.5%	13.3% stricture 3.3% pericarditis	CT use → increased field size and improved OS
Sykes et al,[17] 1998	101 (1985–94)	45–52.5 Gy in 15–16fx	NR	5-y OS 21%	5% stenosis	LRF cause of death in 61.9% (arm 1) vs 41.2%
Randomized altered fractionation						
Shi et al,[18] 1999	85 (1988–90)	1. 68.4 Gy/36fx 2. 41.4 Gy/23fx + 27 Gy/18fx twice a day All ^{60}Co	5-y LRF 79% (arm 1) vs 45% (SS)	5-y OS 15% (arm 1) vs 34% (SS)	Arm 2: increased acute esophagitis (20%) and bronchitis (13%)	
Wang et al,[19] 2012	98 (2004–2007)	1. 64 Gy/32fx 2. 40 Gy/20fx + 24 Gy/16fx twice a day	3-y LRF 58% (arm 1) vs 50%	3-y OS 36% (arm 1) and 43.8% (NS)	Grade 3/4 esophagitis 12% (arm 1) vs 28% (SS)	
Superficial esophageal cancer						
Pasquier et al,[20] 2006	66 (1992–1999)	Median 60 Gy + median 7 Gy/2fx BT boost	CR in 98% 22.7% local failure	5-y OS 35.6% 5-y CSS 76.9%	Grade 3/4: 9%	T1 tumor Nonoperative or refused surgery
Ishikawa et al,[21] 2010	59 (1991–2005)	Median 60 Gy (48–64 Gy) + EB vs BT boost	CR in 88% LRF in 27%	5-y CSS 76% (86% BT boost)	5% treatment-related mortality	T1 tumor Nonoperative or refused surgery
Randomized RT alone vs surgery						
Yu et al,[22] 2006	269 (1998–2002)	1. Surgery alone 2. 50–50.4 Gy at 1.8–2 Gy/fx + 18–21 Gy at 1.5 Gy twice a day	5-y LRF 27.8% (arm 1) vs 57.3% (SS)	5-y OS 34.7% (arm 1) vs 36.9% (NS)	NR	5-y PFS 20.6% (arm 1) and 23.1% (NS)

Abbreviations: BT, brachytherapy; CSS, cause-specific survival; EB, external beam; ESD, equivalent standard dose; LRF, locoregional failure; NR, not reported; NS, not significant; OS, overall survival; RT, radiotherapy; SC, split course; SS, statistically significant; TE, tracheoesophageal.

staging was the only prognostic factor that was significant for survival, with 5-year survival of 42% versus 13%.[17] The use of CT scan was also associated with a significant increase in field size, suggesting that the improved survival may have been caused by better tumor localization.[17] Local control was not reported, but improved ability to target the tumor and exclude patients with metastatic disease may be responsible for improved results in later series of RT alone.[16–22]

CRT

Because of the high rate of local failure, the addition of chemotherapy to RT was investigated in an attempt to improve outcomes (**Tables 2** and **3**).[23–45] Early experience in organ preservation at Wayne State had shown the feasibility of combining the use of chemotherapy and RT in anal cancer, producing pathologic complete responses (pCR) when given preoperatively.[46] With this success in mind, the combination of chemotherapy (5-fluorouracil [5-FU] and mitomycin C or cisplatin) and RT (50–60 Gy) was used preoperatively in esophageal cancer and resulted in a pCR rate of 37% and a 2-year survival of 30%.[47] Because of the good response seen in this initial study, CRT was investigated as a definitive treatment of esophageal cancer. Several early series using various chemotherapy regimens reported promising results, with local failure rates of 27% to 35% and 2-year survival of 29% to 48%.[23–26] One retrospective analysis revealed significant improvements in local control (from 23% to 73%) and 2-year survival (13%–29%) with CRT compared with RT alone.[23]

Early results showing improved local control and survival with CRT led to randomized controlled trials comparing RT alone with concurrent CRT.[34–38,48–51] Most of these trials showed a survival benefit to concurrent CRT, but most of them did not use modern chemotherapy regimens or used split-course RT.[34–37,48–51] Several other randomized trials investigated the use of sequential chemotherapy and RT for locally advanced esophageal cancer and found no benefit in local control or survival but did report increased toxicity.[52–54] Radiation Therapy Oncology Group (RTOG) 8501 compared RT alone (64 Gy) with CRT (50 Gy with 4 cycles of concurrent and adjuvant cisplatin and 5-FU) and revealed a 5-year overall survival benefit to CRT of 26% compared with 0%.[37,38] The CRT arm had a significant improvement in local control from 32% to 54%. However, the CRT arm had 2% treatment-related mortality and an additional 20% of patients experienced grade 4 toxicity, whereas the RT alone arm had no treatment-related mortality and only 3% grade 4 toxicity.[37,38] RTOG 8501 established concurrent CRT as the standard in the nonsurgical management of locally advanced esophageal cancer.

Surgical candidates

Patients with esophageal cancer who are candidates for surgery can receive esophagectomy with or without neoadjuvant or adjuvant therapy or definitive CRT with esophagectomy only if there is persistent or recurrent local disease and the optimal course is controversial. If esophagectomy is to be performed, then neoadjuvant CRT is recommended, because several randomized trials have reported an overall survival benefit for neoadjuvant CRT and this has been confirmed by meta-analysis.[55–59] Two clinical trials[40–43] have randomized patients with locally advanced esophageal cancer to definitive CRT versus neoadjuvant CRT followed by esophagectomy, but the interpretation of these results is unclear. A German trial[40,41] randomized 172 patients with locally advanced SCC of the esophagus to induction chemotherapy (ICT) followed by CRT and then esophagectomy or ICT followed by CRT. Survival for the definitive CRT and surgery arms at 5 and 10 years was 27.9%/17% and 19.2%/12.2%, respectively, and this was not statistically significant.[41] The surgery arm did

Table 2
Selected results of concurrent chemoradiation in the treatment of esophageal cancer: nonrandomized data

Study, Publication Date	Patient Number (Accrual Dates)	Eligibility	CRT	Local Control	Survival	Toxicity	Notes
CRT vs RT							
John et al,[23] 1989	65 (1975–86)	Adenocarcinoma (37%) or SCC of the esophagus, M0	1. RT (1975–83) →56–61 Gy @ 1.8 Gy/fx 2. CRT (1982–86) →41.1 Gy/23fx + 9 Gy/5fx boost after 2.5 wk break c concurrent 4 cycles of 5-FU, MMC, 5-FU–cisplatin	LRF 77% in RT and 27% in CRT (SS)	2-y OS 13% (RT) vs 29% (SS) Median survival 8 mo (RT) vs 11 mo	1 grade 5 pneumonitis in CRT Stomatitis 27% in CRT	Retrospective
CRT alone							
Keane et al,[24] 1985	35 (1980–83)	SCC of esophagus, M0	45–50 Gy/20fx CF or 22.5–25 Gy/10fx x 2 SC Concurrent MMC and 5-FU (1 cycle CF, 2 cycles SC)	2-y LC 29% vs 79% favoring CF	2-y OS 13% vs 48% favoring CF	1 fatal pneumonitis in SC	Improved OS and LC compared with HX controls
Herskovic et al,[25] 1988	22 (1983–85)	SCC of the thoracic esophagus, M0	Cisplatin and 5-FU x 2 cycles c concurrent 30 Gy/15fx → MMC and bleomycin x 1 cycle → 20 Gy/10fx	23% persistent disease 14% additional LRF	Median survival 22 mo	4.5% TRM	18% had salvage esophagectomy
Seitz et al,[26] 1990	35 (1986–89)	SCC of the esophagus, inoperable, M0	Cisplatin and 5-FU x 2 cycles c concurrent 20 Gy/5fx x 2 SC	71% with cCR 25.7% with cPR	2-y OS 41% Median survival 17 mo	5.7% grade 3 nausea 5.7% grade 3 heme	

(continued on next page)

Table 2
(continued)

Study, Publication Date	Patient Number (Accrual Dates)	Eligibility	CRT	Local Control	Survival	Toxicity	Notes
Yu et al,[27] 1995	24 (1987–91)	Adenocarcinoma (12.5%) or SCC of the esophagus	Cisplatin and 5-FU x 3 cycles c concurrent 3 cycles of 20 Gy @ 1.8–2 Gy/fx SC	LF 6% in 17 patients completing therapy	2-y OS 38%	28% TRM (two-thirds sepsis)	
Urba and Turrisi,[28] 1995	27 (1990–92)	Adenocarcinoma (74%) or SCC of the esophagus or GEJ	Carboplatin and 5-FU x 2 cycles c concurrent 40 Gy/ 20fx twice a day SC → Adjuvant carboplatin and 5-FU x 2 cycles	93% of progression outside radiation field 59% palliation of dysphasia	Median survival 6 mo	11% each grade 4 thrombocytopenia and neutropenia 7% grade 3 esophagitis	Unresectable or recurrent after surgery 63% with mets
Gaspar et al,[29] 2000	49 (1992–95)	Adenocarcinoma or SCC of the thoracic esophagus, T1-2, NX-1, M0	Cisplatin and 5-FU x 4 cycles c concurrent 50 Gy/25fx followed by HDR brachytherapy to 15 Gy/3fx (1992–94) but reduced to 10 Gy/2fx (1994–95)	cCR 74% LRF as first site of failure 29%	2-y OS 31%	10% TRM Grade 3/4 toxicity 59%/24%	12% TE fistula
Suntharalingam et al,[30] 2006	37	Adenocarcinoma (76%) or SCC of esophagus or GEJ, M0	Cetuximab, paclitaxel, and carboplatin weekly with concurrent 50.4 Gy/28fx	67% with cCR 43% with pCR	NR	3% grade 4 neutropenia 20% grade 3 esophagitis	

Li et al,[31] 2010	59 (2004–07)	SCC of the esophagus or GEJ	Docetaxel and cisplatin × 2 cycles c concurrent 60–64 Gy at 1.8–2 Gy/fx	71.2% cCR at 6 wk 3-y LRF was 40.4%	3-y OS 36.7% Median survival 22.6 mo	10.2% grade 3 esophagitis. No grade 4/5 toxicity	EUS in 24% 36% with stage IVb c nonregional LNs
Kato et al,[32] 2011	76 (200–2002)	Stage II/III SCC of the thoracic esophagus	Cisplatin and 5-FU × 2 cycles c concurrent 60 Gy/30fx SC → responders received additional 2 cycles of cisplatin & 5-FU	cCR rate of 62.2%	3-y and 5-y OS were 44.7% and 36.8% Median survival 2.8 y	5.3% TRM Grade 3/4 esophagitis and nausea 17% each	11 patients received salvage esophagectomy
Swisher et al,[33] 2011	43 (2003–06)	Adenocarcinoma (73%) or SCC of esophagus or GEJ, > T1N0, M0	Induction 5-FU and cisplatin × 2 cycles → concurrent 5-FU and cisplatin × 1 cycle c concurrent 50.4 Gy/28fx → selective surgical salvage if residual or recurrent local disease with no metastases	46.5% LRF alone and received surgical salvage	1-y OS was 71%	9.8% TRM	EUS used in all patients and PET in some 1-y survival 83% for 15 patients with surgical salvage

Abbreviations: GEJ, gastroesophageal junction; HDR, high-dose-rate; HX, historical; LC, local control; LF, local failure; LN, lymph nodes; LRF, locoregional failure; MMC, mitomycin C; NR, not reported; RT, radiotherapy; SC, split course; SS, statistically significant; TRM, treatment-related mortality.

Table 3
Selected results of concurrent chemoradiation in the treatment of esophageal cancer: randomized data

Study, Publication Date	Patient Number (Accrual Dates)	Eligibility	Treatment Arms	Local Control	Survival	Toxicity	Notes
CRT vs RT							
Araujo et al,[34] 1991	59 (1982–85)	SCC of thoracic esophagus, stage II	1. 5-FU, MMC, and bleomycin c concurrent 50 Gy/25fx 2. 50 Gy/25fx	LF 46.5% (arm 1) vs 74% (NS)	5-y OS 16% (arm 1) vs 6% (NS)	10% severe esophagitis c CRT 61% stenosis, TE fistula in 7 patients c recurrence	
Smith et al,[35] 1999	119 (1982–88)	Stage I/II SCC of the thoracic esophagus	1. 5-FU and MMC x 2 cycles c concurrent 60 Gy/30fx 2. 60 Gy/30fx	NR	2-y OS 27% (arm 1) vs 12% (SS) Median survival 14.8 mo vs 9.2 mo	NR	Patients could receive 40 Gy/20fx → esophagectomy (23 patients from each arm)
Wobbes et al,[36] 2001	211 (1983–89)	SCC, T1-3, N0-N1, M0	1. Cisplatin x 2 cycles c concurrent 20 Gy/5fx x 2 SC RT 2. 20 Gy/5fx x 2 SC RT	Time to LF 10.9 mo (arm 1) vs 6.2 mo (SS)	Median OS 9.6 mo (arm 1) vs 7.9 mo (SS)	6% (arm 1) vs 1% WHO grade 3–4 heme toxicity, no severe toxicity in RT alone	More T3 in arm 1 (20 vs 13%) Closed early because of low accrual
Herskovic et al,[37,38] 1992,1999	121 (1986–90)	Adenocarcinoma (13%) or SCC of esophagus, T1-3, N0-1, M0	1. Cisplatin and 5-FU x 4 cycles c concurrent 30 Gy/15fx regional + 20 Gy/10fx boost 2. 50 Gy regional + 14 Gy boost at 2 Gy/fx	LRF 46% (arm 1) vs 68% (SS)	5-y OS 26% (arm 1) vs 0% (SS)	Severe/life-threatening toxicity 44/20% (arm 1) vs 25/5% (SS) TRM 2% vs 0%	

CRT comparing different radiation dose/fractionation

Study	N (years)	Histology	Treatment	Local control	Survival	Mortality/Toxicity	Comments
Minsky et al,[39] 2002	236 (1995–1999)	Adenocarcinoma (15%) or SCC of esophagus, T1-4, N0-1, M0	1. Cisplatin and 5-FU x 4 cycles c concurrent 50.4 Gy/1.8fx + 14.4 Gy/1.8fx tumor boost 2. Cisplatin and 5-FU x 4 cycles c concurrent 50.4 Gy/1.8fx	LRF/persistent disease 56% (arm 1) vs 52% (NS)	2-y OS 31% (arm 1) vs 40% (NS) Median survival 13 mo (arm 1) vs 18.1 mo	10% (arm 1) vs 2% TRM 7 deaths in high-dose occurred ≤50.4 Gy, 1 fatal fistula after 64.8 Gy	Closed early because of <2.5% chance of survival benefit with higher-dose RT

CRT followed by surgery vs CRT

Study	N (years)	Histology	Treatment	Local control	Survival	Mortality/Toxicity	Comments
Stahl et al,[40,41] 2005,2008	172 (1994–2002)	SCC of upper and mid third esophagus; T3-4, N0-1, M0	Induction 5-FU, cisplatin, and etoposide x 3 cycles then randomized to: 1. 40 Gy/20fx c concurrent cisplatin → esophagectomy 2. Concurrent cisplatin c either 50 Gy20fx + 15 Gy/10fx Hfx boost OR 60 Gy/30fx + HDR boost	2-y LF 36% (arm 1) vs 59% (SS)	3-y OS 31.3% (arm 1) vs 24.4% (NS) Median survival 16.4 vs 14.9 mo 10-y CSS 24.8% vs 12.2% (NS)	TRM 12.8% (arm 1) vs 3.5%	EUS used for staging 33.5% had objective response to induction chemotherapy an independent prognostic factor (HR = 0.3)
Bendenne et al,[42,43] 2007	444 enrolled 259 responders randomized (1993–2000)	Adenocarcinoma (11.2%) or SCC of thoracic esophagus	Concurrent cisplatin and 5-FU x 2 cycles with 15 Gy/5fx x 2 SC or 46 Gy/23fx CF → If response then randomized to: 1. Surgery 2. Concurrent cisplatin and 5-FU x 3 cycles with 15 Gy/5fx SC or 20 Gy/10fx CF	2-y LF 34% (arm 1) vs 43% (SS) 2-y LF 23% for CF and 43% for SC (SS)	2-y OS 34% (arm 1) vs 40% (NS) Median survival 17.7 vs 19.3 mo	3-mo mortality 9.3% (arm 1) vs 0.8%	EUS for staging in some SC RT 67% in arm 1 and 65% in arm 2

(continued on next page)

Table 3
(continued)

Study, Publication Date	Patient Number (Accrual Dates)	Eligibility	Treatment Arms	Local Control	Survival	Toxicity	Notes
CRT comparing different chemotherapy regimens							
Ajani et al,[44] 2008	84 (2001–05)	Adenocarcinoma (66%) or SCC of esophagus or GEJ, > T1N0, M0	1. Induction 5-FU, cisplatin, and paclitaxel x 2 cycles →5-FU and paclitaxel c concurrent 50.4 Gy/28fx 2. Induction cisplatin and paclitaxel x 2 cycles → cisplatin and paclitaxel c concurrent 50.4 Gy/28fx	NR	2-y OS was 56% (arm 1) vs 37% Median survival was 28.7 mo (arm 1) vs 14.9 mo	Grade 3/4 toxicity was 54% (arm 1) vs 60%	EUS used for staging phase II
Conroy et al,[45] 2010	97 (2004–2005)	Adenocarcinoma (17.5%) or SCC of the esophagus, M0, unresectable or inoperable	50 Gy/25fx randomized to concurrent: 1. Oxaliplatin, leucovorin, and 5-FU x 6 q2 wk cycles 2. Cisplatin and 5-FU x 4 q4 wk cycles	cCR in 45% (arm 1) vs 29%	3-y OS 45% (arm 1) vs 29% Median survival 22.7 vs 15.1 mo	Grade 3/4 toxicity was 59.6% (arm 1) vs 62.8%	EUS used for some patients phase II

Abbreviations: CSS, cause-specific survival; HDR, high-dose-rate; HR, hazard ratio; LF, local failure; LRF, locoregional Failure; MMC, mitomycin C; NR, not reported; NS, not significant; RT, radiotherapy; SC, split course; SS, statistically significant; TRM, treatment-related mortality; WHO, World Health Organization.

have improved 2-year local progression-free survival of 64.3% versus 40.7%, but treatment-related mortality was significantly higher at 12.8% versus 3.5%.[40] Fédération Francophone de Cancérologie Digestive (FFCD) 9102 randomized 259 patients with locally advanced esophageal cancer (11.2% AC) to an initial course of CRT and then randomized responders to surgery or further CRT.[42,43] Two-year survival for the definitive CRT arm was not different from surgery at 40% versus 34%.[42] FFCD 9102 also reported improved local control with surgery (66.4% compared with 57%) but had increased 3-month mortality (9.3% vs 0.8%).[42]

The radiation on FFCD 9102 was not standard, because two-thirds of the patients in each arm received split-course radiotherapy. Subsequent analysis revealed significantly worse local control in the split-course patients (56.8% vs 76.7% with CF), but this did not produce a difference in overall survival.[43] Patients on the German trial received 40 Gy of preoperative radiation and less intense chemotherapy than in most other neoadjuvant trials (the CROSS trial did use 41.4 Gy), and the radiation dose received by the split-course patients in FFCD 9102 is also lower than in other neoadjuvant trials.[40,42,57–59] Also, the treatment-related mortality was significantly higher in the surgery arms of the German and FFCD 9102 trials at 9.3 to 12.8% compared with 3.8% to 4.4% in other neoadjuvant CRT trials.[40,42,58–60] For patients with AC of the esophagus, there are no randomized data to compare definitive CRT with trimodality therapy. A recent retrospective analysis of a population-based database revealed that patients who received trimodality therapy compared with definitive CRT had improved 5-year survival of 30% versus 12%.[61] The treatment groups were not balanced, because the trimodality patients were younger and were more likely to have AC; however, multivariate analysis still revealed improved survival with trimodality therapy, with a hazard ratio of 0.66 (0.56–0.77).[61] Both the German and FFCD 9102 trials have criticisms, and surgery is still considered an integral component in the management of patients with esophageal cancer, particularly those with AC.

Response-adapted therapy

Because some patients respond better than others to CRT, efforts have been made to identify prognostic factors to determine if some patients do not benefit from the addition of surgery after CRT. In multiple randomized trials in which neoadjuvant CRT is followed by surgery in an arm, the pCR rate has ranged from 15.6% to 43% in patients who received doses of radiation from 30 Gy to 50.4 Gy **(Table 4)**.[30,47,57–60,62–65] Patients who achieve a pCR after CRT have superior 5-year survival of 50% compared with 22.6% for those who have residual disease at esophagectomy.[66] Timing is also important because there is some evidence that salvage esophagectomy after local progression or recurrence has increased morbidity and mortality compared with patients who receive a planned esophagectomy 4 to 6 weeks after completion of CRT.[67] However, the optimal timing for esophagectomy after completion of CRT is not known, because 1 study found no difference in survival in patients who received esophagectomy either before or after 8 weeks from completion of CRT.[68] Thus, CRT could be given and esophagectomy reserved only for those who have evidence of persistent local disease.

The clinical complete response (cCR) rate often overestimates the pCR rate seen after esophagectomy.[30,64] A positive biopsy on endoscopic ultrasonography (EUS) correlates well to residual disease, with a positive predictive value of 95%, but a negative biopsy on EUS has a low negative predictive value (as low as 31%), with up to 69% of these patients having residual disease on esophagectomy.[69] CT has poor sensitivity and specificity in predicting pCR, but the use of positron emission tomography (PET) imaging to predict response has generated a great deal of interest with

Table 4
pCR response rates to neoadjuvant concurrent CRT

Study, Publication Date	Patient Number (Accrual)	Eligibility	Chemotherapy	Radiation	cCR (%)	pCR (%)	Notes
Steiger et al,[47] 1981	42	SCC of the esophagus	5-FU and either MMC or cisplatin	56–60 Gy	NR	37	35 patients with surgery
Walsh et al,[57] 1996	65 (1990–95)	Adenocarcinoma of the esophagus, M0	5-FU 15 mg/kg/d on days 1–5 and cisplatin 75 mg/m^2 day 7 × 2 cycles with second cycle on week 6	40 Gy in 15 fractions	NR	25	Neoadjuvant arm of phase III trial
Urba et al,[62] 2001	50 (1989–94)	Adenocarcinoma (75%) or SCC of the esophagus or GEJ, M0	Cisplatin 20 g/m^2/d CI on days 1–5, 17–21; 5-FU 300 mg/m^2/d CI on days 1–21; and vinblastine 1 mg/ m^2/d on days 1–4, 17–20	45 Gy in 30 fractions given twice daily	NR	28	Neoadjuvant arm of phase III trial
Lee et al,[63] 2004	51 (1999–2002)	SCC of the esophagus, T2-3N0, T1-3N1, M0	Cisplatin 60 mg/m^2 day 1, 21 and 5-FU 1000 mg/m^2/d CI on days 2–5	45.6 Gy in 38 fractions given twice daily	33	43	Neoadjuvant arm of phase III trial
Burmeister et al,[64] 2005	128 (1994–2000)	Adenocarcinoma (63%) or SCC of the esophagus or GEJ, cT1-3,N0-1, M0	Cisplatin 80 mg/m^2 day 1 and 5-FU 800 mg/m^2/d on days 1–4	35 Gy in 15 fractions	29	16	Neoadjuvant arm of phase III trial. Only 57% completed restaging after CRT

Suntharalingam et al,[30] 2006	37	Adenocarcinoma (76%) or SCC of esophagus or GEJ, M0	Cetuximab 400 mg/m² week 1 then 250 mg/m² weeks 2–6, paclitaxel 50 mg/m² weekly, and carboplatin AUC = 2 weekly	50.4 Gy in 28 fractions	67	43	Phase II
Tepper et al,[58] 2008	30 (1997–2000)	Adenocarcinoma (77%) or SCC of the thoracic esophagus or GEJ, T1-3, N0-1,M0	Cisplatin 100 mg/m² days 1,29 and 5-FU 1000 mg/m²/d CI on days 1–4, 29–32	50.4 Gy in 28 fractions	NRs	40	Neoadjuvant arm of phase III trial
Stahl et al,[65] 2009	60 (200–2005)	Adenocarcinoma of the esophagus, cT3-4NxM0	Cisplatin 50 mg/m² biweekly, 5-FU 2000 mg/m² and leucovorin 500 mg/m² weekly x 6 wk for 2 cycles → Cisplatin 50 mg/m² days 1, 8 and etoposide 80 mg/m² days 3–5 with concurrent	30 Gy in 15 fractions	NR	15.6	Neoadjuvant CRT arm of phase III trial
Van der Gaast et al,[59] 2010	175 (2004–08)	Adenocarcinoma (75.2%) or SCC of the esophagus or GEJ, cT2-3, N0-1,M0	Paclitaxel 50 mg/m² weekly, and carboplatin AUC = 2 wkly x 5 wk	41.4 Gy in 23 fractions	NR	32.6	Neoadjuvant arm of phase III trial
Leichman et al,[60] 2011	93 (2004–08)	Stage II/III adenocarcinoma of the esophagus	Oxaliplatin 85 mg/m² days 1, 15, 29 and protracted-infusion 5-FU 18 mg/m²/d on days 8–43	45 Gy in 25 fractions	NR	28	Phase II

Abbreviations: AUC, area under the curve; cCR, clinical complete response; GEJ, gastroesophageal junction; MMC, mitomycin C.

mixed results (**Fig. 1**).[70–74] PET is useful in detecting interval development of metastatic disease, but in the treatment field a standardized uptake value (SUV) cutoff can miss microscopic disease below the resolution of PET or can be falsely positive because of inflammation from RT. How to best define a response by PET is not known and studies have examined threshold SUV, total lesion glycolosis, tumor volume, and change in maximum SUV (maxSUV).[71–74] PET accuracy for predicting pCR has varied from 34% to 89% in these studies, but change in maxSUV and total lesion glycolosis (multiplying mean tumor volume and mean SUV) seem to be the most promising methods.[71–74] The timing of surgery may also be an important factor, because 1 study reported an increased pCR rate more than 103 days from CRT compared with less than 81 days from CRT, irrespective of RT dose or chemotherapy regimen.[75] One recent study found that patients with PET complete response (PET-CR) treated with definitive CRT had significantly improved survival compared with patients without PET-CR, and the survival was equivalent compared with patients with PET-CR who received esophagectomy. The survival for those patients receiving trimodality therapy was the same in those who had a PET-CR and those who did not have a PET-CR[74]

RTOG 0246 was a phase II study that gave induction cisplatin, 5-FU, and paclitaxel followed by 50.4 Gy with concurrent 5-FU and cisplatin with a 1-year survival goal of

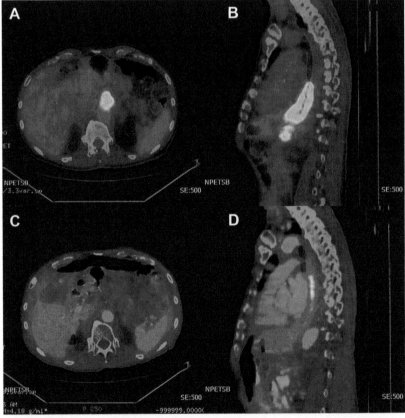

Fig. 1. PET-CT axial (*A*) and sagittal (*B*) slices of a patient with newly diagnosed AC of the distal esophagus with an SUV of 17.5. PET-CT axial (*C*) and sagittal (*D*) slices taken 3 weeks after CRT with SUV of the primary at 3.5.

77.5%.[33] Endoscopic biopsy, EUS, and CT were performed 6 to 8 weeks after completion of CRT and then every 3 months for the first 2 years. PET was encouraged but was optional. Patients would receive salvage esophagectomy if there was any suspicion of local disease and no evidence of metastatic disease. A total of 37 patients received ICT followed by CRT; 18 of these patients underwent selective surgical resection after restaging and 23 patients did not receive esophagectomy (14 because of cCR and 9 because of death or metastases). Only 1 patient, who had a cCR and had requested surgery, was found to have a pCR. Three additional patients received esophagectomy after completion of CRT for suspicion of local recurrence. Treatment-related mortality was 9.8%. The 1-year survival of RTOG 0246 was 71% and will not move on to a phase III trial, but it showed that an organ-preserving approach may be achieved with a more tolerable, effective regimen and more accurate methods to predict response and risk of relapse.[33] However, until further information from prospective studies is obtained, neoadjuvant CRT followed by esophagectomy remains the standard of care in patients who have resectable tumors and are operative candidates.

Radiation Techniques

Radiation treatment planning has evolved considerably since radiotherapy was first used to treat esophageal cancer. Before CT-based treatment planning, simulation was performed by fluoroscopy and fields were largely designed based on bony landmarks. CT-based planning allows for contouring tumor volumes and normal structures and calculating dose to each voxel of a structure. This situation has allowed for more accurate estimation of normal tissue toxicity and dose to the targeted volume. In addition, advances in treatment delivery such as intensity modulated RT (IMRT) have allowed more conformal treatment plans with the goal of minimizing toxicity. Cone beam CT or megavoltage CT with tomotherapy allows the ability to perform daily image guidance to ensure that the target volume is in the treatment field and potentially allows margins for setup error to be reduced. Despite these advances, there is still much to learn about the optimal treatment of esophageal cancer with RT.

Dose and fractionation

A wide range of dose and fractionation schemes have been used in the reported series of patients and randomized trials of radiotherapy for esophageal cancer. Split-course radiotherapy was used frequently before modern treatment planning to reduce treatment toxicity; however, several studies have shown that patients treated with split-course radiotherapy have inferior local control and survival.[24,43] RTOG 8501 established 50 Gy in 25 fractions as the standard dose when treating with concurrent chemotherapy. Intergroup (INT) 0123, attempted to determine if there is a benefit to dose escalation in the setting of CRT.[39] Patients received 4 cycles of cisplatin and 5-FU (2 concurrent and 2 adjuvant) and were randomized to 64.8 Gy in 36 fractions or 50.4 Gy in 28 fractions. Both arms received 50.4 Gy to 5 cm superior and inferior and 2 cm radially beyond the primary tumor. Regional lymph nodes were included. The high-dose arm then received an additional 14.4-Gy cone down to the primary with a 2-cm expansion. INT 0123 enrolled 218 patients, but the trial was stopped after interim analysis revealed that there was no significant difference between the arms, because the 2-year survival was 31% for the high-dose arm and 40% for the low-dose arm.[39] There was no significant difference in local control, but the 10% treatment-related deaths in the high-dose arm was significantly more than the 2% in the low-dose arm. Seven of the 11 treatment-related deaths in the high-dose arm were in patients who had received 50.4 Gy or less, but a separate analysis including only patients receiving the assigned dose still did not reveal a survival benefit to dose escalation.[39] As a result, 50 to 50.4 Gy is the recommended radiotherapy dose when given with concurrent chemotherapy.

Another approach has been to attempt dose escalation with brachytherapy (BT) after a course of external beam RT, but phase II trials have not shown a benefit.[20,76] RTOG 9207 gave 4 cycles of chemotherapy with concurrent 50 Gy in 25 fractions external beam followed by either high-dose-rate (HDR) BT 15 Gy in 3 weekly fractions (later amended to 10 Gy in 2 weekly fractions) or low-dose-rate BT to 20 Gy.[29] One-year survival was 49%, but there was 24% grade 4 toxicity and 10% treatment-related mortality, with a 12% fistula rate. Because of the high rates of toxicity without clear benefit, this regimen was not taken to a phase III trial.[29] Another phase II trial used 3 cycles of induction docetaxel, cisplatin, and 5-FU followed by 45 Gy in 25 fractions external beam RT with concurrent carboplatin. Patients would receive esophagectomy, or if they refused or were unfit for surgery, would receive HDR BT to 15 Gy in 3 weekly fractions.[76] All of the 7 patients treated with HDR BT recurred locally and the trial experienced a 24% TE fistula rate.[76] A BT boost should not be routinely used outside a clinical trial because of the disappointing results of these trials.

LCAF has been used in China for SCC of the esophagus and revealed improved local control and survival compared with CF in 1 randomized trial, but did not improve local control or survival in another trial with shorter follow-up.[18,19] Once RTOG 8501 revealed improved survival with concurrent CRT, another phase III trial was performed that randomized 111 patients to LCAF radiotherapy alone or LCAF radiotherapy with concurrent cisplatin and 5-FU for 4 cycles.[77] The 5-year overall survival and local recurrence rates for the CRT arm were 40% and 33% compared with 28% and 41% in the radiation alone arm, but this was not statistically significant. The CRT arm had increased rates of acute grade 3 and 4 toxicity and acute treatment-related mortality of 46% and 6% compared with 25% and 0%, but there was no difference in late toxicity.[77] No trial has compared LCAF CRT with conventionally fractionated CRT, but the overall treatment-related mortality of 10% for the LCAF CRT arm in this trial suggests that 50 to 50.4 Gy at 1.8 to 2 Gy per fraction should remain the standard at this time.

If a patient's comorbidities preclude the use of chemotherapy and surgery, then 50 to 50.4 Gy in 25 to 28 fractions is still considered the standard dose and fractionation for RT alone. However, local failure in trials of RT alone using daily fractionation is invariably greater than 50%.[10,13,18] A higher dose per fraction may produce greater than 20% 5-year survival, as seen in 1 series, but data on local control are lacking.[17] One randomized trial of LCAF radiotherapy showed improved local control and survival compared with conventionally fractionated RT but with increased acute toxicity.[18] Another series retrospectively compared a hyperfractionated regimen with continuous concomitant boost to 62-Gy to 64-Gy total dose with patients treated with CF and found that the hyperfractionated patients had a 5-year cause-specific survival and locoregional recurrence-free survival of 31.5% and 57.2%, respectively.[16] The use of a hyperfractionated boost or continuous concomitant boost could be considered in patients receiving RT alone, but the possible improvement in local control should be balanced with the likelihood of greater acute toxicity, the patient's performance status, and the logistics of receiving twice-daily RT.

Treatment volume and technique

Esophageal cancer can have submucosal spread cephalad and caudad to the visible tumor. For this reason, radiation clinical trials have added at least an additional 5 cm from gross tumor in the superior and inferior directions to the radiation field edge (location of the 50% isodose line) to ensure that possible submucosal extension is treated.[37,39] With the advent of CT treatment planning, the primary tumor and any clinically positive nodes can be contoured; this is labeled the gross tumor volume (GTV).[78] When contouring the GTV, the radiation oncologist should review and incorporate information from endoscopy, EUS, PET-CT, and other diagnostic studies that may have been performed. PET-CT can also be fused with the planning CT using rigid or deformable registration, or a planning PET-CT in the treatment position can be performed, if available. The use of PET-CT in contouring the GTV may reduce the target volume, intraobserver and interobserver variability, and dose to normal structures.[79] However, the use of PET-CT in treatment planning for esophageal cancer requires more investigation and is the subject of ongoing clinical trials (NCT01156831, NCT00934505). The use of [18F]-fluorothymidine PET (FLT-PET) compared with [18F]-fluorodeoxyglucose PET (FDG-PET) in radiotherapy treatment planning is also being investigated and may be of benefit in more accurately producing a GTV (NCT01243619).[80]

The clinical target volume (CTV) is defined as the GTV plus areas at risk for harboring microscopic disease.[78] The CTV is usually the primary tumor GTV, with an additional 4-cm expansion superior and inferior as well as a 1-cm to 1.5-cm lateral expansion to include the paraesophageal lymph nodes. In addition, any positive lymph nodes in the GTV should also be included in the CTV volume. When creating the CTV, the planning CT should be carefully examined to ensure that at-risk lymph nodes are included, such as the celiac lymph nodes for tumors of the gastroesophageal junction (GEJ) and distal esophagus or the bilateral supraclavicular nodes for tumors of the upper one-third of the esophagus. Elective nodal irradiation is likely particularly important in AC of the esophagus because 81% of patients with pT2-T4 tumors have lymph node metastases.[81] However, 1 small prospective study of 53 patients with SCC staged with CT treated only involved nodes and the primary and found that the rate of isolated out-of-field recurrence was only 8% at 3 years.[82] Although this study suggests that elective nodes may not need to be treated in SCC, these results need to be confirmed and the current practice is to treat at-risk elective nodes to at least 45 Gy.

The planning target volume (PTV) accounts for respiratory motion as well as setup error and should be determined based on patient setup, immobilization, and image guidance (**Fig. 2**).[78] The internal target volume (ITV) is an expansion from the CTV that accounts for variations of the size, shape, and position of the CTV during therapy from respiration, cardiac motion, and peristalsis and can be estimated with four-dimensional CT (4D-CT).[78] The CTV in addition to the ITV and setup error produces

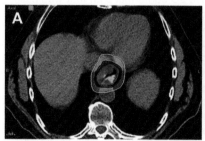 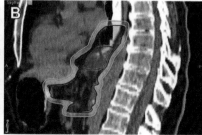

Fig. 2. The GTV (*red*) of an AC of the distal esophagus. The patient was treated on protocol with a CTV (*blue*) expansion 3 cm superior and inferior and 0.5 to 1 cm radially. The lesser curvature and celiac nodes were included in the CTV. The PTV (*green*) was a fixed 1-cm expansion.

the PTV. If 4D-CT is not available, then data from several prospective studies can be incorporated to determine an ITV.[83–85] One study evaluating 4D-CT in 29 patients[83] saw a significant difference in anterior to posterior (A-P) and left to right (L-R) motion in the proximal esophagus, midesophagus, and distal esophagus. Another study evaluated 4D-CT in 30 patients,[84] 25 with distal esophageal tumors, and a 1.5-cm superior to inferior (S-I) and a 0.75-cm radial (A-P and L-R) ITV expansion was found to account for motion of more than 95% of primary tumors; however, this may overestimate motion in tumors of the midthoracic or upper thoracic esophagus. Interfraction (between fractions) motion is greater than intrafraction (during a fraction) motion as measured by CT-on-rails and 12 mm left, 8-mm right, 10-mm posterior, and 9-mm anterior ITV margins were recommended.[85]

To reduce setup error, daily image guidance may be used, if available. To find the optimal frequency of image guidance for esophageal cancer, 25 patients were treated with daily image guidance with megavoltage CT and then 7 less-than-daily image-guided scenarios were evaluated to determine required margins for setup error. Increased frequency of image guidance reduced the setup error; however, even with 60% of fractions being treated with image guidance, there was still substantial setup error because of random setup error.[86] Only daily image guidance could sufficiently reduce PTV margins. Adaptive planning, using data from daily image guidance to customize PTV expansions during the course of treatment, may also allow for reduced dose to normal structures.[87] Further investigation in esophageal tumor motion, image guidance, and margins in esophageal cancer is needed to determine the ideal treatment approach for patients receiving RT for esophageal cancer.

As technology has evolved, two-dimensional (2D) planning has been replaced by three-dimensional (3D) conformal RT because of the ability to increase the dose to the target and reduce the dose to normal structures (**Fig. 3**).[88] IMRT offers even more opportunity to improve conformality, which can reduce the dose to normal structures and offer the ability to escalate dose to the tumor. Multiple dosimetric studies have shown that IMRT can decrease lung dose in the high-dose regions; this can sometimes result in an increased volume of lung receiving lower doses (**Fig. 4**).[89–92] If treating 1 large PTV to 50 to 50.4 Gy, then the theoretic benefit derived from IMRT is modest and the ideal technique for each patient should be evaluated. However, because local failure is still a significant problem with concurrent CRT, further evaluation of dose escalation may be warranted. IMRT with simultaneous integrated boost (SIB) allows for treating a larger volume at risk for harboring microscopic disease at 1.8 to 2.0 Gy per fraction and treating gross disease at 2.2 to 2.3 Gy per fraction concurrently.[90,93] One study compared IMRT plans for the high-dose and low-dose arms of INT 0123 with the low-dose 2D conformal plan that was called for in INT 0123. The 50.4-Gy IMRT plans produced significant reductions in the mean cardiac (33%), lung (25%), and liver (20%) doses compared with the 50.4-Gy 2D plans.[93] The SIB-IMRT plans were able to increase the dose to the GTV by 28% (64.8 Gy) with comparable doses to the normal structures in the 50.4-Gy IMRT plans and significant reductions in the cardiac, lung, and liver doses in the 2D 50.4-Gy plans.[93] With improved treatment techniques, dose escalation may be able to produce improved local control without increased toxicity in patients with esophageal cancer receiving CRT, and this is being investigated in a phase I trial (NCT01102088).

Proton RT offers increased conformality over photon radiotherapy, because there is no exit dose. Dosimetric analyses of proton RT and photon RT with IMRT or 3D conformal techniques have shown that proton RT can reduce the dose to the lungs, heart, and liver.[94,95] Proton RT has been used for esophageal cancer in 1 center in Japan since 1990, and 1 recent study of 19 patients who received various schedules

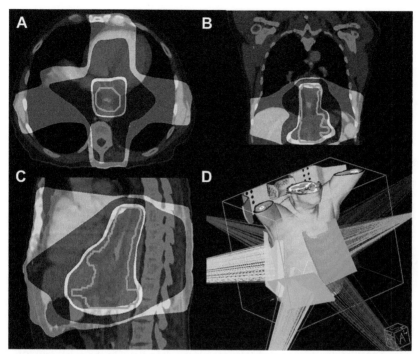

Fig. 3. A 3D conformal plan seen in axial (*A*), coronal (*B*), and sagittal (*C*) slices for a patient with AC of the distal esophagus given 50.4 Gy with concurrent chemotherapy. The PTV is seen in green as well as the volume receiving 100% of the dose (*red*), 95% of the dose (*yellow*), 50% of the dose (*blue*), and 30% of the dose (*white*). The skin rendering with 3D beams is also seen (*D*).

of hyperfractionated concomitant boost proton beam therapy (all treated with a combination of photons and protons) reported 5-year local control and survival of 84.4% and 42.8%.[96] There was 1 grade 3 toxicity, and this compared favorably with the 26% grade 3 or higher toxicity rate in historical controls at the same institution who had been treated with once-daily proton RT.[96] Proton RT does have the potential to further reduce toxicity and potentially escalate dose to the tumor. MD Anderson Cancer Center is planning a phase III randomized controlled trial (NCT01512589) comparing IMRT with proton RT in patients with stage II or III esophageal cancer, with progression-free survival and toxicity burden as the primary outcome measures.

Organs at risk: dose constraints

With modern treatment planning, the dose to normal organs can be accurately measured and incorporated into treatment planning algorithms to attempt to reduce toxicity. The lung can receive substantial dose when treating long portions of the esophagus, and careful attention is required to minimize the risk of radiation pneumonitis (RP), because RP can be an important cause of treatment-related morbidity in patients receiving CRT.[24,33,37] Lung dose constraints are largely derived from results of lung RT, and it is recommended to limit the mean lung dose to less than 20 to 23 Gy and the volume of lung receiving greater than 20 Gy (V20) to less than 30% to 35%.[97] One study of patients who have esophageal cancer receiving CRT used receiver operating characteristics curve analysis to determine that the optimal V20 threshold to

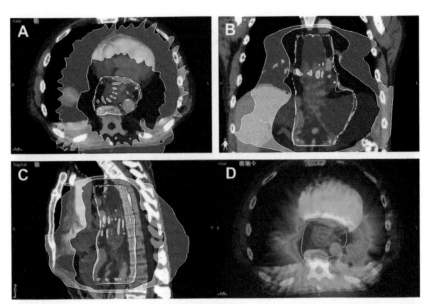

Fig. 4. An IMRT tomotherapy plan seen in axial (*A*), coronal (*B*), and sagittal (*C*) slices for a patient with AC of the distal esophagus given 50.4 Gy with concurrent chemotherapy. Daily megavoltage CT image guidance was used. The PTV is seen in green as well as the volume receiving 100% of the dose (*red*), 95% of the dose (*yellow*), 50% of the dose (*blue*), and 30% of the dose (*white*). Also seen is the dose cloud in the axial view (*D*).

predict the development of RP was 30.5%, with a 17.4% incidence less than this value.[98] There is also evidence that induction and concurrent taxanes increase the risk of RP, and careful attention to reduce lung dose should be taken if a taxane is to be given with RT.[99]

The dose of RT to the heart has been linked to pericarditis, pericardial effusion, and excess cardiac deaths from myocardial infarction, congestive heart failure, cardiomyopathy, or valvular heart disease; however, there is limited information on long-term cardiac toxicity in the setting of CRT for esophageal cancer.[100–106] One study analyzed dose to the entire heart and the pericardium (5-mm shell outside normal heart contour) and found that a mean pericardial dose less than 26.1 Gy and V30 less than 46% significantly reduced the risk of pericardial effusion.[100] In patients treated for Hodgkin lymphoma, dose to the whole heart greater than 30 Gy and dose to 35% of the heart (D35) greater than 38 Gy are associated with excess cardiac mortality.[100,102] RT dose to specific portions of the heart is likely important, as shown by a recent report of patients who have breast cancer treated with RT in Sweden. An increase in stenosis was found in the mid and distal left anterior descending artery and distal diagonal in patients who received high-risk left-sided RT.[103] One population-based study did not find increased cardiovascular mortality in patients who have esophageal cancer treated with RT, and esophageal cancer was the leading cause of mortality.[105] Another single-institution study of patients treated with CRT for esophageal cancer found that a V40 greater than 54% was associated with increased cardiac toxicity and women were 3.57 times more likely to have cardiac toxicity.[106] Care should be taken in attempting to balance the desire to decrease cardiac toxicity with the need to effectively treat the esophageal cancer.

Myelopathy from injury to the spinal cord from radiotherapy can be devastating. As a result, dose limitations for the spinal cord are conservative to minimize the risk of this complication. A dose of 50 Gy at 2 Gy per fraction to the full cross-section of the cord results in a 0.2% incidence of myelopathy, but protocols for CRT in esophageal cancer (RTOG 1010) are generally more conservative and limit the maximum dose to 45 Gy.[107] RT injury to the liver has largely been studied in patients with primary liver cancers or liver metastases, and the risk of liver toxicity is minimized if the whole liver is limited to less than 30 Gy and the mean liver dose less than 32 Gy. There is also evidence that limiting the V30 to less than 60% decreases the risk of liver injury.[108] To minimize acute gastrointestinal toxicity, it is recommended to limit the absolute volume of small bowel receiving 15 Gy or more to less than 120 cm^3 or the peritoneal space volume receiving 45 Gy or more to less than 195 cm^3.[109] Dose constraints to the kidneys vary from protocol to protocol and exact dose limitations are not well defined, but the mean bilateral kidney dose should be limited to less than 18 Gy and the V20 should be less than 32%.[110] If the mean kidney dose to 1 kidney is greater than 18 Gy, then the dose to the contralateral kidney should be further limited to a V6 of less than 30%.[110]

Superficial Esophageal Cancer

Therapeutic options for superficial esophageal cancer (cT1N0) have expanded with the advent of more reliable staging and more advanced endoscopic techniques. Management is based on the risk of lymph node metastases because tumors with low risk of lymphatic spread can be managed with local therapy and operative candidates at higher risk of lymphatic spread are managed by esophagectomy. These candidates include patients with submucosal invasion (SM1-3) who have a 7.5% to 45% risk of lymph node metastases and patients with muscularis mucosa (M3) invasion and lymphovascular invasion who have up to an 18% risk of lymph node metastases.[111,112] Patients with superficial esophageal cancer who are nonoperative candidates and who have contraindications for endoscopic therapies such as endomucosal resection (EMR) or endomucosal dissection (EMD) or cannot be treated adequately with endoscopic therapy alone can receive RT alone or CRT. Several single-institution series have reported acceptable local control and cause-specific survival in patients with superficial esophageal cancer, but these series are almost exclusively in patients with SCC.[20,21,113–115]

In 4 series of patients treated with RT alone for superficial SCC of the esophagus, the 5-year locoregional control and cause-specific survival range from 63% to 79.9% and 76% to 82.1%, respectively.[20,21,113,114] These patients were staged with EUS and CT and then received either BT alone (1 institution for M2 tumors), external beam RT alone (60–66 Gy), or external beam RT with a BT boost (54–60 Gy with variable BT boost). Local failure is most closely related to depth of invasion, with 1 study reporting 5-year locoregional control and cause-specific survival of 75% and 97% for mucosal tumors and 49% and 55% for submucosal tumors.[113] One institution reported on 34 patients with superficial SCC of the esophagus predominantly treated with CRT and found 5-year locoregional control and cause-specific survival to be 81.1% and 91.2%, respectively.[115] Because of the higher risk of local failure in T1b tumors, CRT likely improves local control over RT alone. Some patients in these series who experienced local failure and had refused surgery initially were able to be salvaged with esophagectomy or other local therapy.[20,21,113–115] EMR, EMD, and esophagectomy remain the standard for treatment of superficial esophageal cancer and should be performed in high-volume centers, but RT may be an alternative for the few patients with SCC who are not candidates for these therapies.

Cervical Esophagus

Cancer of the cervical esophagus is uncommon and the histology is greater than 90% SCC. Because cancer of the cervical esophagus can invade the larynx or extend up into the hypopharynx, surgical management can be complex and can require a pharyngolaryngoesophagectomy (PLE), hemithyroidectomy or complete thyroidectomy, and reconstruction with gastric pull-up or free jejunal graft. Early series comparing surgery with RT found that that 5-year survival was 12% to 30% regardless of whether patients received RT alone, surgery alone, or surgery followed by adjuvant RT; however, patients who received surgery had significant treatment-related morbidity and mortality.[116] Because of these results and clinical trials that revealed a benefit to CRT over radiotherapy alone in esophageal cancer and head and neck SCC, CRT is now considered the standard in management of cervical esophageal cancer.[37,117]

Single-institution series of CRT for SCC of the cervical esophagus (largest reported on 50 patients treated with curative intent) have yielded 2-year and 5-year survival rates ranging from 35% to 52% and 19% to 55%, respectively.[118–126] The 1 study with 5-year survival of 55% had 70% of patients with cT1-2N0M0 tumors, whereas most patients in other series had predominantly cT3-4 or N1 tumors.[124] There is a great deal of variability in the dose and fractionation delivered, treatment volumes, and stage of the patients treated. Esophageal cancers are treated with 50 to 50.4 Gy of radiation with concurrent chemotherapy, but 70 Gy is standard in SCC of the head and neck and the optimal dose for the cervical esophagus is unclear at this time. Two series have found improved local control and survival in patients who received greater than 50 or 60 Gy, but another series did not find improved outcomes with 70 Gy compared with 54 Gy.[120,122,123] It is our practice to give 60 to 70 Gy to the primary tumor and involved lymph nodes and give 50 to 56 Gy concurrently to the at-risk nodal volumes. The cervical esophagus has lymph node drainage to the superior mediastinal lymph nodes as well as lower cervical and supraclavicular lymph nodes and it is our practice to include these in the elective nodal volume. In addition, cervical esophageal tumors that invade into the hypopharynx, larynx, or thyroid can acquire the lymph node drainage of these organs and this should be taken into consideration with treatment planning. Further prospective investigation in the optimal treatment of cervical esophageal tumors is needed to improve outcomes, because survival has not significantly changed over the past decade.

Small Cell Carcinoma

Primary small cell esophageal carcinoma (SCEC) is a rare malignancy. Because of the low incidence, no treatment standard has been defined specifically for SCEC. SCEC is highly sensitive to chemotherapy; therefore, most treatments include systemic chemotherapy as part of multimodality therapy.[127–129] However, the role of surgery in locoregional SCEC remains unclear. Most clinicians believe SCEC resembles small cell lung cancer (SCLC); therefore, therapeutic approaches similar to SCLC have been described in the literature.[130,131]

Ku and colleagues[131] reported a case series of 22 patients with SCEC treated at Memorial Sloan-Kettering Cancer Center from 1980 to 2005. Fourteen patients (64%) presented with locoregional SCEC/limited disease (LD). Of the 14 patients with LD, only 3 patients were treated with surgical resection. The other 11 patients with LD received platinum-based ICT. In the ICT group, 7 patients received concurrent CRT, 1 patient had salvage esophagectomy, 2 patients had distant metastases after ICT, and 1 patient had CR after the ICT and underwent prophylactic cranial irradiation.

The median survival for LD was 22.3 months (6 months–11.2+ years). All 3 patients who underwent initial surgical resection developed recurrence (1 locoregional and 2 distant). Of the 7 patients with LD who underwent planned ICT and concurrent CRT without surgery, recurrence occurred in 3 patients (1 locoregional and 2 distant). The median survival for these patients has not been reached.[131]

The data from the case series suggest that patients with LD can achieve long-term survival with ICT followed by consolidative CRT without surgery.[131] Therefore, surgery may not be necessary as part of initial therapy but may be reserved for salvage after documented local failure after chemotherapy or CRT. In contrast, Kuo and colleagues[132] argued in favor of surgical resection followed by adjuvant chemotherapy for patients with LD to improve long-term survival. We are not able to draw a definitive conclusion.

TOXICITY

Regimens of definitive CRT have rates of grade 3 and 4 toxicity of 40% to 60% and 15% to 25% depending on the chemotherapy and RT regimen. More intense chemotherapy regimens have resulted in greater rates of grade 3 and 4 cytopenias and infection, but the rates of grade 3/4 esophagitis are about 20% to 30% with CRT. Treatment-related mortality with definitive CRT is typically 1% to 3%, but has been as high as 10% to 15% in some trials with dose-escalated RT or more intense chemotherapy regimens.[23–45]

Late toxicity from RT includes RP, pericardial effusion, cardiac events, and TE fistula. Patients with symptomatic RP present with shortness of breath, low-grade fever, and decreased oxygen saturation. RP generally manifests within 10 months of CRT.[106] Symptomatic RP can occur in up to 50% to 60% of patients treated with definitive CRT, but the rate of grade 3 to 5 RP is generally around 5% or less.[99] Pericardial effusion can occur in up to 25% of patients treated with CRT but is often not clinically significant.[100] Patients with a malignant TE fistula can be treated with CRT, and about 25% of these close after CRT.[133] Patients with continued or new TE fistula after CRT have a poor prognosis. Rates of TE fistula on modern CRT trials are low, at less than 2%, but some CRT trials with BT boost have produced higher rates of TE fistula, at up to 12%.[29]

FUTURE DIRECTIONS

Current areas of research with respect to definitive CRT in esophageal cancer relate to optimizing the planning, treatment delivery, dose and fractionation, biological therapy, and assessment of which operative candidates may be able to forgo esophagectomy (**Table 5**). Current studies are evaluating the use of FDG-PET and FLT-PET in treatment planning and evaluating treatment response (NCT01156831, NCT01243619). The benefit of IMRT is being evaluated in clinical trials, and MD Anderson Cancer Center is performing a phase I trial investigating the feasibility of an SIB with IMRT with concurrent 5-FU and docetaxel (NCT011020788, NCT00593723). In addition, the benefit of proton therapy will be evaluated in 1 trial randomizing patients to proton therapy or IMRT for esophageal cancer. A phase III dose-escalation trial (CONCORDE) in France is evaluating 40 Gy in 20 fractions with the addition of a 10-Gy or 26-Gy boost with concurrent FOLFOX 4 given in 6 2-week cycles. If local control can be improved by dose escalation without excess toxicity, then this may translate into an overall survival benefit.

Biological therapies targeting cellular proteins or receptors have shown activity in esophageal cancer. With the recent progress in novel therapeutic development, there are strategic attempts to target growth factor-mediated signal pathways in esophageal cancer that regulate cellular response. These signal transduction pathways

Table 5
Ongoing trials of definitive CRT for esophageal cancer

Trial	Eligibility	Target Accrual/Current Accrual (January 2012)	Treatment Arms	Notes
RTOG 0436	Adenocarcinoma or SCC of the esophagus or GEJ, cT1N1M0; T2-4, N0-1, M0; M1a	420/287	50.4 Gy in 28 fractions randomized to concurrent: 1. Cetuximab 400 mg/m^2 day 1 then 200 mg/m^2 weekly on weeks 2–6, paclitaxel 50 mg/m^2 and cisplatin 25 mg/m^2 weekly for 6 wk 2. Paclitaxel 50 mg/m^2 and cisplatin 25 mg/m^2 weekly for 6 wk	Treatment up to physicians if biopsy proved persistent disease after trial therapy
SCOPE 1 (UK)	Adenocarcinoma or SCC of the esophagus or GEJ, cT1-4, N0-1, M0; nonoperative candidate	440/420	50 Gy in 25 fractions starting week 7 randomized to: 1. Cetuximab 400 mg/m^2 day 1 then 250 mg/m^2 weekly on weeks 2–12, cisplatin 60 mg/m^2 day 1 of 21-d cycle for 4 cycles, and capecitabine 650 mg/m^2 by mouth days 1–84 2. Cisplatin 60 mg/m^2 day 1 of 21-d cycle for 4 cycles and capecitabine 650 mg/m^2 by mouth days 1–84	
ACCORD (France)	Adenocarcinoma or SCC of the esophagus or GEJ, cT1-4, N0-1, M0-M1a; nonoperative candidate	266	50 Gy in 25 fractions randomized to concurrent: 1. Oxaliplatin and leucovorin day 1 and 5-FU CI days 1–2 given in 6 2-wk cycles 2. Cisplatin 75 mg/m^2 day 1 and 5-FU 1000 mg/m^2 CI days 1–4 of weeks 1, 5, 8, 11	
CONCORDE (France)	Adenocarcinoma or SCC of the esophagus cT3, N0-N1, M0-M1a Or T1-T2, N0-N1, M0-M1a with a contraindication for surgery	252	Oxaliplatin and leucovorin day 1 and 5-FU CI day 1–2 given in 6 2-wk cycles randomized to concurrent: 1. 40 Gy in 20 fractions with a 10 Gy in 5 fractions boost 2. 40 Gy in 20 fractions with a 26 Gy in 13 fractions boost	
NICE (Brazil)	Adenocarcinoma or SCC of the esophagus or GEJ, cT1-2N1M0 or cT3-4, N0-1, M0, inoperable	104	50.4 Gy in 28 fractions randomized to concurrent: 1. Nimotuzumab 200 mg weekly for 26 wk with cisplatin 75 mg/m^2 day 1 and 5-FU 1000 mg/m^2 CI days 1–4 × 4 cycles 2. Cisplatin 75 mg/m^2 day 1 and 5-FU 1000 mg/m^2 CI days 1–4 × 4 cycles	Phase II/III

may influence growth regulation, apoptosis, angiogenesis, metastatic potential, and increase sensitivity to systemic therapy.[134] In the phase II study by Suntharalingam and colleagues,[30] the addition of the antiepidermal growth factor receptor monoclonal antibody cetuximab to paclitaxel, carboplatin, and radiotherapy was associated with a 67% cCR and 1-year survival rate was ~70%.[135] Because of these encouraging results, the RTOG embarked on a phase III trial, RTOG 0436, testing the addition of cetuximab to cisplatin-definitive and paclitaxel-definitive CRT.

Correlative study with biomarker evaluation is essential, in an attempt to identify niche populations most likely to benefit from a specific therapy. An example of this personalized approach in esophageal AC is trastuzumab in the subset of patients with HER2 overexpression.[136–139] When HER2 positivity was defined as either fluorescence in situ hybridization–positive or immunohistochemistry (IHC) 3+, 33% of patients with distal esophageal AC overexpressed HER2.[136] In the phase III ToGA trial, trastuzumab showed survival benefit in HER2-positive metastatic gastroesophageal AC.[137] The median overall survival was 13.8 months in trastuzumab plus chemotherapy compared with 11.1 months in chemotherapy alone (hazard ratio 0·74; 95% confidence interval 0·60–0·91; $P = 0.0046$). In locoregional disease, RTOG 1010 is an ongoing phase III trial evaluating trastuzumab combined with trimodality treatment in HER2-positive esophageal AC. In this study, maintenance trastuzumab will be given after surgical resection for approximately a year.

The mitogen-activated protein kinases (MAPK) pathway is activated in Barrett-associated dysplasia and AC, and this is a direct consequence of repeated exposure to acid or bile acid reflux. Activation of the MAPK pathway increases proliferation and decreases apoptosis in SEG-1 cells. Sorafenib is a multikinase inhibitor of several known growth regulatory pathways, including the MAPK pathway. Through MAPK inhibition, sorafenib significantly inhibited SEG-1 cell proliferation and reduced cell survival.[140,141] In a phase II trial, sorafenib is being studied in advanced esophageal and GEJ cancer. In the early response observation, Ilson and colleagues[142] reported 1 durable CR and protracted stable disease (>15 months). Of the 14 patients, only 3 (21%) had early disease progression at 2 months. In an attempt to identify correlates of treatment response, phospho-erk (MAPK pathway) is being tested by IHC.

Another area of investigation is determining if some patients who are operable candidates and receive CRT can avoid esophagectomy. The combination of molecular-based imaging, endoscopy, and biomarkers may provide more accurate prognostic information. In addition, biomarkers may be able to better guide therapy, because several recent clinical trials have reported on biomarkers and response to CRT.[60,143–145] One neoadjuvant CRT trial (S0356), with oxaliplatin and 5-FU as the chemotherapy regimen, found that *ERCC-1* gene expression was not associated with pCR rates but was inversely related to progression-free survival and overall survival. Thus, alternate chemotherapy may be beneficial in those with increased *ERCC-1* gene expression.[60] Three other trials have found that DNA repair biomarkers MLH1 and FANCD2 as well as single nucleotide polymorphisms on chromosome 2q36.1 and on STK15 (chromosome 20q13) predict response to CRT (pCR rates) as well as local recurrence and survival.[143–145] Further research is needed using genetic biomarkers to intensify or target therapy for patients with adverse features or to de-escalate therapy for patients with favorable prognosis.

SUMMARY

The management of esophageal cancer requires a multidisciplinary approach and is ideally managed in high-volume centers. Superficial esophageal cancer (cT1N0) is best managed by endoscopic therapy (EMD or EMR) or esophagectomy, but definitive radiotherapy may benefit a small population of patients with SCC and who are not candidates for other therapies. Locally advanced esophageal cancer is best treated with neoadjuvant CRT followed by esophagectomy, but areas of future research include identifying patients who may not benefit from esophagectomy after CRT. Patients who have unresectable disease, are not operative candidates, or refuse surgery should receive definitive CRT and can be expected to have a 2-year survival of 40% to 55%. Patients with a radiographic CR on PET can have a 2-year survival as high as 70%. Improvements in radiotherapy techniques and greater understanding of patient-specific tumor biology may allow tailoring therapy to continue to improve outcomes.

REFERENCES

1. Jemal A, Bray F, Center MM, et al. Global cancer statistics. CA Cancer J Clin 2011;61:69–90.
2. Siegel R, Naishadham D, Jemal A. Cancer statistics, 2012. CA Cancer J Clin 2012;62:10–29.
3. Brown LM, Devesa SS, Chow WH. Incidence of adenocarcinoma of the esophagus among white Americans by sex, stage, and age. J Natl Cancer Inst 2008; 100:1184–7.
4. Cook MB, Chow WH, Devesa SS. Oesophageal cancer incidence in the United States by race, sex, and histologic type, 1977-2005. Br J Cancer 2009;101: 855–9.
5. Edge SB, Byrd DR, Compton CC, et al. AJCC cancer staging manual. 7th edition. New York: Springer; 2010.
6. Gomi K, Oguchi M, Hirokawa Y, et al. Process and preliminary outcome of a patterns-of-care study of esophageal cancer in Japan: patients treated with surgery and radiotherapy. Int J Radiat Oncol Biol Phys 2003;56:813–22.
7. Wouters MW, Gooiker GA, van Sandick JW, et al. The volume-outcome relation in the surgical treatment of esophageal cancer: a systematic review and meta-analysis. Cancer 2012;118(7):1754–63.
8. Appelqvist P, Silvo J, Rissanen P. The results of surgery and radiotherapy in the treatment of small carcinomas of the thoracic esophagus. Ann Clin Res 1979;11: 184–8.
9. Earlam R, Cunha-Melo JR. Oesophageal squamous cell carcinoma: II. A critical review of radiotherapy. Br J Surg 1980;67:457–61.
10. Mantravadi RV, Lad T, Briele H, et al. Carcinoma of the esophagus: sites of failure. Int J Radiat Oncol Biol Phys 1982;8:1897–901.
11. Newaishy GA, Read GA, Duncan W, et al. Results of radical radiotherapy of squamous cell carcinoma of the esophagus. Clin Radiol 1982;33:347–52.
12. Yang ZY, Gu XZ, Zhao S, et al. Long term survival of radiotherapy for esophageal cancer: analysis of 1136 patients surviving for more than 5 years. Int J Radiat Oncol Biol Phys 1983;9:1769–73.
13. De-Ren S. Ten-year follow-up of esophageal cancer treated by radical radiation therapy: analysis of 869 patients. Int J Radiat Oncol Biol Phys 1989;16: 329–34.
14. Okawa T, Kita M, Tanaka M, et al. Results of radiotherapy for inoperable locally advanced esophageal cancer. Int J Radiat Oncol Biol Phys 1989;17:49–54.
15. Petrovich Z, Langholz B, Formenti S, et al. Management of carcinoma of the esophagus: the role of radiotherapy. Am J Clin Oncol 1991;14:80–6.

16. Kikuchi Y. Study on clinical application of multiple fractions per day radiation therapy with concomitant boost technique for esophageal cancer. Hokkaido Igaku Zasshi 1993;68:537–56 [in Japanese].
17. Sykes AJ, Burt PA, Slevin NJ, et al. Radical radiotherapy for carcinoma of the esophagus: an effective alternative to surgery. Radiother Oncol 1998;48:15–21.
18. Shi XH, Yao W, Liu T. Late course accelerated fractionation in radiotherapy of esophageal carcinoma. Radiother Oncol 1999;51:21–6.
19. Wang JH, Lu XJ, Zhou J, et al. A randomized controlled trial of conventional fraction and late course accelerated hyperfraction three-dimensional conformal radiotherapy for esophageal cancer. Cell Biochem Biophys 2012;62:107–12.
20. Pasquier D, Mirabel X, Adenis A, et al. External beam radiation therapy followed by high-dose-rate brachytherapy for inoperable superficial esophageal carcinoma. Int J Radiat Oncol Biol Phys 2006;65:1456–61.
21. Ishikawa H, Nonaka T, Sakurai H, et al. Usefulness of intraluminal brachytherapy combined with external beam radiation therapy for submucosal esophageal cancer: long-term follow-up results. Int J Radiat Oncol Biol Phys 2010;76:452–9.
22. Yu J, Ren R, Sun X, et al. A randomized clinical study of surgery versus radiotherapy in the treatment of resectable esophageal cancer. J Clin Oncol 2006; 24(Suppl 18):4013.
23. John MJ, Flam MS, Mowry PA, et al. Radiotherapy alone and chemoradiation for nonmetastatic esophageal carcinoma. Cancer 1989;63:2397–403.
24. Keane T, Harwood AR, Elhakim T, et al. Radical radiation therapy with 5-fluorouracil infusion and mitomycin C for oesophageal squamous carcinoma. Radiother Oncol 1985;4:205–10.
25. Herskovic A, Leichman L, Lattin P, et al. Chemo/radiation with and without surgery in the thoracic esophagus: the Wayne State experience. Int J Radiat Oncol Biol Phys 1988;15:655–62.
26. Seitz JF, Giovannini M, Padaut-Cesana J, et al. Inoperable nonmetastatic squamous cell carcinoma of the esophagus managed by concomitant chemotherapy (5-fluorouracil and cisplatin) and radiation therapy. Cancer 1990;66:214–9.
27. Yu L, Vikram B, Malamud S, et al. Chemotherapy rapidly alternating with twice-a-day accelerated radiation therapy in carcinomas involving the hypopharynx or esophagus: an update. Cancer Invest 1995;13:567–72.
28. Urba S, Turrisi A. Split-course accelerated radiation therapy combined with carboplatin and 5-flourouracil for palliation of metastatic or unresectable carcinoma of the esophagus. Cancer 1995;75:435–9.
29. Gaspar LE, Winter K, Kocha WI, et al. A phase I/II study of external beam radiation, brachytherapy and concurrent chemotherapy for patients with localized carcinoma of the esophagus (Radiation Therapy Oncology Group Study 9207). Cancer 2000;88:988–95.
30. Suntharalingam M, Dipertrillo T, Akerman P, et al. Cetuximab, paclitaxel, carboplatin and radiation for esophageal and gastric cancer. J Clin Oncol 2006; 24(Suppl 18):4029.
31. Li QQ, liu MZ, Hu YH, et al. Definitive concomitant chemoradiotherapy with docetaxel and cisplatin in squamous esophageal carcinoma. Dis Esophagus 2010;23:253–9.
32. Kato K, Muro K, Minashi K, et al. Phase II study of chemoradiotherapy with 5-fluorouracil and ciplatin for stage II-III esophageal squamous cell carcinoma: JCOG trial (JCOG 9906). Int J Radiat Oncol Biol Phys 2011;81:684–90.
33. Swisher SG, Winter KA, Komaki RU, et al. A phase II study of a paclitaxel-based chemoradiation regimen with selective surgical salvage for resectable

locoregionally advanced esophageal cancer: initial reporting of RTOG 0246. Int J Radiat Oncol Biol Phys 2012;82(5):1967–72.

34. Araujo CM, Souhami L, Gil RA, et al. A randomized trial comparing radiation therapy versus concomitant radiation therapy and chemotherapy in carcinoma of the thoracic esophagus. Cancer 1991;191(67):2258–61.

35. Smith TJ, Ryan LM, Douglass HO, et al. Combined chemoradiotherapy vs. radiotherapy alone for early stage squamous cell carcinoma of the esophagus: a study of the Eastern Cooperative Oncology Group. Int J Radiat Oncol Biol Phys 1998;42:269–76.

36. Wobbes T, Baron B, Paillot B, et al. Prospective randomised study of split-course radiotherapy versus cisplatin plus split-course radiotherapy in inoperable squamous cell carcinoma of the oesophagus. Eur J Cancer 2001;37:470–7.

37. Herskovic A, Martz K, Al-Sarraf M, et al. Combined chemotherapy and radiotherapy compared with radiotherapy alone in patients with cancer of the esophagus. N Engl J Med 1992;326:1593–8.

38. Cooper JS, Guo MD, Herskovic A, et al. Chemoradiotherapy of locally advanced esophageal cancer: long-term follow-up of a prospective randomized trial (RTOG 85-01). JAMA 1999;281:1623–7.

39. Minsky BD, Neuberg D, Kelsen DP, et al. Final report of Intergroup Trial 0122 (ECOG PE-289, RTOG 90-12): phase II trial of neoadjuvant chemotherapy plus concurrent chemotherapy and high-dose radiation for squamous cell carcinoma of the esophagus. Int J Radiat Oncol Biol Phys 1999;43:517–23.

40. Stahl M, Stuschke M, Lehmann N, et al. Chemoradiation with and without surgery in patients with locally advanced squamous cell carcinoma of the esophagus. J Clin Oncol 2005;23:2310–7.

41. Stahl M, Wilke N, Lehmann N, et al. Long-term results of a phase III study investigating chemoradiation with and without surgery in locally advanced squamous cell carcinoma (LA-SCC) of the esophagus. J Clin Oncol 2008;26:4530.

42. Bedenne L, Michel P, Bouche O, et al. Chemoradiation followed by surgery compared with chemoradiation alone in squamous cancer of the esophagus: FFCD 9102. J Clin Oncol 2007;25:1160–8.

43. Crehange G, Maingon P, Peignaux K, et al. Phase III trial of protracted compared with split-course chemoradiation for esophageal cancer: Fédération Francophone de Cancérologie Digestive 9102. J Clin Oncol 2007;25:4895–901.

44. Ajani JA, Winter K, Komaki R, et al. Phase II randomized trial of two nonoperative regimens of induction chemotherapy followed by chemoradiation in patients with localized carcinoma of the esophagus: RTOG 0113. J Clin Oncol 2008; 26:4551–6.

45. Conroy T, Yataghene Y, Etienne PL, et al. Phase II trial of chemoradiotherapy with FOLFOX4 or cisplatin plus fluorouracil in oesophageal cancer. Br J Cancer 2010;103:1349–55.

46. Nigro ND, Vaitkevicius VK, Considine B. Combined therapy for cancer of the anal canal: a preliminary report. Dis Colon Rectum 1974;17:354–6.

47. Steiger Z, Franklin R, Wilson RF, et al. Complete eradication of squamous cell carcinoma of the esophagus with combined chemotherapy and radiotherapy. Am Surg 1981;47:95–8.

48. Earle JD, Gelber RD, Moertel CG, et al. A controlled evaluation of combined radiation and bleomycin therapy for squamous cell carcinoma of the esophagus. Int J Radiat Oncol Biol Phys 1980;6:821–6.

49. Zhang Z. Radiation combined with bleomycin for esophageal carcinoma—a randomized study of 99 patients. Clin J Oncol 1984;6:372–4 [in Chinese].

50. Slabber CF, Nel JS, Schoeman L, et al. A randomized study of radiotherapy alone versus radiotherapy plus 5-fluorouracil and platinum in patients with inoperable, locally advanced squamous cancer of the esophagus. Am J Clin Oncol 1998;21:462–5.

51. Wong RK, Malthaner RA, Zuraw L, et al. Combined modality radiotherapy and chemotherapy in nonsurgical management of localized carcinoma of the esophagus: a practice guideline. Int J Radiat Oncol Biol Phys 2003;55:930–42.

52. Roussel A, Bleiberg H, Dalesio O, et al. Palliative therapy of inoperable oesophageal carcinoma with radiotherapy and methotrexate: final results of a controlled clinical trial. Int J Radiat Oncol Biol Phys 1989;16:67–72.

53. Zhou JC. Randomized trial of combined chemotherapy including high dose cisplatin, and radiotherapy for esophageal cancer. Zhonghua Zhong Liu Za Zhi 1991;13:291–4 [in Chinese].

54. Hishikawa Y, Miura T, Oshitani T, et al. A randomized prospective study of adjuvant chemotherapy after radiotherapy in unresectable esophageal carcinoma. Dis Esophagus 1991;4:85–90.

55. Sjoquist KM, Burmeister BH, Smithers BM, et al. Survival after neoadjuvant chemotherapy or chemoradiotherapy for resectable oesophageal carcinoma: an updated meta-analysis. Lancet Oncol 2011;12:681–92.

56. Kranzfelder M, Schuster T, Geinitz H, et al. Meta-analysis of neoadjuvant treatment modalities and definitive non-surgical therapy for oesophageal squamous cell cancer. Br J Surg 2011;98:768–83.

57. Walsh TN, Noonan N, Hollywood D, et al. A comparison of multimodality therapy and surgery for esophageal adenocarcinoma. N Engl J Med 1996;335:462–7.

58. Tepper J, Krasna MJ, Niedzwiecki D, et al. Phase III trial of trimodality therapy with cisplatin, fluorouracil, radiotherapy, and surgery compared with surgery alone for esophageal cancer: CALGB 9781. J Clin Oncol 2008;26:1086–92.

59. Gaast AV, van Hagan P, Hulshof M, et al. Effect of preoperative concurrent chemoradiotherapy on survival of patients with resectable esophageal or esophagogastric junction cancer: results from a multicenter randomized phase III study. J Clin Oncol 2010;28(Suppl 15):4004.

60. Leichman LP, Gldman BH, Bohanes PO, et al. S0356: a phase II clinical and prospective molecular trial with oxaliplatin, fluorouracil, and external-beam radiation therapy before surgery for patients with esophageal adenocarcinoma. J Clin Oncol 2011;29:4555–60.

61. Mckenzie S, Mailey B, Artinyan A, et al. Improved outcomes in the management of esophageal cancer with the addition of surgical resection to chemoradiation therapy. Ann Surg Oncol 2011;18:551–8.

62. Urba SG, Orringer MB, Turrisi A, et al. Randomized trial of preoperative chemoradiation versus surgery alone in patients with locoregional esophageal carcinoma. J Clin Oncol 2001;19:305–13.

63. Lee JL, Park SI, Kim SB, et al. A single institution phase III trial of preoperative chemotherapy with hyperfractionation radiotherapy plus surgery versus surgery alone for resectable esophageal squamous cell carcinoma. Ann Oncol 2004;15:947–54.

64. Burmeister BH, Smithers BM, Gebski V, et al. Surgery alone versus chemoradiotherapy followed by surgery for resectable cancer of the oesophagus: a randomised controlled phase III trial. Lancet Oncol 2005;6:659–68.

65. Stahl M, Walz MK, Lehmann N, et al. Phase III comparison of preoperative chemotherapy compared with chemoradiotherapy in patients with locally advanced adenocarcinoma of the esophagogastric junction. J Clin Oncol 2009;27:851–6.

66. Scheer RV, Fakiris A, Johnstone PA. Quantifying the benefit of a pathologic complete response after neoadjuvant chemoradiotherapy in the treatment of esophageal cancer. Int J Radiat Oncol Biol Phys 2011;80:996–1001.

67. Swisher SG, Wynn P, Putnam JB, et al. Salvage esophagectomy for recurrent tumors after definitive chemotherapy and radiotherapy. J Thorac Cardiovasc Surg 2002;123:175–83.

68. Kim JY, Correa AM, Vaporciyan AA, et al. Does the timing of esophagectomy after chemoradiation affect outcome? Ann Thorac Surg 2012;93:207–13.

69. Sarkaria IS, Rizk NP, Bains MS, et al. Post-treatment endoscopic biopsy is a poor-predictor of pathologic response in patients undergoing chemoradiation therapy for esophageal cancer. Ann Surg 2009;249:764–7.

70. Westerterp M, van Westreenen HL, Reitsma JB, et al. Esophageal cancer: CT, endoscopic US, and FDG PET for assessment of response to neoadjuvant therapy–systematic review. Radiology 2005;236:841–51.

71. Cerfolio RJ, Bryant AS, Ohja B, et al. The accuracy of endoscopic ultrasonography with fine-needle aspiration, integrated positron emission tomography with computed tomography, and computed tomography in restaging patients with esophageal cancer after neoadjuvant chemoradiotherapy. J Thorac Cardiovasc Surg 2005;129:1232–41.

72. Konski AA, Cheng JD, Goldberg M, et al. Correlation of molecular response as measured by 18-FDG positron emission tomography with outcome after chemoradiotherapy in patients with esophageal carcinoma. Int J Radiat Oncol Biol Phys 2007;69:358–63.

73. Roedl JB, Colen RR, Holalkere NS, et al. Adenocarcinomas of the esophagus: response to chemoradiotherapy is associated with decrease of metabolic tumor volume as measured on PET-CT. Comparison to histopathologic and clinical response evaluation. Radiother Oncol 2008;89:278–86.

74. Monjazeb AM, Riedlinger G, Aklilu M, et al. Outcomes of patients with esophageal cancer staged with [^{18}F] fluorodeoxyglucose positron emission tomography (FDG-PET): can postchemoradiotherapy FDG-PET predict the utility of resection? J Clin Oncol 2010;28:4714–21.

75. Shaikh T, Ruth K, Scott WJ, et al. Effect of increased time from chemoradiation to surgery on the pathologic complete response rate in patients with esophageal cancer. J Clin Oncol 2012;30(Suppl 4):84.

76. Chiarion-Sileni V, Corti L, Ruol A, et al. Phase II trial of docetaxel, cisplatin, and fluorouracil followed by carboplatin and radiotherapy in locally advanced oesophageal cancer. Br J Cancer 2007;96:432–8.

77. Zhao KL, Shi XH, Jiang GL, et al. Late course accelerated hyperfractionated radiotherapy plus concurrent chemotherapy for squamous cell carcinoma of the esophagus: a phase III randomized study. Int J Radiat Oncol Biol Phys 2005;62:1014–20.

78. International Commission on Radiation Units and Measurements. ICRU report 62. Prescribing, recording, and reporting photon beam therapy (Supplement to ICRU report 50). Bethesda (MD): ICRU; 1999.

79. Muijs CT, Beukema JC, Pruim J, et al. A systematic review on the role of FDG-PET/CT in tumour delineation and radiotherapy planning in patients with esophageal cancer. Radiother Oncol 2010;97:165–71.

80. Han D, Yu J, Yu Y, et al. Comparison of (18)F-fluorothymidine and (18)F-fluorodeoxyglucose PET/CT in delineating gross tumor volume by optimal threshold in patients with squamous cell carcinoma of thoracic esophagus. Int J Radiat Oncol Biol Phys 2010;76:1235–41.

81. Meier I, Merkel S, Papadopoulos T, et al. Adenocarcinoma of the esophagogastric junction: the pattern of metastatic lymph node dissemination as a rationale for elective lymphatic target definition. Int J Radiat Oncol Biol Phys 2008;70: 1408–17.
82. Zhao KL, Ma JB, Liu G, et al. Three-dimensional conformal radiation therapy for esophageal squamous cell carcinoma: is elective nodal irradiation necessary? Int J Radiat Oncol Biol Phys 2010;76:446–51.
83. Dieleman EM, Senan S, Vincent A, et al. Four-dimensional computed tomographic analysis of esophageal mobility during normal respiration. Int J Radiat Oncol Biol Phys 2007;67:775–80.
84. Patel AA, Wolfgang JA, Niemierko A, et al. Implications of respiratory motion as measured by four-dimensional computed tomography for radiation treatment planning of esophageal cancer. Int J Radiat Oncol Biol Phys 2009;74: 290–6.
85. Cohen RJ, Paskalev K, Litwin S, et al. Esophageal motion during radiotherapy: quantification and margin implications. Dis Esophagus 2010;23:473–9.
86. Han C, Schiffner DC, Schultheiss TE, et al. Residual setup errors and dose variations with less-than-daily image guided patient setup in external beam radiotherapy for esophageal cancer. Radiother Oncol 2012;102(2):309–14.
87. Hawkins MA, Brooks C, Hansen VN, et al. Cone beam computed tomography-derived adaptive radiotherapy for radical treatment of esophageal cancer. Int J Radiat Oncol Biol Phys 2010;77:378–83.
88. Bedford JL, Viviers L, Guzel Z, et al. A quantitative treatment planning study evaluating the potential of dose escalation in conformal radiotherapy of the oesophagus. Radiother Oncol 2000;57:183–93.
89. Nutting CM, Bedford JL, Cosgrove VP, et al. A comparison of conformal and intensity-modulated techniques for oesophageal radiotherapy. Radiother Oncol 2001;61:157–63.
90. Fu WH, Wang LH, Zhou ZM, et al. Comparison of conformal and intensity-modulated techniques for simultaneous integrated boost radiotherapy of upper esophageal carcinoma. World J Gastroenterol 2004;10:1098–102.
91. Chandra A, Guerrero TM, Liu HH, et al. Feasibility of using intensity-modulated radiotherapy to improve lung sparing in treatment planning for distal esophageal cancer. Radiother Oncol 2007;77:247–53.
92. Mayo CS, Urie MM, Fitzgerald TJ, et al. Hybrid IMRT for treatment of cancers of the lung and esophagus. Int J Radiat Oncol Biol Phys 2008;71:1408–18.
93. Welsh J, Palmer MB, Ajani JA, et al. Esophageal cancer dose escalation using a simultaneous integrated boost technique. Int J Radiat Oncol Biol Phys 2012; 82:468–74.
94. Isacsson U, Lenneras B, Grusell E, et al. Comparative treatment planning between proton and x-ray therapy in esophageal cancer. Int J Radiat Oncol Biol Phys 1998;41:441–50.
95. Welsh J, Gomez D, Palmer MB, et al. Intensity-modulated proton radiotherapy further reduces normal tissue exposure during definitive therapy for locally advanced distal esophageal tumors: a dosimetric study. Int J Radiat Oncol Biol Phys 2011;81:1336–42.
96. Mizumoto M, Sugahara S, Okumura T, et al. Hyperfractionated concomitant boost proton beam therapy for esophageal carcinoma. Int J Radiat Oncol Biol Phys 2011;81:601–6.
97. Marks LB, Bentzen SM, Deasy JO, et al. Radiation dose-volume effects in the lung. Int J Radiat Oncol Biol Phys 2010;76:S70–6.

98. Asakura H, Hashimoto T, Zenda S, et al. Analysis of dose-volume histogram parameters for radiation pneumonitis after definitive chemoradiotherapy for esophageal cancer. Radiother Oncol 2010;95:240–4.

99. McCurdy M, McAleer MF, Wei W, et al. Induction and concurrent taxanes enhance both the pulmonary metabolic radiation response and the radiation pneumonitis response in patients with esophagus cancer. Int J Radiat Oncol Biol Phys 2010;76:816–23.

100. Wei X, Liu HH, Tucker SL, et al. Risk factors for pericardial effusion in inoperable esophageal cancer patients treated with definitive chemoradiation therapy. Int J Radiat Oncol Biol Phys 2008;70:707–14.

101. Hancock SL, Tucker MA, Hoppe RT. Factors affecting late mortality from heart disease after treatment of Hodgkin's disease. JAMA 1993;270:1949–55.

102. Eriksson F, Gagliardi G, Liedberg A, et al. Long-term cardiac mortality following radiation therapy for Hodgkin's disease: analysis with the relative seriality model. Radiother Oncol 2000;55:153–62.

103. Nilsson G, Holmberg L, Garmo H, et al. Distribution of coronary artery stenosis after radiation for breast cancer. J Clin Oncol 2011;30:380–6.

104. Gagliardi G, Constine LS, Moiseenko V, et al. Radiation dose-volume effects in the heart. Int J Radiat Oncol Biol Phys 2010;76:S77–85.

105. Milby AB, Wojcieszynski AP, Apisarnthanarax S, et al. Long-term cardiopulmonary mortality after radiation for locally advanced esophageal cancer. J Clin Oncol 2012;30(Suppl 4):99.

106. Tait LM, Meyer JE, McSpadden E, et al. Cardiac toxicity associated with dose and gender in patients undergoing chemoradiation for esophageal carcinoma. J Clin Oncol 2012;30(Suppl 4):112.

107. Kirkpatrick JP, Van Der Kogel AJ, Schultheiss TE. Radiation dose-volume effects in the spinal cord. Int J Radiat Oncol Biol Phys 2010;76:S42–9.

108. Pan CC, Kavanagh BD, Dawson LA, et al. Radiation-associated liver injury. Int J Radiat Oncol Biol Phys 2010;76:S94–100.

109. Kavanagh BD, Pan CC, Dawson LA, et al. Radiation dose-volume effects in the stomach and small bowel. Int J Radiat Oncol Biol Phys 2010;76:S101–7.

110. Dawson LA, Kavanagh BD, Paulino AC, et al. Radiation-associated kidney injury. Int J Radiat Oncol Biol Phys 2010;76:S108–15.

111. Raja SR, Rice TW, Goldblum JR, et al. Esophageal submucosa: the watershed for esophageal cancer. J Thorac Cardiovasc Surg 2011;142:1403–11.

112. Eguchi T, Nakanishi Y, Shimoda T, et al. Histopathologic criteria for additional treatment after endoscopic mucosal resection for esophageal cancer: analysis of 464 surgically resected cases. Mod Pathol 2006;19:475–80.

113. Murakami Y, Nagata Y, Nishibuchi I, et al. Long-term outcomes of intraluminal brachytherapy in combination with external beam radiotherapy for superficial esophageal cancer. Int J Clin Oncol 2012;17(3):263–71.

114. Ishikawa H, Sakurai H, Tamaki Y, et al. Radiation therapy alone for stage I (IUC T1N0M0) squamous cell carcinoma of the esophagus: indications for surgery or combined chemoradiotherapy. J Gastroenterol Hepatol 2006;21:1290–6.

115. Sasaki T, Nakamura K, Shioyama Y, et al. Treatment outcomes of radiotherapy for patients with stage I esophageal cancer: a single institute experience. Am J Clin Oncol 2007;30:514–9.

116. Mendenhall WM, Sombeck MD, Parsons JT, et al. Management of cervical esophageal carcinoma. Semin Radiat Oncol 1994;4:179–91.

117. Pignon JP, Maitre A, Bourhis J. Meta-analysis of chemotherapy in head and neck cancer (MACH-NC): an update. Int J Radiat Oncol Biol Phys 2007;69:S112–4.

118. Tong DK, Law S, Kwong DL, et al. Current management of cervical esophageal cancer. World J Surg 2011;35:600–7.
119. Chou SH, Li HP, Lee JY, et al. Radical resection or chemoradiotherapy for cervical esophageal cancer? World J Surg 2010;34:1832–9.
120. Huang SH, Lockwood G, Brierley J, et al. Effect of concurrent high-dose cisplatin chemotherapy and conformal radiotherapy on cervical esophageal cancer survival. Int J Radiat Oncol Biol Phys 2008;71:735–40.
121. Uno T, Isobe K, Kawakami H, et al. Concurrent chemoradiation for patients with squamous cell carcinoma of the cervical esophagus. Dis Esophagus 2007;20: 12–8.
122. Wang S, Liao Z, Chen Y, et al. Esophageal cancer located at the neck and upper thorax treated with concurrent chemoradiation: a single institution experience. J Thorac Oncol 2006;1:252–9.
123. Yamada K, Murakami M, Okamoto Y, et al. Treatment results of radiotherapy for carcinoma of the cervical esophagus. Acta Oncol 2006;45:1120–5.
124. Burmeister BH, Dickie G, Smithers BM, et al. Thirty-four patients with carcinoma of the cervical esophagus treated with chemoradiation therapy. Arch Otolaryngol Head Neck Surg 2000;126:205–8.
125. Stuschke M, Stahl M, Wilke H, et al. Induction chemotherapy followed by concurrent chemotherapy and high-dose radiotherapy for locally advanced squamous cell carcinoma of the cervical oesophagus. Oncology 1999;57:99–105.
126. Iop A, Signor S, Fongione S, et al. Radiochemotherapy in the management of locally advanced carcinoma of the cervical esophagus. Proc Am Soc Clin Oncol 2003;22:1324.
127. Casas F, Ferrer F, Farrus B, et al. Primary small cell carcinoma of the esophagus: a review of the literature with emphasis on therapy and prognosis. Cancer 1997; 80:1366–72.
128. Huncharek M, Muscat J. Small cell carcinoma of the esophagus. The Massachusetts General Hospital experience, 1978 to 1993. Chest 1995;107:179–81.
129. Nichols GL, Kelsen DP. Small cell carcinoma of the esophagus. The Memorial Hospital experience 1970 to 1987. Cancer 1989;64:1531–3.
130. Chin K, Shinozaki E, Suenaga M, et al. Irinotecan plus cisplatin for small cell carcinoma of the esophagus: report of 12 cases from single institution experience. Jpn J Clin Oncol 2008;38:426–31.
131. Ku GY, Minsky BD, Rusch VW, et al. Small-cell carcinoma of the esophagus and gastroesophageal junction: review of the Memorial Sloan-Kettering experience. Ann Oncol 2008;19:533–7.
132. Kuo CH, Hsieh CC, Chan ML, et al. Small cell carcinoma of the esophagus: a report of 16 cases from a single institution and literature review. Ann Thorac Surg 2011;91:373–8.
133. Koike R, Nishimura Y, Nakamatsu K, et al. Concurrent chemoradiotherapy for esophageal cancer with malignant fistula. Int J Radiat Oncol Biol Phys 2008; 70:1418–22.
134. Ekman S, Bergqvist M, Heldin CH, et al. Activation of growth factor receptors in esophageal cancer–implications for therapy. Oncologist 2007;12:1165–77.
135. Safran H, Suntharalingam M, Dipetrillo T, et al. Cetuximab with concurrent chemoradiation for esophagogastric cancer: assessment of toxicity. Int J Radiat Oncol Biol Phys 2008;70:391–5.
136. Safran H, Dipetrillo T, Akerman P, et al. Phase I/II study of trastuzumab, paclitaxel, cisplatin and radiation for locally advanced, HER2 overexpressing, esophageal adenocarcinoma. Int J Radiat Oncol Biol Phys 2007;67:405–9.

137. Bang Y, Van Cutsem E, Feyereislova A, et al. Trastuzumab in combination with chemotherapy versus chemotherapy alone for treatment of HER2-positive advanced gastric or gastro-esophageal junction cancer (ToGA): a phase 3, open-label, randomised controlled trial. Lancet 2010;376:687–97.
138. Brien TP, Odze RD, Sheehan CE, et al. HER-2/neu gene amplification by FISH predicts poor survival in Barrett's esophagus-associated adenocarcinoma. Hum Pathol 2000;31:35–9.
139. Grugan KD, Nakagawa H. HER2 amplification in micrometastatic esophageal cancer cells predicts prognosis. Cancer Cell 2008;13:441–53.
140. Keswani RN, Chumsangsri A, Mustafi R, et al. Sorafenib inhibits MAPK-mediated proliferation in a Barrett's esophageal adenocarcinoma cell line. Dis Esophagus 2008;21:514–21.
141. Delgado JS, Mustafi R, Yee J, et al. Sorafenib triggers antiproliferative and pro-apoptotic signals in human esophageal adenocarcinoma cells. Dig Dis Sci 2008;53:3055–64.
142. Ilson D, Janjigian YY, Shah MA, et al. Phase II trial of sorafenib in esophageal and gastroesophageal junction cancer: response observed in adenocarcinoma. J Clin Oncol 2011;29(Suppl 4):41.
143. Pan JY, Ajani JA, Gu J, et al. Associations of Aurora-A (STK15) kinase polymorphisms with clinical outcome of esophageal cancer treated with preoperative chemoradiation. Cancer 2011.
144. Chen PC, Chen YC, Lai LC, et al. Use of germline polymorphisms in predicting concurrent chemoradiotherapy response in esophageal cancer. Int J Radiat Oncol Biol Phys 2012;82(5):1996–2003.
145. Alexander BM, Wang XZ, Niemierko A, et al. DNA repair biomarkers predict response to neoadjuvant chemoradiotherapy in esophageal cancer. Int J Radiat Oncol Biol Phys 2012;83(1):164–71.

Traditional Techniques of Esophagectomy

Brendon M. Stiles, MD*, Nasser K. Altorki, MD

KEYWORDS

- Esophagectomy • Ivor Lewis • Transhiatal • Three-field esophagectomy
- En bloc esophagectomy • Lymph node dissection

KEY POINTS

- Despite the common practice of incorporating chemotherapy or chemoradiotherapy into the treatment paradigm of esophageal cancer, surgical resection remains the cornerstone of most treatment protocols for early stage and locally advanced disease.
- Primary surgical resection should be considered the standard of care for localized esophageal adenocarcinoma.
- Many methods of esophagectomy exist, with no clear consensus as to which technique is superior regarding oncologic outcome.
- Transthoracic approaches to esophagectomy facilitate a more extensive lymph node dissection, while the transhiatal approach is associated with less surgical morbidity.
- The surgeon should balance oncologic principles (surgical margins and adequacy of lymphadenectomy) with the perceived risks of the operative approach on a case-by-case basis.

INTRODUCTION

Esophageal cancer (EC) is the sixth most common cause of cancer deaths worldwide.[1] Treatment of this disease represents a formidable challenge, with an overall survival (OS) of only 10% to 15%. Despite the common practice of incorporating chemotherapy or chemoradiotherapy into the treatment paradigm of EC, surgical resection remains the cornerstone of most treatment protocols for early stage and locally advanced disease.[2] With improvements in surgical techniques and perioperative care, surgical mortality from esophagectomy has decreased steadily over the past three decades. However, considerable controversy exists as to the best surgical approach to EC and to the extent of lymph node dissection necessary during the course of the operation. Although minimally invasive techniques have been used, a variety of traditional surgical approaches are more frequently used. These approaches include transhiatal

Cardiothoracic Surgery, Weill Cornell Medical College, New York-Presbyterian Hospital, 525 East 68th Street, Suite M404, New York, NY 10024, USA
* Corresponding author.
E-mail address: brs9035@med.cornell.edu

Surg Clin N Am 92 (2012) 1249–1263
http://dx.doi.org/10.1016/j.suc.2012.08.001
0039-6109/12/$ – see front matter © 2012 Elsevier Inc. All rights reserved.

(cervical incision and laparotomy); Ivor Lewis (right thoracotomy and laparotomy); McKeown (cervical incision, right thoracotomy, and laparotomy); and left thoracoabdominal. An en bloc dissection, resecting the tumor-bearing esophagus with a wide envelope of adjoining periesophageal tissue, can be performed with any of the transthoracic approaches.

Great variability in technique also exists with regard to the lymphadenectomy, another important component of the surgical strategy. The extent of lymphadenectomy is typically described by fields, with the first, second, and third fields indicating resection of the abdominal, infra-azygous thoracic, and upper thoracic and cervical nodes, respectively. Most surgeons resect nodes from at least the first and second fields, whereas a minority also perform nodal dissection of the third field.

A recent international survey queried high-volume surgeons as to their preferred approaches to esophagectomy.[3] The most common approaches used are the transhiatal (35%–44% of the time) and Ivor Lewis (36%–50% of the time), with variability depending on the location of the primary tumor (**Fig. 1**).[3] A minority of surgeons prefer en bloc (14%–18%) or minimally invasive techniques (3.9–6.5%) during these resections. Only a small percentage performed a three-field lymph node dissection, more frequently for proximal tumors than for gastroesophageal junction tumors, 13% versus 1.3%. Such variability is a reflection of the fact that there are no level 1 data to support the routine use of any one particular technique. In general, the surgical approach should be determined by oncologic principles for individual tumors, balanced against the risk of complications in a patient-specific manner.

TRANSHIATAL ESOPHAGECTOMY

Transhiatal esophagectomy is one of the most common techniques for esophagectomy in North America and Europe. The first attempts at transhiatal resection are credited to Wolfgang Denk of Austria and Alwin von Ach of Germany who used animal models and cadavers.[4,5] Turner[6] is credited with performing the first successful transhiatal esophagectomy in a patient. However, over the next several decades, because of concerns about mediastinal bleeding this technique was not commonly used,

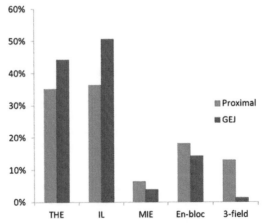

Fig. 1. Surgical approaches used by an international sample of high-volume surgeons (n = 77) for gastroesophageal junction (GEJ) and more proximal esophageal cancers.[3] Multiple responses could be given for each scenario. IL, Ivor Lewis esophagectomy; MIE, minimally invasive esophagectomy; THE, transhiatal esophagectomy.

particularly as transthoracic approaches became more feasible. Orringer and Sloan[7] reintroduced the technique in 1978 as a less morbid alternative to transthoracic resection. It has subsequently been advocated by numerous groups. In the previously mentioned survey, transhiatal esophagectomy was performed in 35% of patients with carcinoma of the proximal esophagus and 44% of patients with carcinoma of the distal third of the esophagus.[3] The procedure entails extirpation of the intrathoracic esophagus without a thoracotomy and advancement of the esophageal substitute, usually a greater curvature gastric tube, to the neck for reconstruction.

Technique

The patient is positioned supine with the neck extended. Arms are tucked and the skin is prepared from the chin to the pubis. The abdominal phase is begun first. A supraumbilical incision is performed from the xiphoid process to the umbilicus. The left lobe of the liver is retracted after division of the left triangular ligament, enhancing hiatal exposure. A table-mounted self-retaining retractor is placed. The peritoneal cavity and stomach are inspected for extramural disease or bulky adenopathy. The right gastroepiploic artery is palpated early to ensure its suitability as a vascular supply to the gastric conduit. The gastrohepatic ligament is opened up to the right crura, with care taken to avoid inadvertent division of any replaced hepatic vessels. The greater omentum is detached from the colon in the avascular plane between it and the mesocolon until the lesser sac is entered. Alternatively the greater omentum is divided at a safe distance from the gastroepiploic arcade to access the lesser sac. With the lesser sac entered, the authors work progressively upward and to the left dividing the gastrocolic and gastrosplenic ligaments, typically dividing the short gastric vessels with a harmonic scalpel or Ligasure device (Covidien, Boulder, CO, USA). When dividing the short gastric vessels, care is taken to maintain the energy source away from the wall of the stomach. High on the greater curvature, posterior peritoneal attachments of the fundus to the diaphragm are divided. The peritoneum overlying the esophageal hiatus is incised to meet the previous dissection. The esophagus can now be encircled with a Penrose drain and retracted upward. Upward retraction is also placed on the underside of the stomach. Attachments of the stomach to the posterior peritoneum overlying the pancreas are sometimes encountered, but are easily divided sharply or with electrocautery. The left gastric vein and artery are then sharply dissected with overlying lymph nodes swept up with the specimen (**Fig. 2**). The artery is then divided at its origin from the celiac axis, typically using a vascular stapler. The vein can either be divided separately first or taken at the same time as the artery if both are cleared of overlying lymph nodes. The stomach is further mobilized from the omentum more distally along the greater curve, again using the harmonic scalpel or Ligasure. Additionally, as one approaches the pylorus it is easy to cause a traction injury to the gastroepiploic vein or artery. Great care must be taken here to preserve the vessels. The authors do not typically perform a Kocher maneuver.

At this point, the cervical phase is begun. A 4-cm collar incision is made, typically within one of the skin creases in the neck. The authors prefer a left-sided neck incision for transhiatal esophagectomy. For transthoracic esophagectomy, the neck is opened on the same side as the thoracotomy. The incision is begun just to the right of the midline and carried leftward over the sternocleidomastoid muscle. The platysma and omohyoid muscles are divided and the sternocleidomastoid muscle is retracted laterally. The trachea and esophagus are retracted medially and the carotid sheath and its contents retracted laterally, typically with the assistance of a self-retaining retractor. If need be, the middle thyroid vein and inferior thyroid artery may be divided

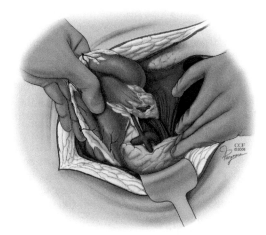

Fig. 2. The celiac axis is dissected easily from the lateral approach. (*Reprinted* with permission, Cleveland Clinic Center for Medical Art & Photography © 2006–2012. All Rights Reserved.)

to facilitate exposure. A sharp dissection using Metzenbaum scissors is then carried posteriorly to the prevertebral fascia. The prevertebral space is then developed bluntly using finger dissection. Subsequently, gentle dissection posterior to the trachea is performed, staying right on the esophagus in the tracheoesophageal groove. The cervical esophagus can then be encircled with a Penrose drain and retracted upward. The esophagus is then bluntly mobilized distally, again keeping the dissection on the esophageal wall.

After the proximal and distal esophagus has been encircled, the transhiatal phase of the operation is begun. Traction is placed on both portions of the esophagus, with careful blunt dissection performed in each direction (**Fig. 3**). Inferiorly and posterior to the esophagus, a hand is inserted through the diaphragmatic hiatus and advanced superiorly. For lower tumors, the mass is carefully dissected free from adjacent structures. The transhiatal dissection then proceeds in a sequential fashion, dividing anterior, posterior, and finally lateral attachments up to the level of the carina. It is essential that the dissection is kept as close to the esophageal wall as possible during the entire mediastinal phase. Lateral esophageal attachments can typically be delivered into the abdomen with a downward raking motion and cauterized or clipped. More commonly, the hiatus is enlarged and at least the lower mediastinal dissection is carried out under direct vision. In the case of lower third and gastroesophageal junction tumors, this maneuver permits a wider dissection around the tumor. Mobilization of the esophagus above the carina is accomplished by keeping the dissection directly on the esophageal wall anteriorly to avoid injury to the membranous trachea (**Fig. 4**). Posterior dissection is carried out in the same manner. Finally, lateral attachments are divided by sliding the index and middle fingers along the sides of the organ. Structures at risk during this maneuver include the arch of the azygos vein and the left recurrent nerve. The proximal esophagus is then delivered into the cervical incision. It is divided sharply and three stay sutures of 3–0 silk are placed proximally to splay it open. The distal end is oversewn and attached to a long 1-in wide Penrose drain. This is then pulled down through the posterior mediastinum and the esophagus delivered into the abdomen. Esophagus and stomach are delivered out of the abdominal incision and any further distal mobilization of the stomach is performed with it on traction.

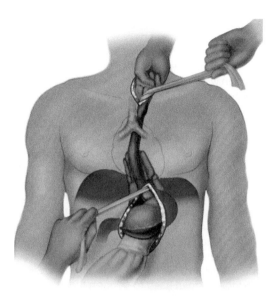

Fig. 3. The initial phase of the distal transhiatal esophageal mobilization is carried out posterior to the esophagus along the prevertebral fascia with the volar aspects of the fingers kept against the esophagus. (*From* Orringer MB. Transhiatal esophagectomy without thoracotomy. Oper Tech Thorac Cardiovasc Surg 2005;10:63; with permission.)

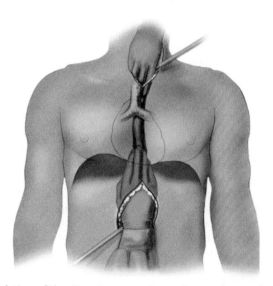

Fig. 4. After completion of the dissection posterior to the esophagus, the anterior esophageal dissection is next performed. The esophagogastric junction is gently retracted inferiorly by the rubber drain encircling the esophagogastric junction, and the surgeon's hand is inserted against the anterior wall of the esophagus palm downward and is advanced upward into the mediastinum. (*From* Orringer MB. Transhiatal esophagectomy without thoracotomy. Oper Tech Thorac Cardiovasc Surg 2005;10:63; with permission.)

While it is maintained on traction, the stomach is transected from the fundus to the third or fourth branch of the left gastric artery using surgical staplers, taking care to obtain an adequate distal margin on the tumor. This preserves a full length of stomach for advancement into the neck. The specimen is handed off. The proximal gastric staple line is then oversewn with 3–0 Lembert silk stitches. A standard pyloromyotomy is then performed bridging approximately 2 cm of stomach and duodenum. It is over-sewn in a transverse fashion using 3–0 silk sutures.

At this point, the gastric conduit is passed into the neck. It is attached to the distal end of the large Penrose drain with two long sutures of different colors to maintain orientation. This attachment is done to the posterior aspect of the stomach so as not to injure the anterior wall to which the anastomosis will be performed. The stomach is then brought up to the cervical incision with a combination of gentle upward traction on the drain, but more importantly with a careful pushing motion from below, maintaining its orientation as it passes transhiatally. Typically, 4 to 5 cm of stomach may be delivered into the neck incision. In a healthy-appearing area of the stomach, several centimeters distal to its tip, the authors then place two 3–0 silk stay sutures. A small vertical gastrotomy is then performed with electrocautery. The posterior wall of the esophagus and anterior wall of the esophagus are then aligned. A 3-cm long, 3.5-mm laparoscopic stapler is then used to perform the posterior wall of the anastomosis. This staple line is then reinforced with several interrupted 3–0 silk sutures placed from the inside of the anastomosis. The anterior wall is then approximated with a single-layer running anastomosis using a 3–0 monofilament absorbable suture, begun at each corner and tied in the middle. Care should be taken to incorporate the esophageal mucosa into each bite. The authors take relatively large bites, at least 5 mm deep on the gastric side. After the anastomosis has been performed, any redundant stomach is retracted into the abdomen. A nasogastric tube is passed carefully under direct palpation and left with its tip terminating above the pylorus. The gastric tube is then secured to the diaphragmatic hiatus anteriorly and posteriorly using long 2–0 silk sutures to prevent intrathoracic herniation of abdominal viscera. A feeding jejunostomy is also routinely placed. The cervical wound is closed loosely, only at the level of the skin. The abdominal fascia is closed with running #1 monofilament absorbable suture and the skin with staples.

TRANSTHORACIC ESOPHAGECTOMY

Transthoracic esophagectomy is the most widely performed approach for cancer of the esophagus worldwide.[3] The procedure can be carried out through a right or left thoracotomy, depending on the preference of the surgeon and the location of the tumor within the esophagus. Generally, a right thoracotomy is required for adequate exposure of tumors in the middle or upper thirds that are anatomically intimately related to the membranous trachea or the arch of the aorta. Tumors located at the gastroesophageal junction or in the lower third of the esophagus can sometimes also be approached through a left thoracotomy incision combined with a left phrenotomy or, alternatively, with a left thoracoabdominal incision.

Ivor Lewis Esophagectomy

Lewis[8] first proposed a combined laparotomy and right thoracotomy approach in 1946. Historically, this was performed as a two-stage procedure with a week separating the laparotomy and thoracotomy. It has since evolved to the standard one-stage procedure in common use today. The patient is positioned supine and an upper midline incision performed. The abdominal phase is carried out in an almost identical fashion to that performed during transhiatal dissection. With a self-retaining retractor in place, the abdomen is explored and the stomach mobilized. Great care is taken in identifying and preserving the right gastroepiploic artery. After all other attachments and blood vessels have been divided and an extensive abdominal lymphadenectomy completed, the distal esophagus is dissected free from its hiatal attachments. The hiatus is manually enlarged so that it may easily accommodate the gastric conduit. Much of the dissection of the distal esophagus can be performed bluntly through the abdomen, again similar to the transhiatal approach. Before completion of the abdominal phase, the authors perform a pyloromyotomy and feeding jejunostomy. The abdomen is then closed and the patient repositioned to a left lateral decubitus position for a right thoracotomy. The authors typically have anesthesia place a double-lumen endotracheal tube before repositioning.

The thoracic phase is performed through a posterolateral thoracotomy through the fifth interspace, sparing the serratus muscle. The right lung is selectively deflated and retracted anteriorly. First, the azygous vein is transected with a thoracoscopic vascular stapler. The pleura overlying the esophagus is opened sharply anterior to the azygous vein. The esophagus is then dissected circumferentially in the region above the tumor. Once free, an umbilical tape is looped around it for traction. The dissection should be carried above the level of the azygous vein superiorly. Inferiorly, the esophagus is dissected from its bed circumferentially to the hiatus. Lymphatics should be ligated or clipped to decrease the incidence of chylothorax.

The stomach is then pulled through the chest through the widened hiatus. It is subsequently divided and tubularized with several fires of a GIA stapler, reinforced with interrupted sutures. The esophagogastric anastomosis can be performed in a variety of ways. Some use an end-to-end anastomotic stapler. The authors prefer to staple the anastomosis posteriorly with a hand sewn anterior closure using a continuous absorbable suture. A nasogastric tube is positioned in the intrathoracic conduit. Any redundant stomach is returned back to the abdomen to straighten the conduit, which helps to ensure proper gastric emptying. The edges of the gastric tube are sutured to the edge of the hiatus to prevent visceral herniation.

McKeown Modification

McKeown[9] described his three-stage variation in 1976. The technique allows for a greater length of the proximal esophagus to be resected and for the anastomosis to be placed in the cervical region. Many surgeons prefer this approach for middle and upper ECs. In the original description the abdominal incision was performed first followed by the thoracotomy from the same modified decubitus position. Most surgeons now perform the right thoracotomy first, especially if there is concern to intrathoracic resectability. The thoracic phase proceeds in the same way as described previously for the Ivor Lewis esophagectomy, except that the proximal esophagus is completely circumferentially mobilized up and into the thoracic inlet. After mobilization of the esophagus, a chest tube is placed and the thoracotomy closed. The double-lumen endotracheal tube is switched to a single-lumen tube after turning the patient to the supine position. The neck is extended and prepared simultaneously with the abdomen to proceed with the abdominal and cervical approaches.

The abdominal procedure is performed first. After the stomach is mobilized as described previously, a right collar incision is performed and the cervical esophagus mobilized. The right-sided incision is preferable because the esophagus has already typically been dissected up into the right thoracic inlet during the thoracic portion of the case. Care is taken to avoid the recurrent laryngeal nerve. The esophagus is transected in the neck and a Penrose drain sutured to the cut specimen end before it is delivered through the mediastinum into the abdomen. After preparation of the gastric tube, the specimen is sent off the field and the gastric conduit advanced into the neck, guided by the Penrose drain. The anastomosis is performed in an identical fashion to the transhiatal approach.

Left Transthoracic Approach

A left transthoracic approach provides excellent exposure of the lower mediastinum, hiatal tunnel, and upper abdomen. Such an approach is well suited for patients with tumors of the lower third of the esophagus and the gastroesophageal junction. However, the authors use it rarely given the excellent exposure afforded by some of the other techniques. The patient is placed in the right lateral decubitus position with the table flexed. Through a straight left lateral thoracotomy, the chest is entered through the sixth interspace. Although others have recommended the division of the costal arch, the authors do not find this necessary for adequate exposure. Its division may increase postoperative discomfort. The mediastinal pleura is incised and the esophagus mobilized and encircled with a Penrose drain. Next, the diaphragm is incised in a semilunar fashion from sternum to spleen to minimize phrenic injury and to facilitate later diaphragmatic closure. The abdomen is explored to assess resectability and the stomach mobilized as previously described. The stomach is then brought through the hiatus. The esophagus is transected 8 to 10 cm proximal to the tumor, and the stomach is divided distally, creating a greater curvature tube for reconstruction. The gastric conduit is passed through the hiatus and the anastomosis performed either in the mediastinum or, preferably, in the neck. The latter is accomplished by bluntly mobilizing the esophagus from underneath the aortic arch and throughout the superior mediastinum. The gastric conduit is then passed underneath the aortic arch and attached to the esophageal stump and safely positioned in the cervical prevertebral space. After closure of the thoracotomy, the patient is placed in a supine position and a small transverse cervical incision is performed, typically on the left. The prevertebral space is entered and esophagus and stomach retrieved for an end-to-side cervical esophagogastrostomy.

En Bloc Esophagectomy

The deep location of the esophagus within the narrow confines of the mediastinum and the lack of a well-defined mesentery have been seen to preclude the application of en bloc resection principles, practiced in most gastrointestinal malignancies, from patients with esophageal carcinoma. Debate therefore exists as to the feasibility and efficacy of radical esophageal resections, with most surgeons favoring more limited transthoracic or transhiatal approaches. However, the authors' group and others advocate an en bloc approach to resection of the esophagus in the hope of altering the natural history of this disease. Logan[10] introduced the en bloc concept in 1963, which was later reintroduced by Skinner[11] in 1979. The basic principle underlying the operation is resecting the tumor-bearing esophagus with a wide envelope of adjoining periesophageal tissue that includes pleural surfaces laterally and pericardium anteriorly. The lymphatics between the esophagus and aorta, including the thoracic duct, are resected en bloc with the esophagus, along with the surrounding mediastinal lymph nodes from the tracheal bifurcation to the hiatus (**Fig. 5**). An upper abdominal lymphadenectomy is also performed that includes the common hepatic, celiac, left gastric, lesser curvature, parahiatal, and retroperitoneal nodes.

An en bloc dissection may be performed with any of the transthoracic approaches. For the three-hole procedure with a cervical anastomosis, the operation is begun in the chest, whereas for an Ivor Lewis esophagectomy the thoracic portion is performed

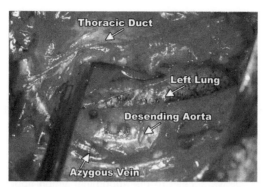

Fig. 5. The lymphatics between the esophagus and aorta, including the thoracic duct, are resected en bloc with the esophagus, along with the surrounding mediastinal lymph nodes from the tracheal bifurcation to the hiatus. (*From* Shields TW, LoCicero J, Reed CE, et al, editors. General thoracic surgery. 7th edition. Philadelphia: Lippincott Williams & Wilkins; 2009, p. 1762; with permission.)

subsequent to the abdominal phase. In the chest, entered through the fifth interspace, the tumor-bearing esophagus is resected en bloc with an envelope of adjoining tissues that includes both pleural surfaces laterally and all lymphovascular tissues wedged dorsally between the esophagus and the spine. The dissection begins by incising the pleura just anterior to the main trunk of the azygous vein throughout its course. The dissection proceeds leftward toward the aortic adventitia, thus mobilizing the thoracic duct throughout its course in the lower and middle mediastinum. The duct is ligated proximally at the aortic hiatus and distally as it crosses to the left side at the level of the aortic arch. Dissection continues anterior to the aorta toward the left pleura, which is incised from the level of the left main bronchus to the diaphragm, completing the posterior mediastinectomy. The anterior dissection begins by division of the azygos vein at its caval junction. Dissection then proceeds along the back of the hilum of the right lung, sweeping all lymphatic tissues, including the subcarinal nodal chain, toward the specimen. For tumors abutting the pericardium, a patch of pericardium is incised en bloc with the specimen, whereas for tumors traversing the esophageal hiatus, a 1-in cuff of diaphragm is resected circumferentially around the tumor. As described, the thoracic en bloc resection therefore includes a complete dissection of the middle and lower mediastinal nodes, including the periesophageal, parahiatal, and subcarinal nodes.

For the abdominal portion of the operation, whether performed before or after the thoracic phase, an aggressive lymph node dissection is also performed by the authors. After entry into the lesser sac and division of the short gastric vessels, the retroperitoneum is incised along the superior border of the pancreas. The retroperitoneal lymphatic and areolar tissues are swept superiorly toward the esophageal hiatus and medially along the splenic artery to the celiac trifurcation. The left gastric artery is divided flush with its celiac origin and the nodes along the common hepatic artery are dissected toward the specimen. This retroperitoneal dissection is bound by the dissected esophageal hiatus superiorly, the hilum of the spleen laterally, and the common hepatic artery and inferior vena cava medially. Finally the lesser curvature and left gastric nodes are included with the specimen as the gastric tube is prepared. After complete mobilization of the gastric conduit and lymphadenectomy, the cancer-bearing specimen is transected proximally and distally and handed off en bloc. The gastric tube is then advanced through the posterior mediastinum and the anastomosis completed as previously described.

THREE-FIELD LYMPH NODE DISSECTION

There is considerable controversy regarding the extent of lymph node dissection necessary during the course of esophagectomy. One view holds that the disease is systemic at the time of diagnosis and that extensive nodal dissection results in potentially higher morbidity with little or no survival benefit. The countervailing opinion holds that a more extensive lymph node dissection permits more accurate staging of patients with EC, eliminates known or occult locoregional disease thereby improving local control, and possibly enhances survival. This view is supported by recent reports suggesting that a greater extent of lymphadenectomy is associated with increased survival for patients with EC.[12–14]

The extent of lymphadenectomy is highly dependent on the surgical approach. The transhiatal approach allows access to the abdominal lymph nodes and to only the lowest periesophageal lymph nodes in the chest. In contrast, most surgeons are able to perform an adequate two-field lymphadenectomy when using transthoracic approaches, which includes resection of the abdominal and the infra-azygous thoracic nodes. Most of the third field upper thoracic and recurrent laryngeal nodes may also be reached from the chest, whereas cervical nodes can only be removed using a neck incision, performed in either a transhiatal or "three-hole" McKeown-type operation **(Fig. 6)**.

The extended lymphadenectomy was introduced by Japanese surgeons, who demonstrated that up to 40% of patients resected by radical two-field esophagectomy developed recurrences in the cervical nodes.[15] They therefore extended their resection to encompass the so-called "third field," including the cervical and superior mediastinal recurrent laryngeal lymph node chains. Much of the third field dissection can be performed from the chest after completely mobilizing the esophagus. Dissection of the nodes in the superior mediastinum includes the nodes along the right and left recurrent laryngeal nerves throughout their mediastinal course. The left recurrent nerve is exposed from the level of the aortic arch to the thoracic inlet and dissected using a "no-touch" technique. Although there is often a paucity of nodal tissue along the left nerve, nodes may often be found along its anterior aspect and carefully excised. The right recurrent nodal chain can be identified by following the vagus nerve back to the origin of the recurrent laryngeal nerve near the base of the right subclavian artery. The right recurrent nodal chain begins at that level and forms a continuous

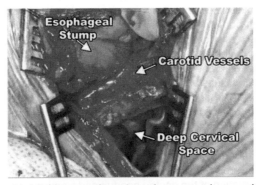

Fig. 6. Most of the third-field upper thoracic and recurrent laryngeal nodes may also be reached from the chest, whereas cervical nodes can only be removed using a neck incision, performed in either a transhiatal or "three-hole" McKeown-type operation. (*Courtesy of Dr Nasser K. Altorki, New York, NY.*)

package that extends through the thoracic inlet to the neck. This packet can be removed en bloc, again using a strict "no-touch" technique. All of these nodes should be appropriately labeled as cervicothoracic nodes, rather than as cervical nodes. When these nodes are positive, or when cervical nodes are apparent on preoperative imaging, they are dissected through the cervical incision, with particular attention to the lower deep cervical nodes located posterior and lateral to the carotid sheath.

RESULTS
Comparison of Transhiatal and Transthoracic Esophagectomy

Several retrospective studies have compared operative mortality and morbidity of transhiatal versus transthoracic esophagectomy. Hulscher and coworkers[16] reviewed the results from 50 series published between 1990 and 1999. In-hospital mortality was 5.7% after transhiatal and 9.2% after transthoracic esophagectomy. Major pulmonary complications were more common in the transthoracic group, 18.7% versus 12.7% (confidence interval [CI], 1.29–1.68), whereas cardiac complications (6.6% vs 19.5%; CI, 0.27–0.41), vocal cord paralysis (3.5% vs 9.5%; CI, 0.27–0.47), and anastomotic leak (7.2% vs 13.6%) were lower in the transthoracic compared with the transhiatal group. Transhiatal esophagectomy was associated with a shorter hospital stay (17.8 days vs 21 days; $P<.0001$). In these studies, there was no clear survival difference after transhiatal versus transthoracic surgical approaches. In the meta-analysis, although the influence of cell type on survival was not specifically examined, there was no statistically significant difference in overall 3- and 5-year survival between the two procedures. Five-year survival was 21.7% for transhiatal and 23% for transthoracic approaches.[16]

The only randomized trial reported to date comparing transthoracic with transhiatal esophagectomy was reported by Hulscher and associates[17] in 2002. The authors randomly assigned 220 patients with adenocarcinoma of the mid to distal esophagus, or adenocarcinoma of the cardia, to either a transhiatal (n = 106) resection or a transthoracic (n = 114) esophagectomy with extended en bloc lymphadenectomy. Although there was no difference in in-hospital mortality (4% vs 2%; $P = .4$), complications were more frequent in the transthoracic group (57% vs 27%; $P<.001$). Median intensive care unit stay (6 vs 2 days) and hospital stay (19 vs 15 days) were longer in the transthoracic group than in the transhiatal group ($P<.001$). This study was powered to detect a 50% relative improvement in survival in favor of the en bloc procedure. Although there was an important trend favoring the transthoracic group in overall (39% vs 29%) and disease-free survival (39% vs 27%) at 5 years, the resultant 25% relative improvement in survival did not achieve statistical significance. There were a significantly greater number of nodes resected with the transthoracic approach (31 vs 16; $P<.001$). A later subgroup analysis subsequently showed that the benefit of en bloc resection was particularly evident in patients with esophageal tumors as opposed to tumors of the gastric cardia.[18] Transthoracic resection resulted in a 14% 5-year survival benefit (51% vs 37% for transhiatal resection). Outcomes could also be assessed and patients subdivided by the number of positive lymph nodes. In patients without any positive nodes and in those with greater than eight metastatic nodes, there was no difference in overall or disease-free survival between the approaches. However, in those patients with one to eight positive nodes, there was an OS difference of 20% favoring the transthoracic approach (39% vs 19%; $P = .05$). The difference in disease-free survival was even more dramatic in this subset of patients, again favoring transthoracic as opposed to transhiatal resection (64% vs 23%; $P = .02$).

Evidence Supporting Extended Lymphadenectomy

No matter the surgical approach, reliable evidence in support of extended lymphadenectomy has been obtained from large population-based registries and multi-institutional observational studies (**Table 1**). Two recent studies analyzed data from the Surveillance Epidemiology and End Results (SEER) database for an association between the total number of lymph nodes removed and OS in EC. Schwarz and Smith[19] analyzed data from approximately 2600 patients with EC treated by esophagectomy, on whom full nodal staging information was available. Multivariate analysis identified that total nodal count, modeled as a continuous variable, was an independent predictor of OS regardless of nodal status (N0 or N1) or tumor histology. The best OS was observed when more than 30 lymph nodes were examined. Using linear regression modeling, the authors calculated a 10% and 3% relative increase in 5-year OS for every 10 extra lymph nodes examined for N0 and N1 patients, respectively. Groth and colleagues[20] also analyzed the SEER database for EC to examine the association between lymph node count and all-cause mortality. Recursive partitioning analysis was used to stratify 4882 patients based on the number of lymph nodes examined. The authors concluded that to maximize all-cause and cancer-specific survival, patients with EC should have at least 30 lymph nodes examined pathologically (hazard ratio 0.58 for cancer specific survival).

In addition to these population-based studies, two large multi-institutional studies were recently reported that examined the association between the number of lymph nodes and survival in patients with EC treated by esophagectomy without preoperative therapy. Peyre and colleagues[12] constructed a database of over 2300 patients with EC from nine esophageal centers worldwide. Cox regression analysis showed that the number of lymph nodes removed was an independent predictor of survival ($P < .0001$). The optimal threshold predicted by Cox regression for this survival benefit was removal of a minimum of 23 nodes. From the Worldwide Esophageal Cancer Collaboration database, Rizk and colleagues[13] reported on 4627 patients with EC with adenocarcinoma and squamous cell carcinoma treated at 13 different institutions worldwide. Risk-adjusted survival was estimated using random survival forests and was averaged for each number of lymph nodes resected. The optimum number of lymph nodes resected were T-classification, N-classification, and cell type dependent. Optimum lymphadenectomy for pN0M0 patient was 10 to 12, 15 to 22, and 31 to 42 for pT1, pT2, and pT3/4 tumors, respectively. For pN+M0 cancers with up to six positive nodes, optimum lymphadenectomy was 10, 15, and 29 to 50 for pT1, T2, and T3/4 tumors, respectively.

Data also exist to support a three-field lymphadenectomy in appropriate clinical circumstances. The authors and others have reported a 25% rate of cervical and recurrent laryngeal nerve lymph node metastases among patients undergoing a three field lymph node dissection, which includes removal of these upper nodal chains.[21,22] The authors have therefore attempted to identify at-risk patients for cervicothoracic nodal metastases and have begun to tailor their nodal dissection to high-risk patients. Variables significantly associated with positive cervical or recurrent laryngeal nodes include squamous cell histology, proximal location, the presence of clinical nodal disease, and higher pT and pN classifications.[21] They therefore advocate dissection of the third field, for all tumors of squamous cell carcinoma histology, and for adenocarcinomas with transmural spread or evidence of nodal disease at lower stations. In this setting, up to a third of patients will have recurrent laryngeal or cervical nodal mestastases.

Table 1
Population or multi-institutional studies supporting extended lymphadenectomy in patients undergoing esophagectomy

Author	Patients	Findings	Recommendations
Schwarz and Smith,[19] 2007: SEER database 1973–2003	5620	Higher total LN count (>30) and negative LN count (>15) associated with improved survival (P<.001); relative increase in overall survival of 4%–5% at 5 y for every 10 LN identified.	Obtain ≥30 LN to optimize staging, survival, and locoregional control
Groth et al,[20] 2010: SEER database 1988–2005	4882 (including patients with neoadjuvant therapy)	Significant difference between stratified LN groups in all-cause (P<.001) and cancer-specific (P = .004) mortality. Cancer-specific morality hazard ratio of 0.58 (confidence interval, 0.44–0.78) with ≥30 LN.	Obtain ≥15 LN to maximize the likelihood of detecting LN metastases; obtain ≥30 LN to optimize cancer-specific mortality
Peyre et al,[12] 2008: Patients from nine international centers before 2002	2303 (surgery alone)	Best threshold of LN removed to maximize survival was 23–29; even when minimum threshold of 23 nodes was achieved, 5-y survival was better after en bloc resection than after lesser types.	To maximize outcome of surgical resection, ≥23 nodes should be removed. En bloc resection is most likely to meet this threshold.
Rizk et al,[13] 2010: Worldwide Esophageal Cancer Collaboration	4627 (surgery alone)	Optimum LN dissection is defined by T classification and histopathologic type; for pN0M0 moderately or poorly differentiated cancers and for all pN+ cancers, 5-y survival improved with increasing LN dissection.	Resect ≥10 LN for pT1, ≥20 LN for pT2, and ≥30 LN for pT3/T4 cancers

Abbreviations: LN, lymph node; SEER, Surveillance Epidemiology and End Results.

PERSPECTIVE

Primary surgical resection should be considered the standard of care for localized esophageal adenocarcinoma. Recent progress in surgical outcomes has been well demonstrated in data from the National Inpatient Sample Database, in which hospital mortality fell from 12.1% in 1998, to 9% in 2002, and to 7% in 2006.[23] This improvement is likely the result of improved surgical technique, but also of improved perioperative care and better patient selection. The results after various surgical approaches suggest that there are only minor substantive differences in mortality, morbidity, or survival between transhiatal and conventional transthoracic esophagectomy. The single randomized trial of transthoracic en bloc esophagectomy versus transhiatal esophagectomy suggests that there may well be a small but significant survival benefit of the transthoracic approach in patients with adenocarcinoma of the middle and distal esophageal thirds, particularly in those with a limited burden of metastatic nodal disease (one to eight positive lymph nodes). These results need to be confirmed by similar trials. The role of three-field lymph node dissection also needs to be further evaluated and more precisely defined, ideally in the context of clinical trials.

SUMMARY

Various possible operative approaches exist to treat patients with EC. Many of the traditional methods of esophagectomy described in this article can also be replicated with minimally invasive techniques. In general, the surgeon should balance oncologic principles (surgical margins and adequacy of lymphadenectomy) with the perceived risks of the operative approach on a case-by-case basis. Although it is tempting to routinely use the same approach to suit individual or institutional practice patterns, there is little doubt that patient-related characteristics and tumor-specific characteristics should play a role in the surgical decision making.

REFERENCES

1. Jemal A, Siegel R, Xu J, et al. Cancer statistics, 2010. CA Cancer J Clin 2010;60: 277–300.
2. DeMeester SR. Adenocarcinoma of the esophagus and cardia: a review of the disease and its treatment. Ann Surg Oncol 2006;13:12–30.
3. Enestvedt CK, Perry KA, Kim C, et al. Trends in the management of esophageal carcinoma based on provider volume: treatment practices of 618 esophageal surgeons. Dis Esophagus 2010;23:136–44.
4. Denk W. Zur radikaloperation des oesophaguskarzinoms. Zentralbl Chir 1913;40: 1065.
5. Dubecz A, Kun L, Stadlhuber RJ, et al. The origins of an operation: a brief history of transhiatal esophagectomy. Ann Surg 2009;249:535–40.
6. Turner G. Excision of the thoracic esophagus for carcinoma. Lancet 1933;2:1315.
7. Orringer MB, Sloan H. Esophagectomy without thoracotomy. J Thorac Cardiovasc Surg 1978;76:643–54.
8. Lewis I. The surgical treatment of carcinomas of the oeshophagus with special reference to a new operation for growths of the middle third. Br J Surg 1946; 34:18.
9. McKeown KC. Total three-stage oesophaectomy for cancer of the oesophagus. Br J Surg 1976;63:259.
10. Logan A. The surgical treatment of carcinoma of the esophagus and cardia. J Thorac Cardiovasc Surg 1963;46:150–61.

11. Skinner DB. En-bloc resection for neoplasms of the esophagus and cardia. J Thorac Cardiovasc Surg 1983;85:59–69.
12. Peyre CG, Hagen JA, DeMeester SR, et al. The number of lymph nodes removed predicts survival in esophageal cancer: an international study on the impact of extent of surgical resection. Ann Surg 2008;248:549–56.
13. Rizk NP, Ishwaran H, Rice TW, et al. Optimum lymphadencectomy for esophageal cancer. Ann Surg 2010;251:46–50.
14. Lee PC, Mirza FM, Port JL, et al. Predictors of recurrence and disease-free survival in patients with completely resected esophageal carcinoma. J Thorac Cardiovasc Surg 2011;141:1196–206.
15. Isono K, Onada S, Okuyama K, et al. Recurrence of intrathoracic esophageal cancer. Jpn J Clin Oncol 1985;15:49–60.
16. Hulscher JB, Tijssen JG, Obertop H, et al. Transthoracic versus transhiatal resection for carcinoma of the esophagus: a meta-analysis. Ann Thorac Surg 2001;72:306–13.
17. Hulscher JB, van Sandick JW, de Boer AG, et al. Extended transthoracic resection compared with limited transhiatal resection for adenocarcinoma of the esophagus. N Engl J Med 2002;347:1662–9.
18. Omloo JM, Lagarde SM, Hulscher JB, et al. Extended transthoracic resection compared with limited transhiatal resection for adenocarcinoma of the mid/distal esophagus: five-year survival of a randomized clinical trial. Ann Surg 2007;246:992–1000.
19. Schwarz RE, Smith DD. Clinical impact of lymphadenectomy extent in resectable esophageal cancer. J Gastrointest Surg 2007;11:1384–94.
20. Groth SS, Virnig BA, Whitson BA, et al. Determination of the minimum number of lymph nodes to examine to maximize survival in patients with esophageal carcinoma: data from the Surveillance Epidemiology and End Results database. J Thorac Cardiovasc Surg 2010;139:612–20.
21. Stiles BM, Mirza F, Port JL, et al. Predictors of cervical and recurrent laryngeal lymph node metastases from esophageal cancer. Ann Thorac Surg 2010;90:1805–11.
22. Lerut T, Nafteux P, Moons J, et al. Three-field lymphadenectomy for carcinoma of the esophagus and gastroesophageal junction in 174 R0 resections: impact on staging, disease-free survival, and outcome: a plea for adaptation of TNM classification in upper-half esophageal carcinoma. Ann Surg 2004;240:962–72.
23. Kohn GP, Galanko JA, Meyers MO, et al. National trends in esophageal surgery: are outcomes as good as we believe? J Gastrointest Surg 2009;13:1900–10.

Minimally Invasive Esophagectomy

Ryan M. Levy, MD, Dhaval Trivedi, MD, James D. Luketich, MD*

KEYWORDS

- Esophagectomy • Esophageal neoplasms • Esophageal surgery
- Thoracic surgery video-assisted • Laparoscopy

KEY POINTS

- Minimally invasive esophagectomy (MIE) has become an established approach for the treatment of esophageal carcinoma.
- In the authors' retrospective series of more than 1000 patients who underwent MIE, overall morbidity, mortality, lymph node harvest, and cancer outcomes were similar to or better than most published series of open esophagectomy.
- The authors' favored approach is a laparoscopic-thoracoscopic Ivor Lewis MIE.
- The Ivor Lewis approach for MIE significantly lowers the incidence of recurrent nerve injury in comparison with approaches requiring a cervical anastomosis.
- In the first randomized controlled trial of MIE versus open esophagectomy, MIE was associated with a shorter hospital stay, fewer pulmonary infections, less vocal cord paralysis, and better short-term quality of life compared with open esophagectomy. Oncologic principles of resection and lymph node retrieval were not compromised using the minimally invasive approach.

INTRODUCTION

Over the past decade, minimally invasive esophagectomy (MIE) has become an accepted approach to treating cancers of the esophagus. When performed at high-volume centers, MIE has been shown to carry similar morbidity, mortality, and oncologic outcomes as open esophagectomy, with the advantages inherent to minimally invasive surgery. MIE techniques have evolved significantly from the initial hybrid approaches of thoracoscopy combined with laparotomy[1–4] to the current MIE, which is performed entirely using laparoscopy and thoracoscopy. Although technically demanding and associated with a significant operator learning curve, MIE is an excellent option for esophageal resection. Advantages include less blood loss, decreased

The authors have nothing to disclose.
Department of Cardiothoracic Surgery, University of Pittsburgh Medical Center, Suite C-800, 200 Lothrop Street, Pittsburgh, PA 15213, USA
* Corresponding author.
E-mail address: luketichjd@upmc.edu

incidence of respiratory complications, shorter of hospital stay, and reduced narcotic requirements.[5–9] In the authors' experience, MIE is also associated with less postoperative pain.

At present, minimally invasive approaches for esophagectomy include laparoscopic transhiatal, laparoscopic-thoracoscopic 3-hole (McKeown), and laparoscopic-thoracoscopic Ivor Lewis esophagectomy. Each of these approaches can be performed with either a lymph node sampling technique or a more complete lymph node dissection. The choice between MIE approaches is, to a large degree, based on surgeon preference. However, the operative approach is at times dictated by the anatomic location of tumor and the margins required for an R0 resection. The choice of operative approach also directly affects postoperative morbidity. Specifically, approaches that include a cervical anastomosis have a higher incidence of anastomotic leak, stricture, recurrent laryngeal nerve injury, and pharyngoesophageal swallowing dysfunction.[10–12] In comparison, transthoracic approaches have a higher incidence of cardiopulmonary complications and more morbid consequences when an anastomotic leak occurs.[13]

The number of lymph nodes sampled at operation has important prognostic and treatment implications. It is also clear that to obtain a more aggressive resection with complete 2-field lymph node dissection, the operation must include thoracic exposure via an Ivor Lewis or McKeown modification.[14–17] A trend toward improved 5-year survival has been observed in subsets of patients with more locally advanced cancers treated with an Ivor Lewis approach.[13,18,19] In addition, local recurrence rates of less than 10% have been reported after complete lymph node dissection using a thoracic approach, compared with local recurrence rates of greater than 40% with transhiatal operations.[20–22] Despite these data, randomized trials comparing transhiatal and transthoracic esophageal resection have not shown significant survival differences between the 2 approaches. However, a trend toward improved long-term survival has been shown after transthoracic resection.[13,19]

The authors previously reported their extensive experience with MIE using a modified McKeown (3-hole) technique.[23,24] These articles demonstrated that MIE could be performed safely with stage-specific survival that was equivalent to previously published open series.[25,26] In light of concerns regarding cervical dissection and anastomosis, the authors' preferred approach is now a completely laparoscopic-thoracoscopic (Ivor Lewis) esophagectomy with abdominal (celiac, left gastric, splenic) and mediastinal (paraesophageal and subcarinal) lymphadenectomy.[27,28] The minimally invasive Ivor Lewis approach works well for most distal esophageal cancers, gastroesophageal junction tumors with gastric cardia extension, and short-to moderate-length Barrett esophagus with high-grade dysplasia. In addition, when there is concern for the length of the gastric conduit, an intrathoracic anastomosis is preferable. In cases of primary gastric tumors with significant lesser curve extension that involve the incisura, the authors prefer a total gastrectomy with roux-en-Y reconstruction. Total laparoscopic and thoracoscopic Ivor Lewis resections should not be performed for upper third or mid-esophageal cancers with significant proximal extension, because of the concern for adequate margin of resection. In this article, the authors describe their current operative technique and present the results and insights that have been attained using this approach.

PREOPERATIVE PLANNING

Preoperative workup is similar to that of patients who will undergo an open esophagectomy. In addition to detailed staging with computed tomography (CT), endoscopic ultrasonography, and positron emission tomography (PET), all patients undergo pulmonary function testing and cardiac evaluation.

SURGICAL TECHNIQUE
Anesthetic Considerations

Anesthetic management during MIE poses specific challenges. Whereas all patients receive an arterial blood pressure monitoring line, central venous catheter placement is not routine. A double-lumen endotracheal tube is placed initially in anticipation of the thoracoscopic phase. In patients with mid-thoracic or upper thoracic tumors, a single-lumen endotracheal tube is initially placed for preoperative bronchoscopy to evaluate airway involvement.

Patients generally require significant volume loading during the laparoscopic phase secondary to the pneumoperitoneum and steep reverse Trendelenburg positioning of the patient. Given the high flow of CO_2 required, the patient can develop significant hypercarbia and acidosis. The surgeon must also be mindful of vasopressors administered by the anesthesiologist, as these agents directly affect the viability of the newly created gastric conduit. Simple measures can be undertaken to help correct these problems. Maneuvers to increase preload include lowering the insufflation pressure, decreasing the degree of reverse Trendelenburg positioning, and further volume loading. In addition to changes in the ventilator settings, hypercarbia can often be corrected by reversing the pneumoperitoneum, allowing the patient time to compensate and clear the excess CO_2. There must be clear and ongoing communication throughout the procedure between the surgeon and the anesthesiologist.

Endoscopic Evaluation

- Esophagogastroscopy is always performed.
- The precise location of the tumor is confirmed.
- Proximal and distal extents are visualized.
- The presence of Barrett esophagus proximal to the tumor margin is noted.
- The stomach is evaluated to confirm suitability for use as a conduit.
- Endoscopic insufflation must be kept to a minimum. Small-bowel dilation can significantly reduce the intra-abdominal domain and add significant difficulty to an already complex surgery.

Laparoscopic Phase

Positioning and laparoscopic port placement

- The patient is initially in the supine position, with arms out and a foot board in place. The surgeon operates from the right side of the table.
- The abdomen is mapped. Both costal margins are outlined. A line is drawn from the xiphoid to the umbilicus. This line is further divided into thirds (**Fig. 1**A).
- Five abdominal ports are used for the gastric mobilization, tube creation, and pyloroplasty (**Fig. 1**B). A sixth port is placed in the right paraumbilical region for placement of the feeding jejunostomy tube.
- The initial port is placed via an open (Hassan) technique in the right paramedian area at the junction of the middle and lower thirds as indicated by the abdominal markings.
- Pneumoperitoneum is set to a pressure of 15 mm Hg.
- Under direct visualization, the left paramedian and left subcostal ports are placed. The left paramedian port now becomes the camera and insufflation port.

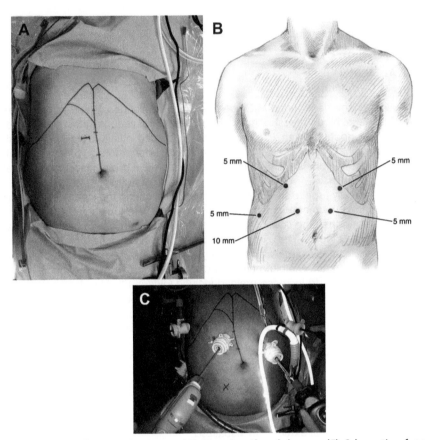

Fig. 1. Laparoscopic port placement. (*A*) Mapping the abdomen. (*B*) Schematic of port placement. (*C*) Intraoperative photo demonstrating port placement. The 10-mm port is placed first in the right mid-abdomen using an open Hassan trocar insertion technique. An additional 5-/11-mm port is placed in the right lower quadrant; this is helpful for retraction during pyloroplasty and creation of a gastric tube. (*B: Courtesy of and* © Heart, Lung and Esophageal Surgery Institute, University of Pittsburgh Medical Center, Pittsburgh, PA; with permission.)

- The assistant then retracts the hepatic flexure to expose the lateral abdominal wall just below the 12th rib. A 5-mm port is placed here and the liver retractor is positioned under the left lobe of the liver.
- A right subcostal 5-mm port is placed.
- All ports should be a hand's breadth apart to avoid unwanted contact between the surgeon and assistant (**Fig. 1**C).
- Skin incisions must be made as small as possible to help ports remain in place and minimize subcutaneous emphysema.

Gastric mobilization

- The abdomen is staged by inspecting the peritoneum, omentum, and liver to rule out any metastatic disease.
- The gastrohepatic ligament is opened.

- The left gastric artery/vein pedicle is identified and traced proximally (**Fig. 2**).
- Lymph nodes suspicious for metastatic involvement are dissected and sent for frozen-section analysis.
- The celiac lymph nodes are examined. A complete lymph node dissection is carried out to include the left gastric and celiac nodes, sweeping all nodal and fatty tissue with the specimen; the nodal dissection is continued along the splenic artery and the superior border of the pancreas. This plane continues cephalad toward the right and left crus, continuous with the preaortic dissection plane into the lower thoracic cavity.
- If the nodes do not appear malignant or are pathologically free of cancer on analysis, dissection of the right crus is initiated to mobilize the lateral aspect of the esophagus.
- The dissection is carried anteriorly and superiorly over the esophagus to expose the anterior hiatus. The phrenoesophageal attachments are transected.
- As the dissection is continued toward the left crus, the fundus of the stomach begins to be mobilized. The medial border of the right crus is then dissected inferiorly until the decussation of the right and left crural fibers is visualized. This maneuver exposes the retroesophageal window and completes the mobilization of the superior portion of the lesser curvature and gastroesophageal junction.
- Posterior mobilization of the stomach is started. After identifying the gastrocolic omentum, the antrum of the stomach is retracted and a window is created in the

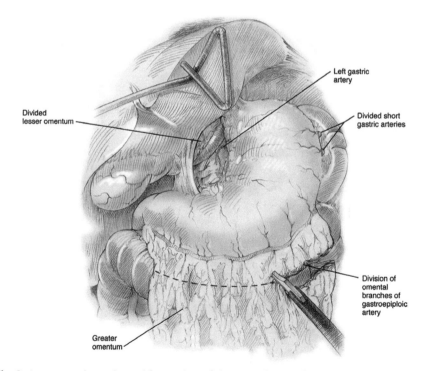

Fig. 2. Laparoscopic staging, with opening of the gastrohepatic ligament and evaluation of left gastric/celiac lymph nodes. (*Courtesy of and* © Heart, Lung and Esophageal Surgery Institute, University of Pittsburgh Medical Center, Pittsburgh, PA; with permission.)

greater omentum, thus allowing access to the lesser sac. The right gastroepiploic arcade must be identified clearly and protected during this mobilization.

- Dissection is carried along the greater curve of the stomach until the end of the gastroepiploic arcade is reached (**Fig. 3**).
- The short gastric vessels are divided with ultrasonic shears (Autosonix; Covidien, Mansfield, MA) or the LigaSure device (LigaSure; Valleylab, Boulder, CO) (**Fig. 4**).
- Once the greater curve of the stomach is mobilized, the fundus is rotated toward the patient's right shoulder to expose retrogastric attachments. These attachments are dissected free toward the lesser curvature until the left gastric artery and vein are encountered.
- The mobilization of the stomach is carried back toward the pyloroantral region. The dissection here must be meticulous, as any injury to the gastroepiploic arcade may render the gastric conduit useless. There are often significant adhesions in the retroantral and periduodenal regions that also need to be dissected to allow for adequate mobilization of the inferior portion of the stomach.
- The pylorus is considered adequately mobilized when it is able to reach the right crus without tension, which may require a partial or complete Kocher maneuver.
- Particular attention to mobilization of the pyloroantral area is needed in patients who have had prior cholecystectomy, pancreatitis, or other biliary tract procedures
- Once the stomach is completely mobilized, the left gastric artery and vein are divided with a vascular load in an Endo GIA stapler (Covidien).
- The pedicle should be completely dissected clean with all nodes swept up into the specimen. Care must be taken not pull up the splenic or hepatic arteries into the stapler.
- At this point, the distal esophagus, gastric fundus, and antrum should be completely mobilized.

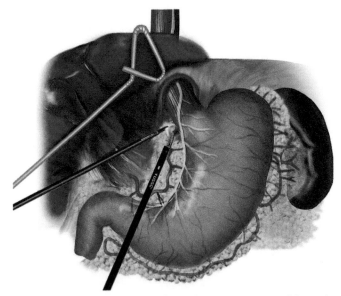

Fig. 3. Laparoscopic staging (continued). The right crus is separated from the esophageal wall/fat pad and the decussation of the crura is identified. Resectability along these tissue planes and along the left crus is confirmed before proceeding to left gastric vascular pedicle ligation and division. (*Courtesy of and* © Jennifer Dallal, MD and James Luketich, MD.)

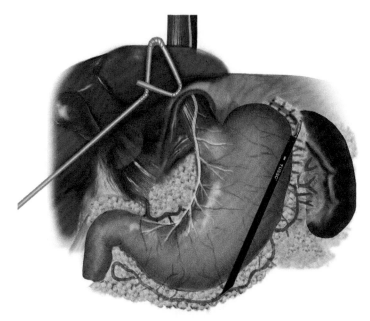

Fig. 4. Division of highest short gastric vessels and dissection along the greater curve of the stomach. (*Courtesy of and* © Jennifer Dallal, MD and James Luketich, MD.)

Creation of gastric tube

- The gastric tube is created before the completion of the pyloroplasty and placement of the feeding jejunostomy tube, thus providing time to assess the viability of the gastric tube as a conduit.
- The first stapler load used for creating the gastric conduit is a vascular load to control bleeding from the adipose tissue and vessels along the lesser curve, above the level of the right gastric artery. No stomach is divided in this initial vascular staple load.
- Subsequent stapler loads consist of purple loads (Endo GIA Reloads with Tri-staple Technology; Covidien). An additional 12-mm port, placed in the right paraumbilical area, is used to assist with the creation of the gastric tube and, subsequently, placement of the jejunostomy tube.
- It is important to stretch the stomach to create a straight conduit. The first assistant grasps the tip of the fundus along the greater curve and gently stretches it toward the spleen. A second grasper is applied through the paraumbilical port to the antral area with a slight downward retraction.
- The stomach is first divided across the antrum with purple staple loads (Endo GIA Reloads with Tri-staple Technology) (**Fig. 5**).
- The staple line is then directed toward the fundus, maintaining a conduit width of 4 to 5 cm, parallel to the greater curvature.
- As the fundus is divided, the graspers are readjusted to keep the stomach on constant stretch.
- The length of the conduit is adjusted if there is concern for tumor extension onto the gastric cardia.
- If there is any concern about the adequacy of the stapled closure, additional reinforcing sutures can be placed; however, this is not generally needed.

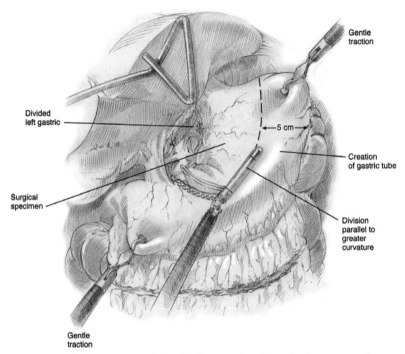

Fig. 5. Creation of the gastric conduit. The first stapler along the lesser curve is a vascular Endo GIA stapler, after which the thick antrum is divided with the purple loads (Endo GIA 45 mm), fired sequentially. The antrum and the fundus are pulled in opposite directions to provide adequate tension during the creation of the gastric conduit. (*Courtesy of and* © Heart, Lung and Esophageal Surgery Institute, University of Pittsburgh Medical Center, Pittsburgh, PA; with permission.)

- The right gastric vessels are preserved. The conduit is observed while the pyloroplasty in completed.

Pyloroplasty

- The pyloroplasty is started by clearly identifying the pylorus.
- Stay sutures are placed on the superior and inferior aspects of the pylorus with 2-0 Surgidac suture (Covidien) using the Endostitch device (Covidien).
- Once the pylorus has been placed on stretch, the anterior wall is transected with ultrasonic shears.
- The pyloroplasty is closed transversely in a Heineke-Mikulicz fashion using simple, interrupted 2-0 Surgidac sutures (**Fig. 6**). Care must be taken to include mucosa with each suture, as it will generally retract and lead to a suboptimal closure. A total of 4 to 6 sutures are generally required.
- At the conclusion of the abdominal portion of the operation, a small omental patch is placed over the pyloroplasty.
- In patients who have received neoadjuvant chemotherapy with radiation, a pedicled omental flap to wrap the anastomosis in the chest is created. A 3-cm wide, 8- to 10-cm long omental pedicle, originating from the upper greater curve of the gastric conduit, is dissected free.

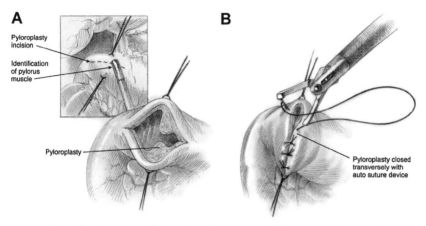

Fig. 6. Creation of pyloroplasty (*A*) and vertical closure (*B*) in a Heineke-Mikulicz fashion. (*Courtesy of and* © Heart, Lung and Esophageal Surgery Institute, University of Pittsburgh Medical Center, Pittsburgh, PA; with permission.)

Placement of feeding jejunostomy tube

Using a percutaneous catheter kit, a feeding jejunostomy tube (10F catheter) is placed in the left lower quadrant (**Fig. 7**).

- The greater omentum is retracted out of the pelvis to expose the underlying transverse colon, which is then retracted superiorly toward the hiatus to expose the ligament of Treitz.
- After tracing the jejunum distally for 30 to 40 cm from the ligament of Treitz, a loop of small bowel (antimesenteric border) is tacked to the anterior abdominal wall using the Endostitch device. The 12-mm trocar previously placed in the right

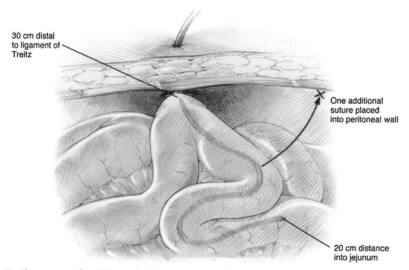

Fig. 7. Placement of a 10F needle jejunostomy catheter and an antitorsion stitch 3 to 4 cm distally along the antimesenteric border. (*Courtesy of and* © Heart, Lung and Esophageal Surgery Institute, University of Pittsburgh Medical Center, Pittsburgh, PA; with permission.)

paraumbilical region is used as the operating port while the camera is switched to the 11-mm port in the right paramedian area.

- The feeding tube is passed into the jejunum using the Seldinger technique under direct laparoscopic vision.
- Proper placement of the catheter is confirmed by observing distension of the jejunum as air is insufflated into the needle catheter.
- To prevent leakage from the enterotomy site, the jejunum is tacked to the abdominal wall using an additional Endostitch in a purse-string fashion.
- An antitorsion stitch is placed approximately 3 to 4 cm distal to the insertion site.

Preparation for thoracoscopic phase

- The most superior portion of the gastric tube is stitched to the specimen. It is important to keep the stomach aligned correctly so that during the mobilization of the conduit into the chest, it does not twist in the abdomen. This alignment is ensured by suturing the greater curvature along the short gastric vessels to the staple line of the proximal gastric remnant (**Fig. 8**).

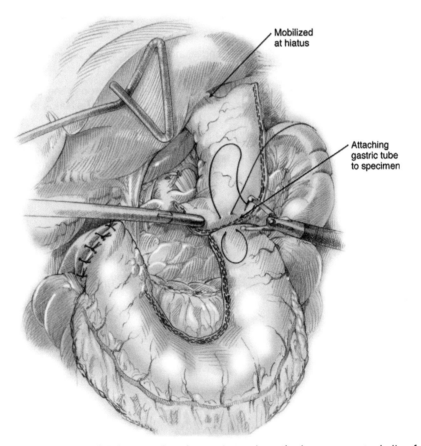

Mobilized
at hiatus

Attaching
gastric tube
to specimen

Fig. 8. The gastric conduit is secured to the specimen along the lesser curve staple line for proper orientation during the thoracoscopic portion with a horizontal U-stitch. (*Courtesy of and* © Heart, Lung and Esophageal Surgery Institute, University of Pittsburgh Medical Center, Pittsburgh, PA; with permission.)

- If an omental flap has been created, the distal end is sutured to the conduit tip.
- The viability of the conduit is confirmed and staple line checked for hemostasis. Clips can be applied to the staple line as needed.
- The laparoscopic portion of the procedure is completed by pushing the specimen and attached gastric tube into the lower mediastinum. The proximal gastric cardia (specimen side) along with the sutured conduit tip is gently placed through the hiatus, taking care to maintain the orientation of the conduit (**Fig. 9**).
- If the hiatus appears wide, the crura are reapproximated with an Endostitch to avoid potential herniation of the conduit into the chest at a later time.
- The pyloroplasty is covered with a patch of omentum, and a final inspection for bleeding in the abdomen is made. The liver retractor is removed.
- The initial cut-down port is removed, and the fascia is closed under laparoscopic visualization using a Carter-Thomason suture passer device.
- Finally, the surgeon places a nasogastric tube into the mid-esophagus.

Thoracoscopic Phase

Positioning and port placement

The patient is turned to the left lateral decubitus position for the thoracoscopic phase. Correct placement of the double-lumen endotracheal tube is confirmed. The operating surgeon stands on the right side of the table (facing the patient's back) while the assistant stands on the left side of the table.

Five thoracoscopic ports are used (**Fig. 10**).

- A 10-mm camera port is placed in the eighth or ninth intercostal space, just anterior to the mid-axillary line.

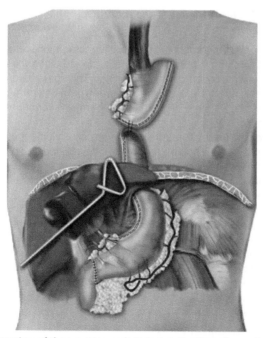

Fig. 9. Proper orientation of the gastric conduit during the thoracoscopic part of the procedure. (*Courtesy of and* © Jennifer Dallal, MD and James Luketich, MD.)

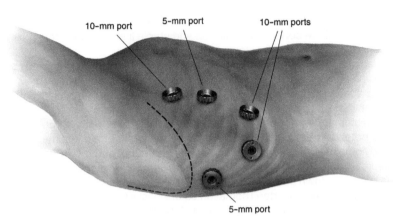

Fig. 10. Thoracoscopic port placement. (*From* Tsai WS, Levy RM, Luketich JD. Technique of minimally invasive Ivor Lewis esophagectomy. Oper Techn Thorac Cardiovasc Surg 2009;14:176–92; with permission.)

- The working port is a 10-mm port placed in the eighth or ninth intercostal space, posterior to the posterior axillary line.
- Another 10-mm port is placed in the anterior axillary line at the fourth intercostal space, through which a fan-shaped retractor aids in retracting the lung to expose the esophagus.
- A 5-mm port is placed just inferior to the tip of the scapula for the surgeon's left hand.
- A final 5-mm port is placed at the sixth rib, at the anterior axillary line, for suction by the assistant.

Diaphragm retraction, mobilization of the thoracic esophagus, and removal of the esophagogastric specimen

- The first step in the thoracoscopic phase is placement of a retraction stitch on the diaphragm. A 48-inch, 0 Surgidac suture is placed using the Endostitch device through the central tendon of the diaphragm. The suture is brought out through the lateral chest wall at the level of the insertion of the diaphragm through a small stab incision. This maneuver retracts the diaphragm inferiorly, exposing the distal esophagus in the chest.
- Mobilization of the thoracic esophagus begins by dividing the inferior pulmonary ligament up to the inferior pulmonary vein. When taking down the inferior pulmonary ligament, it is important to dissect onto the pericardium to expose a relatively avascular plane and the medial aspect of the dissection.
- The inferior pulmonary vein is retracted anteriorly and the dissection is carried superiorly along the pericardium to the level of the subcarinal lymph nodes.
- Level VII lymph nodes are dissected en bloc with the esophagus.
- The posterior, membranous wall of the right mainstem bronchus is at risk during this mobilization and should be clearly identified. Asking the anesthesiologist to remove the suction catheter out of the right mainstem bronchus can be helpful in visualizing the bronchus, as it prevents it from collapsing.
- With the lung retracted anteriorly, the pleura lying anterior to the esophagus is incised to the level of the azygos vein (**Fig. 11**) After the azygos vein is isolated and freed from the mediastinal pleura, it is divided with a vascular load of the Endo GIA stapler. The vagus nerve is transected to prevent any traction injuries to the recurrent nerve during the mobilization of the esophagus.

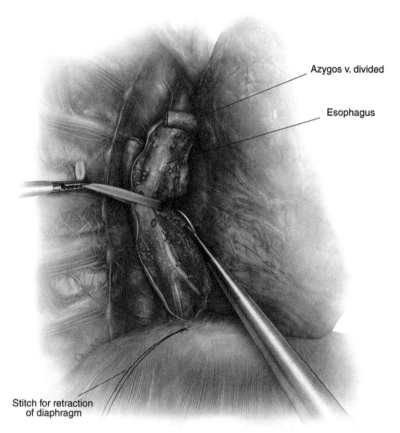

Azygos v. divided

Esophagus

Stitch for retraction
of diaphragm

Fig. 11. Thoracoscopic esophageal mobilization. The lung is retracted anteriorly and the pleura along the esophagus is excised. The subcarinal lymph nodes are excised en bloc along with the specimen. (*From* Tsai WS, Levy RM, Luketich JD. Technique of minimally invasive Ivor Lewis esophagectomy. Oper Techn Thorac Cardiovasc Surg 2009;14:176–92; with permission.)

- Above the azygos, dissection is done close to the esophagus. The mobilization is continued proximally above the azygos; the extent depends on the tumor location.
- Attention is turned to mobilizing the esophagus laterally.
- The pleura is divided superficially along the posterior groove to the esophagus to avoid injury to the thoracic duct and the underlying aorta. The thoracic duct is not routinely resected with the specimen. Lymphatics and aortoesophageal vessels are controlled with endoclips and subsequently divided with the ultrasonic shears. A careful thoracic duct ligation should be considered if there are any concerns over trauma to the duct.
- The lateral dissection is carried from above the azygos vein to the gastroesophageal junction and the deep margin of the dissection is the contralateral pleura, which is occasionally entered to remove a bulky tumor. If the esophagus is difficult to dissect, a Penrose drain may be placed around the esophagus to provide traction to pull the esophagus out of its mediastinal bed.
- With the esophagus mobilized medially and laterally, the specimen is pulled into the chest with the attached gastric conduit. Extreme care must be taken to

maintain the proper orientation of the gastric conduit with the staple line facing the lateral chest wall (staple line facing up in lateral position). This alignment is mandatory to avoid spiraling or twisting of the conduit.

- The stitch between the specimen and conduit is cut and the tip of the conduit is tacked to the diaphragm with an Endostitch to prevent it from slipping down into the abdomen.
- The specimen is retracted anteriorly and superiorly from the esophageal bed, and the mobilization completed off the contralateral pleura.
- Above the level of the azygos vein, the dissection plane moves onto the wall of the esophagus to avoid injury to the recurrent laryngeal nerve. Lymph nodes above the azygos vein are not routinely harvested.
- When the esophagus is completely mobilized, a 4-to 5-cm mini-thoracotomy is made between the surgeon's working port and the tip of the scapula. The ribs are not spread. A wound protector (Applied Medical, Rancho Santa Margarita, CA) is placed to protect the skin and chest wall from trocar implants.
- The esophagus is transected at or above the level of the azygos vein using Endo Shears (Covidien) at a level appropriate for the tumor while the nasogastric tube is pulled back.
- The specimen is removed through the wound protector and sent to Pathology for analysis of the margins.

Creation of gastroesophageal anastomosis

- Creation of the esophagogastric anastomosis starts with securing the anvil of an EEA stapler (Covidien) into the proximal esophagus. The authors' standard approach is to use a 28-mm EEA stapler in an attempt to minimize the risk of stricture and decrease the need for postoperative dilations. On rare occasion, a Foley balloon catheter may be used to dilate the proximal esophagus if difficulty is encountered when placing the 28-mm anvil. If the Foley balloon catheter fails, a 25-mm stapler may be used.
- Two purse-string sutures are placed using a 2-0 Endostitch to secure the anvil into the proximal esophagus. The first stitch can be technically challenging, as the anvil has a tendency to migrate out of the proximal esophagus (**Fig. 12**). All layers of the esophagus must be included in the purse-string sutures to ensure complete rings after EEA firing.
- The gastric conduit is pulled further into the chest and the tip of the gastric conduit is opened on the right side of the staple line using ultrasonic shears.
- The EEA stapler is placed through the wound protector and positioned in the conduit. The stapler spike is brought out along the greater curve of the gastric conduit to dock with the anvil.
- Before creating the anastomosis, the amount of conduit that will lie in the chest is carefully estimated. It is a common mistake to bring an excess stomach into the chest with the intent of minimizing tension on the anastomosis. A redundant conduit above the diaphragm can lead to significant problems with conduit emptying. In addition, ensuring proper orientation of the stomach is critical to prevent twisting.
- Once the stapler has been fired, the excess gastric tip (the gastrostomy through which the stapler was placed) is trimmed using sequential loads of an articulating linear stapler (**Figs. 13** and **14**).
- If an omental flap was harvested, it is now wrapped around the anastomosis.
- The chest is thoroughly irrigated and inspected for hemostasis.

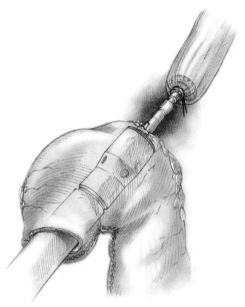

Fig. 12. Creation of esophagogastric anastomosis. The anvil is secured in the proximal esophagus with 2 purse-string sutures. The EEA stapler is introduced into the conduit via a gastrostomy and is docked with the anvil, keeping the conduit aligned with the lesser curve staple line facing the camera. (*Courtesy of and* © Heart, Lung and Esophageal Surgery Institute, University of Pittsburgh Medical Center, Pittsburgh, PA; with permission.)

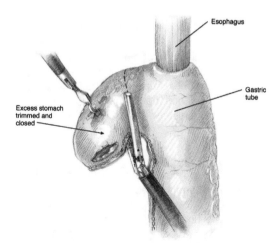

Fig. 13. The gastrostomy is closed with the Endo GIA stapler and this part of the stomach is sent as the final gastric margin. Care is taken that this staple line does not encroach too close to the circular EEA staple line. A Jackson-Pratt drain is left in the esophageal bed posterior to the anastomosis. (*Courtesy of and* © Heart, Lung and Esophageal Surgery Institute, University of Pittsburgh Medical Center, Pittsburgh, PA; with permission.)

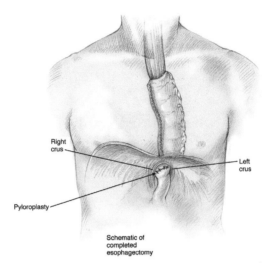

Fig. 14. Completed reconstruction. (*Courtesy of and* © Heart, Lung and Esophageal Surgery Institute, University of Pittsburgh Medical Center, Pittsburgh, PA; with permission.)

Drain placement and closure

- A 10-mm Jackson-Pratt drain is placed posteriorly along the anastomosis and a chest tube is directed posteriorly toward the apex.
- The nasogastric tube is advanced past the anastomosis under thoracoscopic visualization.
- The gastric conduit is sutured to the right crus with a single 2-0 Endostitch to prevent delayed herniation of the conduit.
- A multilevel intercostal nerve block can be performed to aid in postoperative pain management.
- The mini-thoracotomy site is closed in multiple layers.
- Particular attention is paid to securing the Jackson-Pratt drain with multiple sutures to the skin.
- Once the patient is turned to the supine position, the oropharynx and nasopharynx are thoroughly suctioned of all secretions.
- The double-lumen endotracheal tube is exchanged for a single-lumen tube. Through this, an adult bronchoscope is used to suction all secretions. At this time, both right and left mainstem bronchi are examined for any evidence of airway injury.

Postoperative Care

- Patients generally spend the first postoperative day in the intensive care unit (ICU). Most patients will spend 1 week in the hospital.
- The nasogastric tube is removed on postoperative day 2 and trickle tube feeds are started through the jejunostomy tube.
- An esophagram is obtained on day 3 or 4, provided the patient has a good cough and adequate pulmonary toilet.
- Oral intake is initiated if the esophagram is negative for leak. The initial diet consists of 1 to 2 oz (28–57 g) of clear liquids per hour. This diet is quickly advanced to full liquids, no more than 3 to 4 oz (85–113 g) per hour along with cycled tube feeds.

- The Jackson-Pratt drain is pulled back a few centimeters on day 5 and is secured in place. It is removed at the first postoperative clinic visit.

DISCUSSION

Minimally invasive techniques have evolved significantly over the past decade. At the University of Pittsburgh, the authors have now performed more than 1000 minimally invasive esophagectomies. In the initial cases a totally laparoscopic approach was used, similar to that described by DePaula and colleagues[29] and Swanstrom and Hansen.[30] They soon transitioned to a laparoscopic-thoracoscopic McKeown approach (thoracoscopic mobilization of the intrathoracic esophagus, laparoscopic gastric tube creation, and a cervical anastomosis). This technique resolved several technical shortcomings of the laparoscopic transhiatal approach, including better visualization of periesophageal tissues and a more complete mediastinal lymphadenectomy. The authors performed more than 500 esophagectomies with this modified McKeown technique and demonstrated reduced perioperative morbidity and mortality in comparison with many open series.[23]

Perhaps the most significant technical concern with the modified McKeown MIE is the cervical dissection and associated recurrent laryngeal nerve injury. Postoperative dysfunction in pharyngeal transit and swallowing, even in the absence of recurrent nerve injury, are not infrequent after cervical dissection. Moreover, as described in open series using a cervical anastomosis, anastomotic stricture and leak occurs with increased frequency.[31] These concerns prompted the authors' more recent experience with a completely thoracoscopic-laparoscopic Ivor Lewis esophagectomy (as described herein).[27] There is a steep operator learning curve associated with the minimally invasive Ivor Lewis approach, but the omission of a cervical dissection reduces the rate of recurrent nerve injury to near zero. With a chest anastomosis, pharyngeal transit and oropharyngeal swallowing dysfunction should be improved as well.

The authors recently reviewed their experience of more than 1000 MIEs performed at the University of Pittsburgh Medical Center over a 15-year period.[28] Modified McKeown MIE was performed electively in 481 patients and Ivor Lewis MIE in 530. By 2006 Ivor Lewis MIE was the authors' preferred approach, thus the majority of patients in the last 5 years of the study period underwent Ivor Lewis MIE. The median length of stay (8 days) and ICU stay (2 days) were similar between the 2 approaches. The median number of lymph nodes resected was 21. The overall operative mortality was 1.7%. Overall morbidity, mortality, lymph node harvest, and cancer outcomes for the entire cohort were similar or better than most published series of open esophagectomy. The Ivor Lewis MIE group had both a significantly lower incidence of recurrent nerve injury (1%) and a significantly lower operative mortality rate (0.9% at 30 days) than the modified-McKeown MIE group.[28]

During MIE, thoracoscopic port placement is critical, as poorly positioned trocars can cause difficulty in performing a safe and complete dissection. In addition, both blood and lung can obscure visualization of the esophagus, which lies at the dependent aspect of the operative field. Prone positioning has been described as an alternative approach to facilitate operative exposure and address other technical concerns. Compared with open series, low rates of anastomotic leak (3%), low mortality (1.5%), and equivalent stage-specific survival have been shown with the thoracoscopic prone approach.[32] Described advantages of the prone position include the need for fewer ports, favorable surgeon ergonomics, improved exposure (lungs and blood do not obscure the operative view because of the effects of gravity), and improved ventilation in the prone position. Potential disadvantages include a longer setup time, thoracoscopic views unfamiliar to most surgeons, difficult airway management, and difficulty of open conversion (posterior thoracotomy) in the case of massive hemorrhage.[33] The prone position is a safe alternative to the decubitis position with potentially fewer complications, but the technique has yet to gain favor among thoracic surgeons.[34] In addition, no randomized data are currently available and long-term results are lacking.

MIE has been compared with open esophagectomy in multiple series in the literature. Nagpal and colleagues[6] performed a meta-analysis of 12 studies with a total of 672 patients, including patients who underwent open eosphagectomy, hybrid MIE, and MIE. The investigators concluded that MIE was associated with better operative and postoperative outcomes. MIE patients had less blood loss and shorter ICU and hospital stays. In addition, the MIE group had a 50% decrease in morbidity with a significantly lower incidence of respiratory complications in comparison with the open esophagectomy group. There was no significant difference in anastomotic leak rate, anastomotic stricture rate, gastric conduit ischemia, chyle leak, vocal cord palsy, or 30-day mortality. In their subgroup analysis, the investigators found that even patients who underwent one stage of their esophagectomy (hybrid MIE) minimally invasively (eg, laparotomy with thoracoscopy or laparoscopy with thoracotomy) had significantly less blood loss and fewer respiratory complications compared with patients who underwent open esophagectomy. Oncologic outcomes, as assessed by lymph node retrieval, were comparable in all 3 groups.[6] Dantoc and colleagues[35] performed a meta-analysis looking at oncologic outcomes and 5-year mortality in patients undergoing open esophagectomy versus MIE. This review included 17 case-controlled studies with 1586 patients. Lymph node yield was significantly higher ($P = .03$) in the MIE group, median 16 nodes (range 5.7–33.9), as compared with the open group, median 10 nodes (range 3–32.8). The 5-year survival rates were similar in the MIE group (12.5%–67%) and the open group (16%–57%; $P = .33$). The investigators concluded that MIE provides oncologic outcomes equivalent to those of open esophagectomy.

While the safety and feasibility of minimally invasive esophagectomy have been demonstrated in single-institution studies and meta-analyses, the results of large, prospective, multicenter trials investigating MIE are only now emerging. E2202 is phase II study that was coordinated by the Eastern Cooperative Oncology Group (ECOG). The primary objective of this multicenter trial was to evaluate the safety, feasibility, and outcomes following MIE in a multi-institutional setting. Sixteen credentialed sites in the United States enrolled patients with biopsy-proven high-grade dysplasia or esophageal cancer of the mid-esophagus or distal esophagus. Esophagectomy was performed using either a modified McKeown MIE or an Ivor Lewis MIE. A total of 106 patients were eligible for the preliminary analysis. Protocol surgery was completed in 99 of 106 patients (93%). The perioperative mortality was 2%. Median ICU and hospital stay were 2 and 9 days, respectively. Adverse events included anastomotic leak (7.8%) and pneumonia (4.9%). At a median follow-up of 19 months, the estimated 3-year overall survival was 50%.[36] This phase II study demonstrated that MIE is safe and feasible, with low perioperative morbidity and mortality and good oncologic results, and suggests that MIE can be adopted by other centers with appropriate expertise in open esophagectomy and minimally invasive surgery.

Recently, the results of the first randomized controlled trial comparing open esophagectomy and MIE, the TIME trial, were published.[8] After randomization, 56 patients were assigned to the open esophagectomy group and 59 to the MIE group. MIE was performed with the patient in the prone position. There was significantly less blood loss during MIE than during open esophagectomy, and hospital stays were shorter for patients who underwent MIE (11 days vs 14 days for open esophagectomy). Patients who underwent MIE had significantly fewer pulmonary infections than patients who underwent open esophagectomy (9% within 2 weeks of MIE compared with 29% after open esophagectomy). Short-term quality of life, assessed 6 weeks after surgery, was significantly better after MIE than after open esophagectomy. Completeness of resection, the number of lymph nodes retrieved, and perioperative mortality (30-day and in-hospital) were similar between the 2 approaches.

SUMMARY

MIE has become an established approach for the treatment of esophageal carcinoma. At the University of Pittsburgh, the authors now predominantly perform a laparoscopic-thoracoscopic Ivor Lewis esophagectomy. Perioperative morbidity and mortality are comparable with their previously established MIE approach with cervical anastomosis while essentially eliminating recurrent nerve injury, limiting the length of the gastric conduit required, and allowing a more aggressive gastric resection margin. Recent data from other publications suggest that lymph node yields may be improved. Multicenter trials currently under way, ECOG E2202 and the TIME trial,[8,36] will help further define the benefits of MIE.

REFERENCES

1. McAnena OJ, Rogers J, Williams NS. Right thoracoscopically assisted oesophagectomy for cancer. Br J Surg 1994;81:236–8.
2. Collard JM, Lengele B, Otte JB, et al. En bloc and standard esophagectomies by thoracoscopy. Ann Thorac Surg 1993;56:675–9.
3. Peracchia A, Rosati R, Fumagalli U, et al. Thoracoscopic esophagectomy: are there benefits? Semin Surg Oncol 1997;13:259–62.
4. Cuschieri A. Endoscopic subtotal oesophagectomy for cancer using the right thoracoscopic approach. Surg Oncol 1993;2(Suppl 1):3–11.
5. Verhage RJ, Hazebroek EJ, Boone J, et al. Minimally invasive surgery compared to open procedures in esophagectomy for cancer: a systematic review of the literature. Minerva Chir 2009;64:135–46.
6. Nagpal K, Ahmed K, Vats A, et al. Is minimally invasive surgery beneficial in the management of esophageal cancer? A meta-analysis. Surg Endosc 2010;24: 1621–9.
7. Sgourakis G, Gockel I, Radtke A, et al. Minimally invasive versus open esophagectomy: meta-analysis of outcomes. Dig Dis Sci 2010;55:3031–40.
8. Biere SS, van Berge Henegouwen MI, Maas KW, et al. Minimally invasive versus open oesophagectomy for patients with oesophageal cancer: a multicentre, open-label, randomised controlled trial. Lancet 2012;379:1887–92.
9. Narumiya K, Nakamura T, Ide H, et al. Comparison of extended esophagectomy through mini-thoracotomy/laparotomy with conventional thoracotomy/laparotomy for esophageal cancer. Jpn J Thorac Cardiovasc Surg 2005;53:413–9.
10. Hulscher JB, Tijssen JG, Obertop H, et al. Transthoracic versus transhiatal resection for carcinoma of the esophagus: a meta-analysis. Ann Thorac Surg 2001;72: 306–13.
11. Martin RE, Letsos P, Taves DH, et al. Oropharyngeal dysphagia in esophageal cancer before and after transhiatal esophagectomy. Dysphagia 2001;16:23–31.
12. Easterling CS, Bousamra M 2nd, Lang IM, et al. Pharyngeal dysphagia in postesophagectomy patients: correlation with deglutitive biomechanics. Ann Thorac Surg 2000;69:989–92.

13. Hulscher JB, van Sandick JW, de Boer AG, et al. Extended transthoracic resection compared with limited transhiatal resection for adenocarcinoma of the esophagus. N Engl J Med 2002;347:1662–9.

14. Greenstein AJ, Litle VR, Swanson SJ, et al. Effect of the number of lymph nodes sampled on postoperative survival of lymph node-negative esophageal cancer. Cancer 2008;112:1239–46.

15. Altorki NK, Zhou XK, Stiles B, et al. Total number of resected lymph nodes predicts survival in esophageal cancer. Ann Surg 2008;248:221–6.

16. Veeramachaneni NK, Zoole JB, Decker PA, et al. Lymph node analysis in esophageal resection: American College of Surgeons Oncology Group Z0060 trial. Ann Thorac Surg 2008;86:418–21.

17. Wolff CS, Castillo SF, Larson DR, et al. Ivor Lewis approach is superior to transhiatal approach in retrieval of lymph nodes at esophagectomy. Dis Esophagus 2008; 21:328–33.

18. Rizzetto C, DeMeester SR, Hagen JA, et al. En bloc esophagectomy reduces local recurrence and improves survival compared with transhiatal resection after neoadjuvant therapy for esophageal adenocarcinoma. J Thorac Cardiovasc Surg 2008;135:1228–36.

19. Omloo JM, Lagarde SM, Hulscher JB, et al. Extended transthoracic resection compared with limited transhiatal resection for adenocarcinoma of the mid/distal esophagus: five-year survival of a randomized clinical trial. Ann Surg 2007;246: 992–1000.

20. Lerut T, Coosemans W, Decker G, et al. Extended surgery for cancer of the esophagus and gastroesophageal junction. J Surg Res 2004;117:58–63.

21. Hulscher JB, van Sandick JW, Tijssen JG, et al. The recurrence pattern of esophageal carcinoma after transhiatal resection. J Am Coll Surg 2000;191:143–8.

22. Thomson IG, Smithers BM, Gotley DC, et al. Thoracoscopic-assisted esophagectomy for esophageal cancer: analysis of patterns and prognostic factors for recurrence. Ann Surg 2010;252:281–91.

23. Luketich JD, Alvelo-Rivera M, Buenaventura PO, et al. Minimally invasive esophagectomy: outcomes in 222 patients. Ann Surg 2003;238:486–94.

24. Luketich JD, Schauer PR, Christie NA, et al. Minimally invasive esophagectomy. Ann Thorac Surg 2000;70:906–11.

25. Kent MS, Schuchert M, Fernando H, et al. Minimally invasive esophagectomy: state of the art. Dis Esophagus 2006;19:137–45.

26. Nguyen NT, Roberts P, Follette DM, et al. Thoracoscopic and laparoscopic esophagectomy for benign and malignant disease: lessons learned from 46 consecutive procedures. J Am Coll Surg 2003;197:902–13.

27. Bizekis C, Kent MS, Luketich JD, et al. Initial experience with minimally invasive Ivor Lewis esophagectomy. Ann Thorac Surg 2006;82:402–6.

28. Luketich JD, Pennathur A, Awais O, et al. Outcomes after minimally invasive esophagectomy: review of over 1000 patients. Ann Surg 2012;256(1):95–103.

29. DePaula AL, Hashiba K, Ferreira EA, et al. Laparoscopic transhiatal esophagectomy with esophagogastroplasty. Surg Laparosc Endosc 1995;5:1–5.

30. Swanstrom LL, Hansen P. Laparoscopic total esophagectomy. Arch Surg 1997; 132:943–7.

31. Rizk NP, Bach PB, Schrag D, et al. The impact of complications on outcomes after resection for esophageal and gastroesophageal junction carcinoma. J Am Coll Surg 2004;198:42–50.

32. Palanivelu C, Prakash A, Senthilkumar R, et al. Minimally invasive esophagectomy: thoracoscopic mobilization of the esophagus and mediastinal

lymphadenectomy in prone position—experience of 130 patients. J Am Coll Surg 2006;203:7–16.

33. Jarral O, Purkayastha S, Athanasiou T, et al. Thoracoscopic esophagectomy in the prone position. Surg Endosc 2012;26(8):2095–103.

34. Feng M, Shen Y, Wang H, et al. Thoracolaparoscopic esophagectomy: is the prone position a safe alternative to the decubitus position? J Am Coll Surg 2012;214(5):838–44.

35. Dantoc MM, Cox MR, Eslick GD. Does minimally invasive esophagectomy (MIE) provide for comparable oncologic outcomes to open techniques? A systematic review. J Gastrointest Surg 2012;16:486–94.

36. Luketich JD, Pennathur A, Catalano PJ, et al. Results of a phase II multicenter study of MIE (Eastern Cooperative Oncology Group Study E2202). J Clin Oncol 2009;27(Suppl):15s [abstract: 4516].

Esophageal Reconstruction with Alternative Conduits

Jenifer L. Marks, MD, Wayne L. Hofstetter, MD*

KEYWORDS

- Esophageal replacement • Conduit • Jejunum • Reconstruction • Supercharged
- Esophagectomy • Colon interposition • Jejunal interposition

KEY POINTS

- Both the colon and supercharged pedicled jejunum are acceptable options for esophageal reconstruction when the stomach is not available.
- It is useful to be adept at all reconstruction options so as to individualize treatment as indicated.
- Inherent advantages of jejunum are the relative lack of diverticular and malignant disease progression observed with an aging patient.
- The major relevant drawback for the long-segment jejunal interposition remains the complexity and potential side effects of the microvascular augmentation.
- The small bowel also seems to require fewer reoperations for dilatation, redundancy, and stasis compared with historical data on the colon.

INDICATIONS

A jejunal or colonic conduit is indicated for any long-segment esophageal replacement caused by active or prior cancer, prior operative interventions with complications requiring resection or diversion, or in the setting of discontinuity caused by rupture.[1,2] The patient's past medical and surgical history dictates which organs are available as options for reconstruction. There is some debate in the literature over which organ is better for reconstruction; however, there is no consensus and often surgeon experience, hospital resources, and preferences dictate which is used.

SURGICAL TECHNIQUE
Long-Segment Supercharged Jejunal Conduit

Preoperative evaluation
Routine preoperative evaluation is necessary when planning a supercharged jejunal conduit for esophageal replacement. A complete history and physical should be

The authors have no relevant disclosures.
Funding: The Carl and Ginny Edwards and the Stuart and Flora Mason family foundations contributed to the completion of this project.
Department of Thoracic and Cardiovascular Surgery, University of Texas MD Anderson Cancer Center, 1400 Hermann Pressler Drive, Houston, TX 77030–4008, USA
* Corresponding author.
E-mail address: whofstetter@mdanderson.org

performed, taking note of any previous abdominal, thoracic, or sternal incisions because they may alter the surgical plan and position of the conduit. In the setting of esophageal cancer, complete staging should be performed, including esophago-gastroduodenoscopy/endoscopic ultrasonography and positron emission tomography/computed tomography (PET/CT) to confirm disease stage. A CT chest/abdomen/pelvis with contrast should be obtained to evaluate for any radiographic abnormalities of the small bowel, mesentery, or major abdominal vessels. Consultation with a plastic surgeon in addition to the esophageal surgeon is necessary when planning a supercharged jejunal conduit. Thorough preoperative patient education and counseling should be provided that focuses on postoperative expectations, dietary modifications, and lifestyle modifications that will be necessary following the procedure. In contrast to a colon interposition, there is no need for presurgical preparation of the bowel when the jejunum is used. If, however, there are worries about the viability of the small bowel as a useable conduit, it is worth preparing the colon as another alternative.

Surgical procedure

The patient is positioned supine with a shoulder roll in place and the head turned slightly to the right. The left neck, chest, and abdomen are prepped into the field. At least 1 leg should be prepped into the field for possible harvest of a saphenous vein graft.

Abdomen

An upper midline incision is made and the ligament of Treitz identified along with the proximal jejunum. A complete lysis of adhesions should be performed and any prior feeding jejunostomy or gastrostomy should be taken down and the bowel repaired. Transillumination of the proximal jejunal mesentery delineates the individual jejunal vessels and their arcades. The first vessel is left in place and the conduit is generally based on the second to fourth jejunal vessels. No vessels are divided at this time; the proposed pedicle for supercharging is identified and marked with a marking pen for future dissection (**Fig. 1**). Attention is now turned toward the route through which the conduit will pass. The transmediastinal position of the conduit is determined in part by the indication for reconstruction. Because reversal of discontinuity is a frequent indication, the posterior mediastinum is not an option in these situations. Therefore, a supercharged jejunal conduit is most often placed in the retrosternal position or, less often, subcutaneously on the anterior chest. We think that the microvascular anastomoses and subsequent lie of the conduit is best with the conduit in the retrosternal position. Also, if local/regional recurrence in the posterior mediastinum is a factor or the need for radiation exists, the conduit should be placed away from this field.

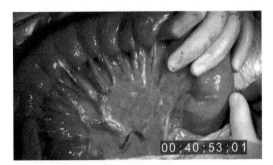

Fig. 1. Marking of the jejunal vessels for later division.

Neck

A left cervicotomy incision is made starting 2 cm below the sternal notch proceeding upwards and lateral along the anterior border of the sternocleidomastoid (SCM). Before fully exposing the esophagus, the left hemimanubrium, head of clavicle, and medial aspect of the first rib are removed to increase the space available in the thoracic inlet for the conduit and microvascular anastomosis to the internal thoracic vessels. This removal also alleviates points of bony compression on the conduit that may lead to mesenteric congestion, vascular compromise, or late dysphagia and stricture formation. The clavicular head of the SCM is separated from the clavicle using electrocautery and the sternal notch exposed. The posterior aspect of the manubrium, clavicle, and first rib must be carefully dissected to avoid injury to the innominate and subclavian vessels. Care must also be taken when freeing the inferior aspect of the clavicle, first rib, and lateral manubrium so as not to injure the internal thoracic vessels that will be used as donor vessels for the microvascular augmentation.

A saw or rongeur can then be used to remove the hemimanubrium, clavicular head, and medial aspect of the first rib. The internal thoracic vessels are approximately 1 cm lateral to the edge of the manubrium and should be identified and protected during the bony removal. The posterior aspect of the sternum should be freed as much as possible from the top because this is the superior aspect of the tunnel through which the conduit will pass.

The esophagus is exposed by retracting the SCM and carotid sheath laterally and the trachea medially. The omohyoid muscle may need to be divided. Retraction on the trachea should only be performed with a sponge or finger to avoid compression injury to the recurrent laryngeal nerve (RLN). The esophagus can be encircled with a Penrose and blunt dissection used to fully mobilize the esophagus down into the thoracic cavity if still in its native position. If the patient is already in discontinuity, the esophagostomy should be taken down and the esophagus positioned in the neck where it will lie for the anastomosis. The end of the esophagostomy generally requires trimming back to healthy mucosa for creation of the anastomosis.

Retrosternal tunnel

The retrosternal tunnel for the conduit is then created from the abdomen. The posterior aspect of the sternum is identified and blunt dissection used to create the space proceeding superiorly until the dissection from the cervical incision has been reached. A laparotomy pad can be placed within the tunnel for hemostasis if needed. The tunnel should be large enough to accommodate the conduit without any narrowing or points of compression from adjacent soft tissue. The conduit will later be tacked to this exit point from the chest to prevent herniation of the conduit or abdominal contents. A measuring device is used at this point to carefully measure the distance needed to traverse the thoracic cavity and allow for a tension free anastomosis in the neck. The distance measured is then used to locate where the distal aspect of the conduit will be. The conduit should lie in as straight a line as possible with no redundancy or large mesenteric loops in the bowel. This position is critical to the formation of a straight, well-functioning jejunal interposition.

Conduit creation and passage

At this point, the proximal pedicle of the jejunum, usually the second jejunal vessel, is divided close to its origin from the superior mesenteric artery (shown in **Fig. 2** just before dividing) and the bowel divided a few centimeters proximal to this. The next jejunal vascular pedicle, usually the third, is also divided close to its origin. The fourth branch is left intact as the vascular pedicle that feeds the distal flap but the mesentery

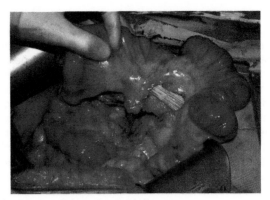

Fig. 2. Isolation of jejunal pedicle to be divided.

is opened up around the vessels to create length in the conduit adequate to reach the neck. The mesentery between the second and third vessels is divided all the way to the mesenteric border of the bowel to allow the jejunum to unfurl and straighten (**Fig. 3**). This step is the key that removes the redundant S loops from the bowel and allows the conduit to lie in a straight mediastinal course. It is also the step that results in ischemia to the most proximal portion of the small bowel creating the need for vascular augmentation.

If a jejunogastric anastomosis is to be constructed, the length is measured to the posterior wall of the stomach and the distal aspect of the jejunum divided at the appropriate length. If a Roux limb is to be performed for reconstruction, the distal jejunum does not require division.

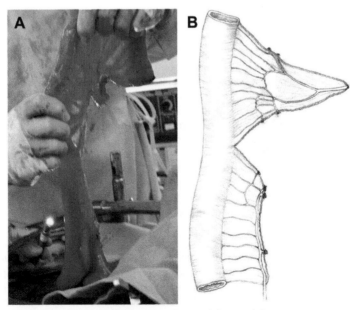

Fig. 3. (*A, B*) Opening of jejunal mesentery for straight conduit course.

After measuring the dividing the bowel and mesentery, the conduit is passed retro-colic for a posterior mediastinal reconstruction, or often antecolic for a retrosternal reconstruction. The conduit is placed within a plastic bag to allow passage through the mediastinum. The plastic bag provides protection for small vessels as the conduit is pulled through the chosen mediastinal route. Marking sutures placed on opposite sides of the proximal bowel limb or some alternative means should be used to ensure that no twisting of the conduit occurs as it is pulled through the mediastinum. Care must be taken to avoid excess traction on the conduit, which can lead to tearing of the mesentery and result in ischemic areas. Once positioned in the neck, the recipient vessels are prepared and the vascular augmentation is performed. The venous anastomosis is typically performed with a 2-mm or 4-mm coupling device using either the internal mammary vein or the jugular vein. Saphenous vein grafts can be used if there is a length discrepancy for the venous augmentation. The arterial anastomosis is then performed under the operating microscope, directly to the donor vessel.

An indicator flap is created using the most proximal 2 to 3 cm of jejunum. The prox-imal 2 to 3 cm of the jejunum and its intact mesentery are separated from the main conduit and set aside to be externalized at the completion of the procedure as an indi-cator flap (**Fig. 4**).

Reconstruction
The esophagojejunal anastomosis is performed via a hand-sewn or stapled technique. A stapled functional end-to-end anastomosis may be performed with a posterior linear staple line between the esophagus and jejunal conduit followed by hand-sewn or stapled closure of the hood (modified Collard or Orringer technique). As an alternative, the circular stapling device may be used, but care must be taken to avoid a blind pouch that will lead to a pseudo-Zenker's phenomenon.

The abdominal reconstruction is performed by either creating a Roux limb and distal jejunojejunal anastomosis or via a jejunogastric anastomosis low on the posterior wall of the stomach. A Roux limb is used more frequently because there is no remaining stomach available for reconstruction. If a stomach anastomosis is used, we advocate a two-thirds gastrectomy to avoid gastric stasis issues created by a vagotomized

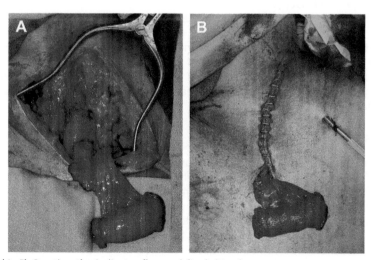

Fig. 4. (*A, B*) Creating the indicator flap and final skin closure.

stomach. A feeding jejunostomy is routinely created. If there is remaining stomach that is not in continuity with the conduit (ie, a Roux limb was created), a drainage procedure at the pylorus should be performed.

When closing the neck incision, the indicator flap should be positioned at the inferior aspect of the wound in a straight course to avoid compromising the blood supply. Once a drain is placed and the wound closed, 1 or both ends of the indicator segment should be opened to allow for drainage of secretions. This flap is left externalized as a monitor for the perfusion of the proximal bowel segment until just before discharge. At that point, it can be amputated at the bedside.

Intraoperative and Postoperative Management

This is a procedure of long duration with several operative teams involved. The patient and operating room should be kept warm throughout the procedure. Intravenous fluids should be optimized to help avoid fluid overload in the immediate postoperative period. Many patients are able to be extubated on the evening of postoperative day 0 if the operation was uneventful. Early extubation is essential for pulmonary toilet and normal postoperative progression of ambulation should be encouraged.

Vasopressors should be avoided if possible and fluid given for blood pressure support. Blood pressure should be maintained at preoperative systolic levels, because this is the perfusion pressure the bowel is used to receiving. Tube feeds are generally begun on postoperative day 3 and slowly advanced as bowel function tolerates. Careful postoperative observation by an experienced team, aggressive pulmonary toilet, early mobilization, and optimal pain control are factors that lead to an uneventful postoperative course.

Complications

Most of the complications seen after a supercharged jejunal interposition are similar to those seen after esophagectomy. Bowel ischemia resulting in conduit loss is infrequent. Thrombosis or diminished flow through the vascular anastomosis may occur and, if perfusion is compromised, the vascular augmentation should be revised to avoid graft loss. The indicator flap serves as a guide to the viability of the conduit and should be monitored frequently. Suspicion of conduit ischemia should prompt evaluation via endoscopy.

Nonobstructive mesenteric ischemia is another complication that can occur at or downstream from the feeding jejunostomy. Patients experience pain with the initiation of tube feedings as the vascular demand increases with bowel function. If symptoms occur, the tube feeds should be held and the patient resuscitated with intravenous fluids and monitored for signs of bowel ischemia. Other complications such as bleeding, aspiration pneumonia, RLN damage, and stricture formation are managed using standard techniques.

RESULTS

Data presented recently update a 10-year experience from MD Anderson Cancer Center.[3] The database was combined with the experience from The Methodist Hospital where all of the surgical participants were trained at MD Anderson and have 4 years of independent programmatic growth. Sixty patients received a supercharged jejunal conduit, largely for reconstruction related to previous discontinuity or gastroesophageal junction tumor extending so low into the stomach that it precluded use of that organ as a conduit option. Postoperative complications included 18 (30%) patients with pneumonia, 19 (31.7%) patients had an anastomotic leak, 9 (15%) required intervention (others were managed conservatively), and 4 (6.7%) patients experienced graft loss. Most patients (88%) were able to return to an oral diet with complete independence from supplemental nutrition after jejunal reconstruction. Thirty-day mortality, including in hospital mortality, was 5% with a 90-day mortality of 10%. These results represent a group of high-risk patients, 42% of whom were undergoing reversal of discontinuity. Given these results, we prefer a supercharged jejunal conduit for esophageal reconstruction only when the stomach is not available, not as a primary option.

Short-Segment Jejunal Interposition

When only a segment of the distal esophagus needs reconstruction, a short-segment jejunal interposition, referred to as the Merendino procedure, is a good option. The mesentery of the jejunum is mobile enough to allow creation of a short-segmental conduit, based on an in situ vascular pedicle that is passed retrogastric and anastomosed with the distal esophagus and proximal stomach. Little additional preoperative evaluation is necessary for this procedure. Routine history and physical should identify any previous abdominal operations or small bowel disorders that might affect operative plans. Imaging in addition to a CT of the chest/abdomen is not necessary. This operation was initially described as treatment of severe gastroesophageal reflux but is no longer performed often for this indication.

Operative technique

An upper midline incision is made and, if necessary, a lysis of adhesions performed. The proximal jejunum and its mesentery are inspected and an area chosen with good length for transposition. The vascular pedicle for the piece of jejunum to be transposed is identified and freed as a pedicle from its surrounding mesentery. The length of bowel needed for reconstruction is determined by examining the diseased segment of esophagus that requires replacement, and the bowel is transected after isolating the vascular pedicle. It is acceptable, and often necessary, to divide a single branch of the jejunal vessels coming off the superior mesenteric artery to achieve length for reconstruction. Perfusion of the graft via arcades in the mesentery is generally robust. The mobilized jejunum is then passed in a retrocolic and retrogastric position and placed near the hiatus in an isoperistaltic manner to replace the esophageal defect. The mesentery and bowel are then inspected for any tension or points of compression along their route. If the appearance and lie of the conduit are satisfactory, the esophagojejunal anastomosis can then be performed with the EEA stapler or a hand-sewn technique. This anastomosis is in the mediastinum and often difficult to visualize. It is critical to be certain that enough jejunal and mesenteric length are mobilized to render the anastomosis tension free. The jejunogastric anastomosis is then performed high on the posterior wall of the stomach near the greater curvature in a nonvagotomized stomach, or to the gastric remnant after two-thirds gastrectomy in a fully vagotomized patient. This type of replacement can also be performed as a Roux-en-Y when a total gastrectomy is necessary. The jejunojejunal anastomosis is performed using standard techniques.

The mesenteric defect should be closed in a way that does not put any tension on the transposed segment. A feeding jejunostomy should be considered in these patients based on the discretion of the operating surgeon and the indication for the procedure. Circumstances that might increase the possibility of perioperative complications requiring prolonged nil-by-mouth status should prompt placement of a feeding jejunostomy.

Colon

The colon is another option for esophageal reconstruction when the stomach is not available. The right or the left colon may be used for reconstruction and can provide an adequate length to reach the pharynx. The transverse colon is part of the conduit whether it is used in conjunction with the right or left colon. A left colon graft is based on the ascending branch of the left colic artery, whereas the middle colic vessels are the primary blood supply for a right colon graft. If colon is chosen to replace the esophagus, we generally use an isoperistaltic left colon conduit given the better size match to the native esophagus and thicker wall compared with the right colon. If the patient has an extended life expectancy, some think the colon to be a better reconstruction choice than the stomach because it is resistant to peptic strictures and provides a barrier to reflux into the proximal esophagus.

Preoperative evaluation
Preoperative evaluation is similar to that for a jejunal conduit, with special attention paid to the colonic vessels. A CT angiogram should be obtained to identify and delineate the vascular supply to right and left colon, including marginal arteries connecting the left and middle colic arcades, known as the arc of Riolan (**Fig. 5**). Previous abdominal operations or bowel resections may limit use of the colon if vessels have already been sacrificed or if the mesentery is scarred and foreshortened. In those situations, a formal angiogram may be beneficial. In addition to a CT scan, a colonoscopy or double contrast barium enema should be obtained to rule out any primary colonic lesions, diverticular disease, or vascular malformations. Patients should be placed on a liquid diet and given a mechanical bowel prep 24 to 48 hours before the operation to remove bulky stool from the conduit.

Surgical procedure
This article describes esophageal replacement with a left colon conduit because it is used more often than the right colon. Reasons for this include generally a better size match, its ability to be placed as an isoperistaltic conduit, and avoidance of the terminal ileum and cecum as part of the conduit. The left colon is completely mobilized from the retroperitoneum and the greater omentum is removed from the transverse

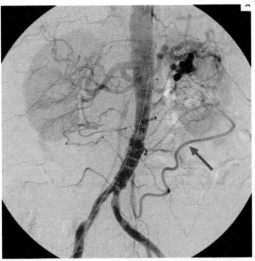

Fig. 5. Angiogram of arc of Riolan (*arrow*). (*Courtesy of* Dr Donna D'Souza, Minneapolis, MN.)

colon. Great care is taken to preserve the mesenteric vessels at all times during mobilization and to identify the ascending branch of the left colic artery, because this serves as the vascular pedicle for the conduit. The mesentery may be transilluminated to facilitate identification of the mesenteric vessels. The middle colic artery also needs to be identified in the transverse colon mesentery.

An umbilical tape is used to approximate the length of colon needed for reconstruction by measuring the distance from 5 cm below the xiphoid process to the angle of the jaw if the conduit will be placed in the posterior mediastinum. For a retrosternal conduit, the measurement should be extended to the earlobe. After determining the length of colon needed for transposition, isolation of the vascular pedicle is initiated by opening the transverse mesocolon on the right side of the middle colic vessels. The mesentery is also opened on both sides of the left colic artery. Small bulldog clamps are placed on the middle colic vessels that will be ligated and they are left in place for 5 to 10 minutes to confirm graft viability. The vascular arcade communicating with the right colic arterial system is also clamped or ligated to ensure that all arterial flow to the potential conduit is derived from the ascending branch of the left colic artery. If the graft continues to appear healthy after vascular isolation, the left branch of the middle colic artery is ligated and divided at its origin from the superior mesenteric artery. The length of colon needed is then confirmed and the bowel is then transected at the appropriate level (**Fig. 6**).

The conduit is placed in a retrogastric position and passed through the posterior mediastinum, retrosternal, or subcutaneous route to its final position in the left neck. A plastic bag should again be used when passing the conduit to protect the mesentery and ensure a straight and untwisted course through the mediastinum. If using the retrosternal route, the ipsilateral hemimanubrium, clavicular head, and medial aspect of the first rib should be removed as described earlier for a jejunal conduit.

After mobilizing the esophagus as previously described, the esophagocolonic anastomosis can be hand sewn or performed with the use of stapling devices. The cologastric anastomosis should be performed high on the posterior aspect of the greater curvature after two-thirds gastrectomy. This method helps to avoid pooling of food material in the conduit, which occurs if the anastomosis is placed low on the posterior wall of the stomach (known as a saddlebag deformity). A short portion of the intra-abdominal conduit is positioned and secured in place near the hiatus and serves as a barrier to the reflux of gastric conduits back into the thoracic portion of the conduit, and tacking sutures to the diaphragm helps to prevent conduit and

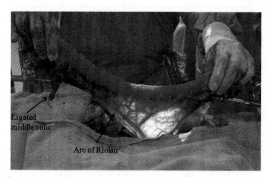

Fig. 6. Prepared left colon conduit with transillumination of mesentery.

abdominal content herniation through the hiatus. The anastomosis is then performed such that there is no excess length of conduit within the mediastinum or abdomen. The colocolonic anastomosis completes continuity of the bowel and a feeding jejunostomy tube is placed.

Complications

Early complications associated with colonic conduits are secondary to vascular or anastomotic problems. There is no indicator flap with a colonic conduit so the patient must be monitored carefully for any signs of conduit ischemia. There are 3 colonic anastomoses with this reconstruction and a leak may occur from any 1 or more if ischemia or tension is present. Leaks in the neck are generally managed with opening the neck incision and allowing wide drainage. An intra-abdominal leak may require more aggressive measures and possibly reexploration if less invasive means of managing the leak are unsuccessful. Late complications include senescent lengthening and/or dilation of the colon, which can lead to stasis, reflux, and regurgitation that often require revisional surgery to correct.

Results

The literature on colon interposition for esophageal reconstruction shows good short-term and long-term results (**Table 1**). Rates of anastomotic leak range from 0% to 28%, whereas, reported rates of graft loss are 0% to 9.4%. Reported rates of perioperative mortality vary widely, from 0% to 17% and inherently reflect the different patient populations in need of esophageal reconstruction. Results published by experienced centers are not significantly different than that seen with gastric pull-up procedures. However, there is a need for late reoperation in up to 30% of patients for conduit redundancy, dilation, and associated stasis. Limited functional data exist comparing swallowing function with colon compared with jejunal grafts but it is thought that jejunal conduits maintain peristalsis after transposition and therefore may lead to better functional outcomes.[4,15]

| Table 1 | | | | |
| Selected published series of esophageal replacement with colon or supercharged jejunum | | | | |
Colon Conduits	**N**	**Leak**	**Graft Loss (%)**	**Perioperative Mortality (%)**
Isolauri et al,[4,5] 1987	248	4	3	16
Demeester et al,[6] 1988	92	4.3	7.6	5
Cerfolio et al,[7] 1995	32	3.3	9.4	9.4
Fujita et al,[8] 1997	53	28	5.7	17
Popovici[9] 2003	347	6.9	1.4	4.6
Knezevic et al,[10] 2007	336	9.2	2.4	4.1
Mine et al,[11] 2009	95	13	0	5.3
Klink et al,[12] 2010	43	30	9	16
Hagen et al,[13] 2001	72	13	5.6	5.6
Supercharged Jejunal Conduits				
Hirabayashi et al,[14] 1993	14	14.3	0	0
Ascioti et al,[1] 2005	26	26.9	7.7	0
Blackmon et al,[3] 2012	60	31.7	6.7	5

SUMMARY

Both the colon and supercharged pedicled jejunum are acceptable options for esophageal reconstruction when the stomach is not available. There are technical aspects unique and critical to the success of each operation and most surgeons prefer 1 technique rather than others given past experiences. Inherent advantages of jejunum are the relative lack of diverticular and malignant disease progression observed with an aging patient. The small bowel also seems to require fewer reoperations for dilation, redundancy, and stasis compared with historical data on the colon. The major relevant drawback for the long-segment jejunal interposition remains the complexity and potential side effects of the microvascular augmentation. We find that it is useful to be adept at all reconstruction options so as to individualize treatment as indicated.

REFERENCES

1. Ascioti A, Hofstetter W, Miller M, et al. Long-segment, supercharged, pedicled jejunal flap for total esophageal reconstruction. J Thorac Cardiovasc Surg 2005;130:1391–8.
2. Swisher S, Hofstetter W, Miller M. The supercharged microvascular jejunal interposition. Semin Thorac Cardiovasc Surg 2007;19:56–65.
3. Blackmon S, Correa A, Skoracki R, et al. Super-charged pedicled jejunal interposition for esophageal replacement: a 10 year experience. Annals of Thoracic Surgery, in Press.
4. Isolauri J, Reinikainen P, Markkula H. Functional evaluation of interposed colon in esophagus. Manometric and 24-hour pH observations. Acta Chir Scand 1987;153:21–4.
5. Isolauri J, Markkula H, Autio V. Colon interposition in the treatment of carcinoma of the esophagus and gastric cardia. Ann Thorac Surg 1987;43:420–4.
6. DeMeester T, Johansson K, Franze I, et al. Indications, surgical technique, and long-term functional results of colon interposition or bypass. Ann Surg 1988;208:460–74.
7. Cerfolio R, Allen M, Deschamps C, et al. Esophageal replacement by colon interposition. Ann Thorac Surg 1995;59:1382–4.
8. Fujita H, Yamana H, Sueyoshi S, et al. Impact on outcome of additional microvascular anastomosis–supercharge–on colon interposition for esophageal replacement: comparative and multivariate analysis. World J Surg 1997;21:998–1003.
9. Popovici Z. A new philosophy in esophageal reconstruction with colon. Thirty-years experience. Dis Esophagus 2003;16:323–7.
10. Knezevic JD, Radovanovic NS, Simic AP, et al. Colon interposition in the treatment of esophageal caustic strictures: 40 years of experience. Dis Esophagus 2007;20:530–4.
11. Mine S, Udagawa H, Tsutsumi K, et al. Colon interposition after esophagectomy with extended lymphadenectomy for esophageal cancer. Ann Thorac Surg 2009; 88:1647–53.
12. Klink CD, Binnebösel M, Schneider M, et al. Operative outcome of colon interposition in the treatment of esophageal cancer: a 20-year experience. Surgery 2010;147:491–6.
13. Hagen J, DeMeester S, Peters J, et al. Curative resection for esophageal adenocarcinoma: analysis of 100 en bloc esophagectomies. Ann Surg 2001;234(4):520–30.
14. Hirabayashi S, Miyata M, Shoji M, et al. Reconstruction of the thoracic esophagus, with extended jejunum used as a substitute, with the aid of microvascular anastomosis. Surgery 1993;113:515–9.
15. Chen H, Rampazzo A, Gharb B, et al. Motility differences in free colon and free jejunum flaps for reconstruction of the cervical esophagus. Plast Reconstr Surg 2008;122:1410–6.

Complications of Esophagectomy

Daniel Raymond, MD, FACS

KEYWORDS

- Esophagectomy • Postoperative complication • Morbidity

KEY POINTS

- Esophageal resection and replacement remains a formidable challenge for all health care providers.
- Pulmonary complications are almost uniformly recognized as the most frequent complication following esophagectomy and have been implicated in nearly two-thirds of postoperative mortalities.
- The impact of respiratory complications on outcome certainly warrants significant attention by all surgeons.
- The overall morbidity rates following an esophagectomy are generally reported to be in the 50% to 60% range; however, interpretation of this number epitomizes the challenges in interpretation of the literature.

Esophageal resection and replacement remains a formidable challenge for all health care providers. The challenges of removal of this relatively simple organ traversing 3 distinct anatomic zones in the body (neck, chest, and abdomen) and reconstitution of the gastrointestinal tract has led to considerable variation in technique. Currently, the Society of Thoracic Surgery General Thoracic Surgery Database (**Box 1**) lists 14 different methods of performing esophagectomy. This highlights the variability that exists today and underscores the challenges of quantifying and comparing outcomes. Numerous variables, including etiology of disease, patient demographics, comorbidities, disease stage, treatment variables, surgeon experience, intraoperative variables, and health center differences, should be considered when discussing operative complications.

MORTALITY

The mortality rate after esophagectomy, usually defined as in-hospital or 30-day postoperative mortality, ranges anywhere from 0%[1] to 22%,[2] depending on the variables mentioned in the previous paragraph. Mortality has clearly been linked to surgical

Thoracic & Cardiovascular Surgery, Cleveland Clinic Foundation, 9500 Euclid Avenue, J4-402, Cleveland, OH 44195, USA
E-mail address: raymond3@ccf.org

Surg Clin N Am 92 (2012) 1299–1313
http://dx.doi.org/10.1016/j.suc.2012.07.007
0039-6109/12/$ – see front matter © 2012 Elsevier Inc. All rights reserved.

Box 1
Partial list of esophagectomy techniques with associated CPT codes

- Transhiatal: total esophagectomy, without thoracotomy, with cervical esophagogastrostomy (43107)
- Three hole: total esophagectomy with thoracotomy; with cervical esophagogastrostomy (43112)
- Ivor Lewis: partial esophagectomy, distal two-thirds, with thoracotomy and separate abdominal incision (43117)
- Thoracoabdominal: partial esophagectomy, thoracoabdominal approach (43122)
- Minimally invasive 3-hole esophagectomy
- Minimally invasive esophagectomy, Ivor Lewis approach
- Minimally invasive esophagectomy, abdominal and neck approach
- Total esophagectomy without thoracotomy; with colon interposition or small intestine reconstruction (43108)
- Total esophagectomy with thoracotomy; with colon interposition or small intestine reconstruction (43113)
- Partial esophagectomy, cervical, with free intestinal graft, including microvascular anastomosis (43116)
- Partial esophagectomy, with thoracotomy and separate abdominal incision with colon interposition or small intestine (43118)
- Partial esophagectomy, distal two-thirds, with thoracotomy only (43121)
- Partial esophagectomy, thoracoabdominal with colon interposition or small intestine (43123)
- Total or partial esophagectomy, without reconstruction with cervical esophagostomy (43124)

Data from Listing Available at: www.sts.org.

---

volume. Metzger and colleagues[2] performed a meta-analysis of 13 studies evaluating the impact of surgical volume on mortality after esophagectomy, revealing a greater than threefold increase in median mortality rate when comparing low-volume centers (<5 cases per year; 18.0% median mortality) to high-volume centers (>20 cases per year; 4.9% median mortality). Similarly, Rodgers and colleagues[3] identified surgical volume as a significant predictor of mortality in a retrospective review of the Nationwide Inpatient Sample database including 3243 esophagectomies. Additional variables in this study predicting mortality included age, sex, race, and peripheral vascular disease. Notably absent from this list, owing to availability of data, is a preoperative assessment of nutritional status and/or functional status, which has been demonstrated by others to have a strong influence on postoperative mortality.[4,5] **Table 1** lists the mortality rates following esophagectomy in a random selection of relatively high-volume studies.

PULMONARY COMPLICATIONS

Pulmonary complications are almost uniformly recognized as the most frequent complication following esophagectomy and have been implicated in nearly two-thirds of postoperative mortalities.[6] Bailey and colleagues[7] reported an overall morbidity rate of 49.5% in a 10-year review of 1777 esophagectomies performed in the Department of Veterans Affairs system. The most common complication was respiratory in origin, including pneumonia (21.4%), reintubation (16.2%), and ventilator

Table 1			
Mortality rate following esophagectomy from selected studies			
	Year	n	Mortality Rate, %
Bailey et al[7]	2003	1777	9.8
Orringer et al[38]	2007	—	—
Group I	1976–98	1063	4.0
Group II	1998–2006	944	1.0
Rodgers et al[3]	2007	3243	11.4
Lin et al[5]	2004	170	12.4
Kuo et al[61]	2001	—	—
High volume	—	674	2.5
Low volume	—	519	9.2
Varghese et al[62]	2011	1505	7.6
Atkins et al[6]	2004	379	5.8
Tandon et al[11]	2001	168	10.4
Gockel et al[63]	2005	424	6.7
Togo et al[21]	2010	378	3.4

dependency for more than 48 hours (21.8%). Similarly, Avendano and colleagues[8] retrospectively evaluated a single-surgeon 6-year experience and identified significant pulmonary complications in 36.1% of patients. Of these patients, pneumonia occurred in 90.0% and was associated with a 35.0% mortality rate in comparison with an overall mortality rate of 11.5%. Further multivariate analysis of preoperative factors correlating with duration of mechanical ventilation identified preoperative chemoradiotherapy ($r = 0.30$; $P = .02$), forced vital capacity ($r = -0.43$; $P<.01$) and forced expiratory volume in 1 second (FEV_1) ($r = -0.34$; $P = .02$) as significant predictors. Although the study did not identify a particular threshold of pulmonary impairment that placed a patient population at excessive risk, patients with a preoperative FEV_1 less than 65% had significantly longer durations of mechanical ventilation and length of stay. Alternatively, Bartels and colleagues[4] used a vital capacity less than 90% and a P_{ao2} (arterial partial pressure of oxygen) less than 70 mmHG to identify patients with compromised pulmonary function that related to an increased risk of postoperative mortality in their composite scoring system.

In their efforts to identify strategies to reduce postoperative complications, Atkins and colleagues[6] identified age ($P = .002$) and pneumonia ($P = .0008$) as independent factors associated with mortality in a multivariate analysis of 379 patients undergoing esophagectomy. Patients with pneumonia were noted to have an almost sevenfold increase in mortality (20.0% vs 3.1%) in this study and it was considered the principal cause of death in 54.5% of all mortalities. Further investigation evaluated the swallowing function in this population. Pneumonia occurred in 8.8% of patients with a normal swallow study or delayed gastric emptying as opposed to 38.6% in patients with evidence of aspiration or anastomotic leak. Clearly, diminished airway protection in the perioperative period contributes to respiratory complications in patients undergoing an esophagectomy.[9,10] Efforts directed at airway protection including aspiration precautions, identification of recurrent nerve injury and postoperative assessment by a multidisciplinary "swallow" team may bear significant fruit. Additional factors clearly play a role, including preoperative aspiration in patients with impaired swallowing and preoperative malnutrition. In a retrospective, single-center review of 168 patients undergoing esophagectomy, Tandon and colleagues[11] reported a 44.0% rate of respiratory complications including acute respiratory distress syndrome (ARDS) in 14.5%. Notably, the mortality rate in the ARDS population was 50.0% in comparison to 3.5% in the remainder of the population. Furthermore, multivariate analysis identified several significant factors in the development of ARDS, including low body mass index (BMI) (0.58; confidence interval [CI] 0.41–0.82; $P = .004$), anastomotic leak (22.52; CI 3.16–160.36; $P = .002$), hypoxemia index (1.76; CI 1.26–2.47; $P = .001$), smoker (9.95; CI 1.07–92.7; $P = .04$), and postoperative fluid requirement (2.98; CI 1.16–7.67, $P = .04$).

The impact of respiratory complications on outcome certainly warrants significant attention by all surgeons. Protocols, including experienced staff, set in place at high-volume centers may be one reason to explain overall improvement in outcomes in such centers. Recognition of patients at risk for aspiration is imperative during the critical period of anesthetic induction. Careful attention to surgical technique with regard to conduit perfusion, conduit tunneling, construction of the anastomosis, and gastric outlet procedures in addition to avoidance of recurrent laryngeal nerve injury all remain vital considerations. The choice of approach may also have an impact on respiratory complications. Hulscher and colleagues[12] randomized 220 patients to a transthoracic versus a transhiatal approach for mid-distal esophageal cancers. Comparison of outcomes revealed a significantly higher rate of pulmonary complication in the transthoracic group (57% vs 27%, $P<.001$), as well as an increased time requiring mechanical ventilation. Notably the transthoracic route did result in a greater number of lymph nodes resected (31 ± 4 vs 16 ± 9; $P<.001$), but this did not translate into a significant improvement in 5-year survival (transthoracic 39%; CI 20–38 vs transhiatal 29%; CI 30–48). The trend, however, did favor a transthoracic approach. Respiratory complications from selected studies are listed in **Table 2**.

CARDIOVASCULAR COMPLICATIONS

Cardiovascular complications can include of broad group of events that are variably defined and reported in the literature. Atrial fibrillation remains a common complication following thoracic operations. Atkins and colleagues[6] reported a 13.7% rate of arrhythmia following an esophagectomy in a single-center, retrospective review of 379 patients. These findings were similar to the 11.5% rate of arrhythmia noted by Seely and colleagues[13] in their review including 258 patients undergoing esophagectomy. Murthy and colleagues[14] performed a more focused review of 921 patients undergoing esophagectomy at The University of Hong Kong, Queen Mary Hospital, and identified a 22% rate of atrial fibrillation. When patients were matched with controls without atrial fibrillation, there were significantly higher rates of pulmonary complications, renal failure, a 6.0-fold increase in anastomotic leak rates, and

Table 2					
Respiratory complications following esophagectomy from selected studies					
	Year of Publication	n	Pneumonia, %	Reintubation, %	Ventilator Dependency >48 h, %
Bailey et al[7]	2003	1777	21.4	16.2	21.8
Avendano et al[8]	2002	61	32.8	19.7	19.7
Atkins et al[6]	2004	379	15.8	6.1	4.7
Tandon et al[11]	2001	168	17.8	NA	23.8

Abbreviation: NA, not available.

3.7-fold increase in mortality among patients who developed atrial fibrillation. In addition, atrial fibrillation has been associated with increased length of stay and greater cost following thoracic surgery.[15] Clearly, the concept of prevention remains very attractive for reduction of morbidity, mortality, and cost. Underlying this, however, is a lack of understanding regarding the role of atrial fibrillation as a causative factor of postoperative morbidity rather than an indicator of autonomic tone and physiologic stress, which is the true determinant of morbidity. Furthermore, a concern regarding conduit perfusion among patients undergoing esophagectomy is particularly important when considering periods of relative hypotension precipitated by atrial fibrillation. The risks and benefits of prophylaxis against atrial fibrillation was investigated in the PeriOperative IShcemic Evaluation (POISE) trial[16] in which perioperative beta-blockade was linked to a decreased risk of perioperative myocardial infarction and atrial fibrillation but an increased risk of stroke and 30-day mortality.

In several large series, myocardial infarction is reported to occur in 1.1% to 3.8% of patients undergoing esophagectomy.[6,7,13] Although perioperative beta-blockade has been a commonly accepted practice, the recent results of the POISE trial[16] have generated some measure of caution. Familiarity with the American College of Cardiology/American Heart Association guidelines[17] for the Perioperative Cardiovascular Evaluation and Care of Noncardiac Surgical Patients remains an essential guide for all surgeons to appropriately risk stratify patients and provide quality postoperative care. Esophagectomy is classified as an intermediate-risk procedure for which guidance is provided on preoperative testing and perioperative heart rate control. Again, a unique feature of esophagectomy is the compromised perfusion to the neo-esophagus and thus the enhanced susceptibility to malperfusion, which may affect the overall morbidity associated with the use of prophylactic chronotropic agents not seen in other noncardiac surgeries.

The American College of Chest Physicians Guidelines on the Prevention of Venous Thromboembolism[18] classified esophagectomy as a high-risk procedure and thus recommends postoperative thromboprophylaxis with low molecular weight heparin, unfractionated subcutaneous heparin 3 times daily, or fondaparinux. Alternatively, some would classify esophagectomy as high risk for bleeding, especially in the setting of blunt mediastinal dissection, and thus justify mechanical means of thromboprophylaxis only. Further complicating the matter is the frequent use of neuraxial anesthesia, which limits the use of perioperative anticoagulants for thromboprophylaxis.[19] Unfortunately, a paucity of data exist to help clarify these issues and therefore clinical practice varies. Bailey and colleagues[7] report a postoperative deep venous thrombosis rate of 0.9% and pulmonary embolus rate of 0.7%. Atkins and colleagues[6] reports a combined rate of 2.4%. Clearly, the esophagectomy patient population is high risk, for it typically has several established risks for venous thromboembolism, including cancer, advanced age, smoking, bedrest, and neoadjuvant therapy. Thus, an aggressive prophylactic regimen is justified. The concern regarding postoperative bleeding and the limitations of neuraxial anesthesia may limit this approach.

RECURRENT LARYNGEAL NERVE INJURY

Recurrent nerve injury, usually on the left, often occurs during dissection of the cervical esophagus. **Table 3** lists rates of recurrent laryngeal injury reported in various published series. Not surprisingly, recurrent nerve injury is associated with the site of the anastomosis. In a meta-analysis of cervical versus thoracic anastomoses for esophagectomy, Biere and colleagues[20] demonstrated a significant increase in risk with the cervical anastomosis (odds ratio [OR] 7.14; CI 1.75–29.14; $P = .006$). Togo

Table 3
Recurrent laryngeal nerve injury rates following esophagectomy from selected studies

	Year of Publication	n	Recurrent Laryngeal Nerve Injury Rate, %
Atkins et al[6]	2004	379	2.1
Orringer et al[38]	2007	—	—
Group I	1976–98	1063	7.0
Group II	1998–2006	944	2.0
Hulscher et al[12]	2002	—	—
Transhiatal	—	106	13.0
Transthoracic	—	114	21.0
Gockel et al[64]	2005	424	15.7
Altorki et al[65]	2002	88	6.0

and colleagues[21] were further able to demonstrate a significant relationship between recurrent nerve injury, postoperative swallowing disorder, and pneumonia ($P<.001$).

Principles for the avoidance of this complication include precise knowledge of cervical esophageal anatomy, maintaining the plane of dissection as close as possible to the esophagus, and avoidance of metal or rigid retractors along the tracheo-esophageal groove. Once nerve injury is suspected, laryngoscopy and swallow evaluation should immediately be undertaken. The author advocates aggressive management of this condition with vocal cord injection for temporary medialization to enhance postoperative pulmonary toilet and prevent aspiration. Recurrent nerve injury can recover with time, especially if the nerve remains intact. Baba and colleagues[22] report spontaneous recovery rate of 41.2% in their retrospective series including 51 with vocal cord paralysis after esophagectomy. If the problem persists, permanent vocal cord medialization should be considered. Notably in Baba and colleagues' series,[22] 36.7% of patients who did not have spontaneous remission within a year experienced a significant decline in their performance status.

CHYLOTHORAX

Chyle consists of lymphocytes, fat, protein, and electrolytes and flows via the thoracic duct at approximately 2 to 4 L per day. Injury to the lymphatic system during esophagectomy can result in clinically significant chyle leak at rates reported to be between 0% and 8% (**Table 4**) and can carry an associated mortality of up to 50%.[23] The diagnosis of a chyle leak is generally based on an increase in chest tube output with enteral alimentation and change in nature of the output to a milky appearance. Pleural fluid triglyceride level higher than 110 mg/dL or presence of chylomicrons is generally

Table 4
Rates of chylothorax following esophagectomy from selected studies

	Year of Publication	n	Chylothorax Rate, %
Orringer et al[38]	2007	2029	1.0
Atkins et al[6]	2004	379	0.79
Avendano et al[8]	2002	61	8.2
Merigliano et al[26]	2000	1787	1.1
Bolger et al[23]	1991	537	2.0

diagnostic of a chyle leak.[24] Once diagnosis is confirmed, management includes elimination of enteral nutrition with consideration for parenteral nutrition support, close observation of chest tube output, octreotide, and fluid resuscitation. In a retrospective analysis of 23 patients with chyle leak following esophagectomy, Dugue and colleagues[25] demonstrated a 61% success rate with conservative management, whereas Merigliano and colleagues[26] identified a 36% rate in their retrospective series. Furthermore, in the Dugue and colleagues[25] report, chyle output was significantly greater on day 5 in those patients who failed conservative management (23 vs 6.7 mL per kg; $P<.001$) and an output of greater than 10 mL/kg on day 5 after onset had a sensitivity of 86% and specificity of 100% in identifying those patients who would fail conservative management.

Early surgical intervention is now favored by many surgeons, given the high mortality associated with the resultant immunologic and nutritional depletion in an already compromised patient population.[26] Where available, preoperative lymphangiogram and percutaneous embolization/disruption of the thoracic duct can yield excellent success rates but is highly dependent on the experience of the interventionalist.[27,28] Surgical intervention is directed by the hemithorax involved based on chest tube output, although generally right video-assisted thoracoscopic surgery (VATS) or a thoracotomy is required for access to the thoracic duct. Attempts can be made to identify the source of the leak by administering cream or vegetable oil enterally before the procedure, although this should be coordinated with the anesthesia team. If the leak can be identified, the duct should be ligated proximally and distally using ties or clips. If the leak is not identified, mass ligation of all tissue between the spine and the aorta, including the azygous vein, is performed as caudal as possible in the right hemithorax. Pleurodesis may also be entertained at this time to prevent effusion recurrence.

CONDUIT-RELATED DISORDERS
Anastomotic Leak

Ischemia and deinnervation are inherent to the creation of the neo-esophagus during esophagectomy. Compromised conduit perfusion at the site of anastomosis, quantified by Boyle and colleagues[29] as up to a 70% reduction in blood flow, results in impaired healing and thus the predisposition to leak. The variety of techniques available for performance of esophagectomy preclude any definitive conclusions; however, several variables have been implicated in the ultimate integrity of the anastomosis: anastomotic technique, anastomotic location, conduit location, and conduit selection. **Table 5** lists the reported rates of anastomotic leaks following esophagectomy from selected studies. Anastomotic techniques include hand sewn (single vs double layer) and stapled (circular vs linear) with surgeon experience likely being the most important determinant at present. In a meta-analysis of 4 randomized controlled trials, Beitler and colleagues[30] demonstrated no difference in anastomotic leak rates (stapled 9% vs hand sewn 8%; $P = .67$), but did reveal a higher rate of stricture formation in the circular stapled group (27% vs 16%; $P<.02$). In the 1990s, a hybrid linear stapled technique was reported by Collard and colleagues,[31] which demonstrated a 65% increase in the anastomotic cross-sectional area. Orringer and colleagues[32] subsequently reported 114 consecutive patients with a similar hybrid technique that revealed a reduction in anastomotic leak rate to 2.7% from 10.0% to 15.0%. Additionally, Ercan and colleagues[33] at the Cleveland Clinic retrospectively compared the modified Collard technique with a standard hand-sewn anastomosis in 274 patients. Using a propensity-matched analysis, they revealed freedom from anastomotic leak was not statistically significant between groups (stapled 96% vs sewn

Table 5
Anastomotic leak rates following esophagectomy from selected studies

	Year of Publication	n	Anastomotic Leak Rate, %
Atkins et al[6]	2004	379	14.0
Seely et al[13]	2010	52	9.6
Orringer et al[38]	2007	2007	12.0
Hulscher et al[12]	2002	—	—
Transhiatal	—	106	14.0
Transthoracic	—	114	16.0
Briel et al[42]	2004	393	10.9
Merritt et al[66]	2011	138	12.3[3,7,38,61,62]
van Heijl et al[53]	2010	607	10.7

89%; P = .09); however, freedom from cervical wound infection (stapled 92% vs sewn 71%; P = .001) and freedom from anastomotic dilation (stapled 34% vs sewn 10%; $P<.0001$) were improved in the stapled group.

Anastomotic location (cervical vs thoracic) remains a highly debated subject in the thoracic literature. Theoretically, the cervical location is associated with a higher overall leak rate; however, the anatomic confines of the neck and thoracic inlet limit the resultant surrounding contamination and, thus, morbidity. Additionally, a cervical anastomosis performed with a transhiatal approach can avoid the morbidity of thoracotomy. The thoracic anastomosis, owing potentially to shorter conduit length requirements and less tension, has a lower leak rate. On the other hand, the morbidity of pleural and mediastinal soilage is theoretically higher. Biere and colleagues[20] performed a meta-analysis of trials comparing cervical and thoracic anastomoses including 4 randomized trials. Recurrent laryngeal nerve injury (OR 7.14; 95% CI 1.75–29.14; $P<.001$) and anastomotic leak (OR 3.43; 95% CI 1.09–10.78; P = .03) were associated with a cervical anastomosis in multivariate analysis, whereas pulmonary complications, stricture formation, tumor recurrence, and mortality were not. Additionally, using the Surveillance, Epidemiology, and End Results (SEER) database, Chang and colleagues[34] performed a retrospective cohort review comparing 225 transhiatal resections to 643 transthoracic resections. The unadjusted anastomotic complication rate, identified by need for postoperative endoscopic dilation, was higher (43.1% vs 34.5%; P = .02) in the transhiatal group. Notably, there was no significant difference in risk-adjusted 5-year survival between groups. Proponents of thoracic anastomoses[35–37] have further demonstrated mortality for intrathoracic leaks similar to that of cervical leaks and attributed concerns regarding higher mortality to outdated data and concepts extrapolated from the treatment of Boerhaave syndrome. At present, the choice of anastomotic location remains clinician dependent. The cervical anastomosis does appear to be associated with a higher leak rate, which may translate into a higher rate of postoperative stricture and dysphagia. This does not, however, appear to translate into a worsened overall survival. Additionally, individual reports, such as Orringer and colleagues remarkable 3% leak rate,[38] following cervical esophagogastric anastomosis emphasizes the importance of surgeon experience and awareness of outcomes.

Orthotopic placement of the neo-esophagus in the posterior mediastinum is generally preferred by most thoracic surgeons. Urschel and colleagues[39] previously performed a meta-analysis of trials comparing the posterior mediastinal route and the retrosternal route and were unable to demonstrate any difference in postoperative morbidity. Other series, however, have revealed a higher anastomotic leak rate in the retrosternal route, likely attributable to increased length requirements for the conduit, as well as compression.[38,40,41] Conduit choice may also affect anastomotic integrity, although most surgeons presently prefer the stomach because of its ease of preparation, a robust blood supply, and sufficient length. Alternative conduits, including colon and jejunum, are typically chosen only out of necessity. Briel and colleagues[42] previously reported significantly lower anastomotic complication rates in patients undergoing colonic interposition when compared with gastric conduits. Others, however, have reported higher anastomotic complication rates associated with colonic interposition,[38,40,43] which again emphasizes the importance of surgeon experience, as these were centers that preferred the gastric conduit.

CONDUIT ISCHEMIA

Although relative conduit ischemia is essentially inherent to esophagectomy, ischemia requiring further surgical intervention is reported at a variable rate. Orringer and colleagues[38] reported a 2% rate of gastric tip necrosis requiring takedown of the intrathoracic stomach and cervical esophagostomy. Bailey and colleagues[7] reported a 0.8% rate of "graft failure," although the definition is unclear. Griffin and colleagues[44] reported a 1% rate of gastric conduit ischemia requiring reintervention. Gastric necrosis was reported as the underlying cause of death in 2 (22%) of the 9 mortalities in the study. Endoscopic evaluation of conduits by Briel and colleagues[42] identified conduit ischemia in 9.2% of patients in their retrospective review. Mortality rates rose roughly fourfold in patients experiencing conduit ischemia, which was also noted to be a significant risk factor for development of an anastomotic leak (OR 5.5; 95% CI 2.5–12.1).

FUNCTIONAL CONDUIT DISORDERS

"Normal" digestive function is reported in fewer than 20% of patients following esophagectomy.[45,46] Functional conduit disorders contribute significantly to poor postoperative digestive function after an esophagectomy and include dumping syndrome, delayed gastric emptying, dysphagia, and esophageal reflux. Dumping occurs in up to 50% of patients following esophagectomy with 1% to 5% having disabling symptoms.[47] Most have early symptoms (**Table 6**), characterized by gastrointestinal and vasomotor symptoms occurring 10 to 30 minutes after eating, theoretically because of rapid transit of hyperosmolar gastric contents into the small bowel. Late symptoms occurring 1 to 3 hours after a meal are reported in 25% of patients[48] and are attributed to hypoglycemia secondary to a profound insulin response to a carbohydrate challenge. Management generally begins with dietary alterations, including reduction in carbohydrate intake, especially simple sugars, increased frequency and decreased size of meals, and fluid restriction around meals to slow gastric transit. Octreotide may be considered in patients refractory to dietary modification.

Delayed gastric emptying occurs in up to 50% of patients following an esophagectomy[47] secondary to truncal vagotomy performed during resection. Vagal sparing procedures[49] can be performed for Barrett esophagus with high-grade dysplasia and intramucosal carcinoma. This precludes an effective lymph node dissection, but improves the rate of postoperative dumping and weight loss. More recently, others have questioned the necessity of a pyloroplasty or pyloromyotomy. Lanuti and colleagues[50] evaluated 242 patients who underwent an esophagectomy, comparing those with and without pyloromyotomy. Pyloromyotomy did not reduce the incidence of gastric outlet obstruction, pneumonia, respiratory failure, anastomotic stricture, or

Table 6 Dumping syndrome symptoms/signs		
Early Dumping		**Late Dumping**
Gastrointestinal	*Vasomotor*	
Abdominal Fullness	Flushing	Perspiration
Abdominal Cramping	Headache	Tremulousness
Diarrhea	Diaphoresis	Hunger
Nausea	Syncope	Tachycardia
Vomiting	Fatigue	Decreased arousal
Borborygmi	Palpitations	
	Pallor	

Data from Donington JS. Functional conduit disorders after esophagectomy. Thorac Surg Clin 2006;16(1):53–62.

mortality, or reduce the length of stay. Gastric outlet obstruction was furthermore successfully managed with pyloric dilation in 96.7% of patients. Urschel and colleagues[51] further performed a meta-analysis of 553 patients in 9 randomized clinical trials evaluating the need for pyloric drainage procedures. They identified a reduced rate of early postoperative gastric outlet obstruction among patients who had a pyloric drainage procedure, but there was no significant effect on other outcomes, including mortality, anastomotic leak, pulmonary morbidity, nutritional symptoms, or long-term gastric emptying. Proponents of gastric outlet procedures emphasize the low morbidity of the procedure and potential benefits with regard to early pulmonary complications. Opponents emphasize the long-term benefits of an intact pylorus, including diminished biliary reflux, diminished dumping, avoidance of complications at the site of the procedure, and the ability to address gastric outlet issues endoscopically. More recently, botulinum toxin has been injected into the pylorus,[52] thus achieving, theoretically, a temporary gastric outlet procedure that may achieve the early benefits of a gastric outlet procedure while avoiding later complications. Further data are necessary, including larger trials for more definitive conclusions.

Dysphagia can occur in up to 65% of patients following esophagectomy,[1] with only 3% to 4% experiencing severe dysphagia.[47] The most common etiology is an anastomotic stricture, although conduit functional disorders, anatomic obstruction, and tumor recurrence also contribute. Dysphagia and anastomotic stricture are not uniformly reported or defined and are often based on subjective reporting by the patient. In a retrospective evaluation of 607 patients undergoing esophagectomy at a single center, van Heijl and colleagues[53] identified stricture formation in 41.7% at a median of 74 days postoperatively. A history of cardiovascular disease, gastric tube compared with colonic interposition, and anastomotic leakage were identified as factors predictive of stricture formation on multivariate analysis. Interestingly, in this study, patients were identified based on dysphagia limiting intake to semisolids and liquids and was subsequently assessed endoscopically. Alternatively, Williams and colleagues[1] performed endoscopy on all patients reporting dysphagia postoperatively (66%). Strictures were characterized as minimal to mild (luminal diameter >12 mm and 9–12 mm respectively) in 48% of patients and moderate to severe (luminal diameter 5–8 mm and <5 mm respectively) in 52% of patients. All patients experienced symptomatic improvement with subsequent endoscopic dilation and 77% had sustainable relief of dysphagia following a median of 2 dilation sessions.

In comparison, van Heijl and colleagues[53] reported a median of 5 dilations, which is likely attributable to the severity of stricture, given the more stringent indications for endoscopy. Interestingly, Williams and colleagues[1] reported a higher rate of dysphagia following a hand-sewn technique as opposed to a linear stapled anastomosis, although this did not correlate with the degree of stenosis identified on endoscopy.

Reflux of gastric and duodenal contents following esophagectomy with gastric conduit reconstruction is reported in 60% to 80% of patients.[54] Yuasa and colleagues[55] performed 24-hour pH and bilirubin monitoring on 25 patients following Ivor Lewis esophagectomy and identified 3 patterns of reflux: (1) acid and duodeno-gastroesophageal reflux (16%), (2) acid reflux only (12%), and (3) duodenogastroesophageal reflux only (28%). Dresner and colleagues[56] similarly reported a 42% rate of acid reflux and an 83% rate of bile reflux in their analysis of 20 patients following esophagectomy. Furthermore, 47% of patients developed columnar metaplasia in the esophageal remnant, raising concern for development of a second malignancy. Further study by Wolfsen and colleagues[57] identified recurrent Barrett metaplasia in 18% (8/45) of patients undergoing surveillance endoscopy following esophagectomy for completely resected high-grade dysplasia or localized adenocarcinoma. One of these patients developed high-grade dysplasia and 2 developed adenocarcinoma on subsequent evaluation.

Several factors have been noted to contribute to postoperative reflux. Conduit choice is an important factor and a reason some surgeons use to support the use of the colon. Loss of natural antireflux mechanisms, conduit motility, intra-abdominal to intrathoracic pressure gradients, pyloric drainage procedures, position of the anastomosis, and recovery of acid secretion in the gastric conduit are all likely contributing factors that can be controlled by a host of technical and clinical maneuvers with limited success.[54] Treatment with proton pump inhibitors, motility agents, and endoscopic evaluation certainly is justified in the symptomatic patient.

DIAPHRAGMATIC HERNIA

Hernia at the hiatal defect created for the neo-esophagus is a challenging problem. Price and colleagues[58] identified 15 (0.69%) patients with hiatal hernia following esophagectomy in a review of 2182 patients from a single center. Fourteen patients underwent trans-abdominal repair and 1 through the left chest. There was no difference between the Ivor Lewis and transhiatal approaches (0.92% vs 0.83%). The median time that elapsed between the initial operation and the hernia repair was 21 months. Median hospital stay following repair was 10 days, with a 60% morbidity rate and no mortalities. Kent and colleagues[59] additionally noted a higher rate of diaphragmatic hernia formation in minimally invasive procedures (2.8% vs 0.8%). Generally speaking, diaphragmatic hernia repair should be considered in all patients unless small and asymptomatic, or in patients who are at prohibitive risk for surgical intervention.[58]

SUMMARY

The overall morbidity rates following an esophagectomy is generally reported in the 50% to 60% range[7,13,60]; however, interpretation of this number epitomizes the challenges in interpretation of the literature. Often this term is not defined or uniformly reported, and therefore the reader is left unable to compare outcomes between studies. For instance, Avendano and colleagues[8] report an 87% rate of atelectasis or pleural effusion that was not considered clinically important. Atkins and colleagues,[6] on the other hand, report a 10.6% rate of effusion/empyema. Notably, the methods section states that effusions were counted only if specific intervention was required. Certainly, either method of reporting is legitimate; however, without clearly stated, standardized definitions and uniform reporting, it is difficult to draw meaningful conclusions. The solution to this problem is the participation in a prospective, standardized outcomes reporting system, such as the Society of Thoracic Surgery National Database, which permits participants to compare risk-adjusted outcomes with their peers to identify means of improving outcomes and preventing complications.

REFERENCES

1. Williams VA, Watson TJ, Zhovtis S, et al. Endoscopic and symptomatic assessment of anastomotic strictures following esophagectomy and cervical esophagogastrostomy. Surg Endosc 2008;22(6):1470–6.
2. Metzger R, Bollschweiler E, Vallbohmer D, et al. High volume centers for esophagectomy: what is the number needed to achieve low postoperative mortality? Dis Esophagus 2004;17(4):310–4.
3. Rodgers M, Jobe BA, O'Rourke RW, et al. Case volume as a predictor of inpatient mortality after esophagectomy. Arch Surg 2007;142(9):829–39.
4. Bartels H, Stein HJ, Siewert JR. Preoperative risk analysis and postoperative mortality of oesophagectomy for resectable oesophageal cancer. Br J Surg 1998;85(6):840–4.
5. Lin FC, Durkin AE, Ferguson MK. Induction therapy does not increase surgical morbidity after esophagectomy for cancer. Ann Thorac Surg 2004;78(5):1783–9.
6. Atkins BZ, Shah AS, Hutcheson KA, et al. Reducing hospital morbidity and mortality following esophagectomy. Ann Thorac Surg 2004;78(4):1170–6.
7. Bailey SH, Bull DA, Harpole DH, et al. Outcomes after esophagectomy: a ten-year prospective cohort. Ann Thorac Surg 2003;75(1):217–22.
8. Avendano CE, Flume PA, Silvestri GA, et al. Pulmonary complications after esophagectomy. Ann Thorac Surg 2002;73(3):922–6.
9. Heitmiller RF, Jones B. Transient diminished airway protection after transhiatal esophagectomy. Am J Surg 1991;162(5):442–6.
10. Martin RE, Letsos P, Taves DH. Oropharyngeal dysphagia in esophageal cancer before and after transhiatal esophagectomy. Dysphagia 2001;16(1):23–31.
11. Tandon S, Batchelor A, Bullock R, et al. Peri-operative risk factors for acute lung injury after elective oesophagectomy. Br J Anaesth 2001;86(5):633–8.
12. Hulscher JB, van Sandick JW, de Boer AG, et al. Extended transthoracic resection compared with limited transhiatal resection for adenocarcinoma of the esophagus. N Engl J Med 2002;347(21):1662–9.
13. Seely AJ, Ivanovic J, Threader J, et al. Systematic classification of morbidity and mortality after thoracic surgery. Ann Thorac Surg 2010;90(3):936–42.
14. Murthy SC, Law S, Whooley BP, et al. Atrial fibrillation after esophagectomy is a marker for postoperative morbidity and mortality. J Thorac Cardiovasc Surg 2003;126(4):1162–7.
15. Vaporciyan AA, Correa AM, Rice DC, et al. Risk factors associated with atrial fibrillation after noncardiac thoracic surgery: analysis of 2588 patients. J Thorac Cardiovasc Surg 2004;127(3):779–86.
16. Devereaux PJ, Yang H, Yusuf S, et al. Effects of extended-release metoprolol succinate in patients undergoing non-cardiac surgery (POISE trial): a randomised controlled trial. Lancet 2008;371(9627):1839–47.

17. Fleisher LA, Beckman JA, Brown KA, et al. ACC/AHA 2007 guidelines on perio-perative cardiovascular evaluation and care for noncardiac surgery: executive summary: a report of the American College of Cardiology/American Heart Association Task Force on Practice Guidelines. Circulation 2007;116(17):1971–96.

18. Geerts WH, Bergqvist D, Pineo GF, et al. Prevention of venous thromboembolism: American College of Chest Physicians Evidence-Based Clinical Practice Guidelines (8th Edition). Chest 2008;133(Suppl 6):381S–453S.

19. Horlocker TT, Wedel DJ, Rowlingson JC, et al. Regional anesthesia in the patient receiving antithrombotic or thrombolytic therapy: American Society of Reg Anesth Pain Med Evidence-Based Guidelines (Third Edition). Reg Anesth Pain Med 2010;35(1):64–101.

20. Biere SS, Maas KW, Cuesta MA, et al. Cervical or thoracic anastomosis after esophagectomy for cancer: a systematic review and meta-analysis. Dig Surg 2011;28(1):29–35.

21. Togo S, Li J, Wei X, et al. Complications and mortality after esophagectomy for esophageal carcinoma: risk factor analysis in a series of 378 patients. Chirurgie Thoracique Cardio-Vasculaire 2010;14:25–8 [in French].

22. Baba M, Natsugoe S, Shimada M, et al. Does hoarseness of voice from recurrent nerve paralysis after esophagectomy for carcinoma influence patient quality of life? J Am Coll Surg 1999;188(3):231–6.

23. Bolger C, Walsh TN, Tanner WA, et al. Chylothorax after oesophagectomy. Br J Surg 1991;78(5):587–8.

24. Staats BA, Ellefson RD, Budahn LL, et al. The lipoprotein profile of chylous and nonchylous pleural effusions. Mayo Clin Proc 1980;55(11):700–4.

25. Dugue L, Sauvanet A, Farges O, et al. Output of chyle as an indicator of treatment for chylothorax complicating oesophagectomy. Br J Surg 1998;85(8):1147–9.

26. Merigliano S, Molena D, Ruol A, et al. Chylothorax complicating esophagectomy for cancer: a plea for early thoracic duct ligation. J Thorac Cardiovasc Surg 2000;119(3):453–7.

27. Boffa DJ, Sands MJ, Rice TW, et al. A critical evaluation of a percutaneous diagnostic and treatment strategy for chylothorax after thoracic surgery. Eur J Cardiothorac Surg 2008;33(3):435–9.

28. Cope C, Salem R, Kaiser LR. Management of chylothorax by percutaneous catheterization and embolization of the thoracic duct: prospective trial. J Vasc Interv Radiol 1999;10(9):1248–54.

29. Boyle NH, Pearce A, Hunter D, et al. Intraoperative scanning laser Doppler flowmetry in the assessment of gastric tube perfusion during esophageal resection. J Am Coll Surg 1999;188(5):498–502.

30. Beitler AL, Urschel JD. Comparison of stapled and hand-sewn esophagogastric anastomoses. Am J Surg 1998;175(4):337–40.

31. Collard JM, Romagnoli R, Goncette L, et al. Terminalized semimechanical side-to-side suture technique for cervical esophagogastrostomy. Ann Thorac Surg 1998;65(3):814–7.

32. Orringer MB, Marshall B, Iannettoni MD. Eliminating the cervical esophagogastric anastomotic leak with a side-to-side stapled anastomosis. J Thorac Cardiovasc Surg 2000;119(2):277–88.

33. Ercan S, Rice TW, Murthy SC, et al. Does esophagogastric anastomotic technique influence the outcome of patients with esophageal cancer? J Thorac Cardiovasc Surg 2005;129(3):623–31.

34. Chang AC, Ji H, Birkmeyer NJ, et al. Outcomes after transhiatal and transthoracic esophagectomy for cancer. Ann Thorac Surg 2008;85(2):424–9.

35. Crestanello JA, Deschamps C, Cassivi SD, et al. Selective management of intrathoracic anastomotic leak after esophagectomy. J Thorac Cardiovasc Surg 2005; 129(2):254–60.
36. Martin LW, Hofstetter W, Swisher SG, et al. Management of intrathoracic leaks following esophagectomy. Adv Surg 2006;40:173–90.
37. Sarela AI, Tolan DJ, Harris K, et al. Anastomotic leakage after esophagectomy for cancer: a mortality-free experience. J Am Coll Surg 2008;206(3):516–23.
38. Orringer MB, Marshall B, Chang AC, et al. Two thousand transhiatal esophagectomies: changing trends, lessons learned. Ann Surg 2007;246(3):363–72.
39. Urschel JD, Urschel DM, Miller JD, et al. A meta-analysis of randomized controlled trials of route of reconstruction after esophagectomy for cancer. Am J Surg 2001;182(5):470–5.
40. Collard JM, Tinton N, Malaise J, et al. Esophageal replacement: gastric tube or whole stomach? Ann Thorac Surg 1995;60(2):261–6.
41. Ngan SY, Wong J. Lengths of different routes for esophageal replacement. J Thorac Cardiovasc Surg 1986;91(5):790–2.
42. Briel JW, Tamhankar AP, Hagen JA, et al. Prevalence and risk factors for ischemia, leak, and stricture of esophageal anastomosis: gastric pull-up versus colon interposition. J Am Coll Surg 2004;198(4):536–41.
43. Davis PA, Law S, Wong J. Colonic interposition after esophagectomy for cancer. Arch Surg 2003;138(3):303–8.
44. Griffin SM, Shaw IH, Dresner SM. Early complications after Ivor Lewis subtotal esophagectomy with two-field lymphadenectomy: risk factors and management. J Am Coll Surg 2002;194(3):285–97.
45. Headrick JR, Nichols FC 3rd, Miller DL, et al. High-grade esophageal dysplasia: long-term survival and quality of life after esophagectomy. Ann Thorac Surg 2002; 73(6):1697–702.
46. McLarty AJ, Deschamps C, Trastek VF, et al. Esophageal resection for cancer of the esophagus: long-term function and quality of life. Ann Thorac Surg 1997; 63(6):1568–72.
47. Donington JS. Functional conduit disorders after esophagectomy. Thorac Surg Clin 2006;16(1):53–62.
48. Burt M, Scott A, Williard WC, et al. Erythromycin stimulates gastric emptying after esophagectomy with gastric replacement: a randomized clinical trial. J Thorac Cardiovasc Surg 1996;111(3):649–54.
49. Peyre CG, DeMeester SR, Rizzetto C, et al. Vagal-sparing esophagectomy: the ideal operation for intramucosal adenocarcinoma and Barrett with high-grade dysplasia. Ann Surg 2007;246(4):665–71.
50. Lanuti M, de Delva PE, Wright CD, et al. Post-esophagectomy gastric outlet obstruction: role of pyloromyotomy and management with endoscopic pyloric dilatation. Eur J Cardiothorac Surg 2007;31(2):149–53.
51. Urschel JD, Blewett CJ, Young JE, et al. Pyloric drainage (pyloroplasty) or no drainage in gastric reconstruction after esophagectomy: a meta-analysis of randomized controlled trials. Dig Surg 2002;19(3):160–4.
52. Martin JT, Federico JA, McKelvey AA, et al. Prevention of delayed gastric emptying after esophagectomy: a single center's experience with botulinum toxin. Ann Thorac Surg 2009;87(6):1708–13.
53. van Heijl M, Gooszen JA, Fockens P, et al. Risk factors for development of benign cervical strictures after esophagectomy. Ann Surg 2010;251(6): 1064–9.
54. Aly A, Jamieson GG. Reflux after oesophagectomy. Br J Surg 2004;91(2):137–41.

55. Yuasa N, Sasaki E, Ikeyama T, et al. Acid and duodenogastroesophageal reflux after esophagectomy with gastric tube reconstruction. Am J Gastroenterol 2005;100(5):1021–7.
56. Dresner SM, Griffin SM, Wayman J, et al. Human model of duodenogastro-oesophageal reflux in the development of Barrett's metaplasia. Br J Surg 2003; 90(9):1120–8.
57. Wolfsen HC, Hemminger LL, DeVault KR. Recurrent Barrett's esophagus and adenocarcinoma after esophagectomy. BMC Gastroenterol 2004;4:18.
58. Price TN, Allen MS, Nichols FC 3rd, et al. Hiatal hernia after esophagectomy: analysis of 2,182 esophagectomies from a single institution. Ann Thorac Surg 2011;92(6):2041–5.
59. Kent MS, Luketich JD, Tsai W, et al. Revisional surgery after esophagectomy: an analysis of 43 patients. Ann Thorac Surg 2008;86(3):975–83.
60. Shen KR, Harrison-Phipps KM, Cassivi SD, et al. Esophagectomy after anti-reflux surgery. J Thorac Cardiovasc Surg 2010;139(4):969–75.
61. Kuo EY, Chang Y, Wright CD. Impact of hospital volume on clinical and economic outcomes for esophagectomy. Ann Thorac Surg 2001;72(4):1118–24.
62. Varghese TK Jr, Wood DE, Farjah F, et al. Variation in esophagectomy outcomes in hospitals meeting Leapfrog volume outcome standards. Ann Thorac Surg 2011;91(4):1003–9.
63. Gockel I, Exner C, Junginger T. Morbidity and mortality after esophagectomy for esophageal carcinoma: a risk analysis. World J Surg Oncol 2005;3:37.
64. Gockel I, Kneist W, Keilmann A, et al. Recurrent laryngeal nerve paralysis (RLNP) following esophagectomy for carcinoma. Eur J Surg Oncol 2005;31(3):277–81.
65. Altorki N, Kent M, Ferrara C, et al. Three-field lymph node dissection for squamous cell and adenocarcinoma of the esophagus. Ann Surg 2002;236(2):177–83.
66. Merritt RE, Whyte RI, D'Arcy NT, et al. Morbidity and mortality after esophagectomy following neoadjuvant chemoradiation. Ann Thorac Surg 2011;92(6):2034–40.

Quality of Life After an Esophagectomy

Sartaj S. Sanghera, MD[a], Steven J. Nurkin, MD[a],
Todd L. Demmy, MD[b],*

KEYWORDS

• Esophagectomy • Quality of life • Esophageal cancer

KEY POINTS

- Esophagectomy is no longer the standard approach for high-grade dysplasia, and data are emerging that early invasive cancers may also be managed by endoscopic therapies without compromising survival.
- A more complete understanding of the postoperative health-related quality of life (HR-QOL) may enable the treating surgeon to perform more informed patient selection and better tailor the delivery of intraoperative and perioperative care.
- Esophagectomy performed in the setting of trimodality therapy remains the best option for potentially curative treatment of esophageal cancer.
- For early neoplasia detected during the course of surveillance, organ-preserving endoscopic therapies present an attractive alternative to esophagectomy.
- Although the assessment of HR-QOL as an outcome measure has improved over the last 2 decades, significant limitations remain.

INTRODUCTION

Esophageal cancer is a challenging clinical problem. Its incidence is rising largely from the increasing diagnosis of adenocarcinoma in the setting of intestinal metaplasia.[1,2] Longevity remains disappointingly low, with 5-year overall survival uniformly around 30% among all patients undergoing a potentially curative resection.[3] Esophagectomy, generally performed in the setting of multimodality therapy, offers the best chance of a cure.[4] In the past 2 decades, better multimodality therapies including surgical technique refinements have reduced perioperative mortality. Most specialized, high-volume centers now claim 30-day operative mortality rates of less than 5%.[5-7] However, the operation continues to cause severe physiologic stress, with morbidity rates

[a] Department of Surgical Oncology, Roswell Park Cancer Institute, University at Buffalo, Elm and Carlton Streets, Buffalo, NY 14263, USA; [b] Department of Thoracic Surgery, Roswell Park Cancer Institute, University at Buffalo, Elm and Carlton Streets, Buffalo, NY 14263, USA
* Corresponding author.
E-mail address: todd.demmy@roswellpark.org

Surg Clin N Am 92 (2012) 1315–1335
http://dx.doi.org/10.1016/j.suc.2012.07.001
0039-6109/12/$ – see front matter © 2012 Elsevier Inc. All rights reserved.
surgical.theclinics.com

approaching 50%.[8,9] Predictably, this seriously impairs the patient's physical, social, and emotional functioning.

It has long been argued that common outcome measures of cancer therapy (like survival) do not describe the effectiveness of the intervention adequately.[10,11] This is especially true for aggressive neoplasms with low cure rates like esophageal cancer. The limited survival, coupled with high associated morbidity of therapeutic interventions, makes study of residual QOL of paramount importance to patients and their treating surgeons.[12] A more complete understanding of the postoperative health-related quality of life (HR-QOL) may enable the treating surgeon to perform more informed patient selection and better tailor the delivery of intraoperative and perioperative care.

The common use of surveillance endoscopies in the setting of Barrett esophagus has yielded many early carcinomas for which rapidly evolving endoscopic therapeutic modalities have challenged traditional treatments.[13,14] Esophagectomy is no longer the standard approach for high-grade dysplasia, and data are emerging that early invasive cancers may also be managed by endoscopic therapies without compromising survival.[15] Given accurate assignment of early stage status, traditional outcome measures such as overall and disease-free survival will likely be too similar to compare new technologies. Less conventional parameters, like cost-effectiveness and HR-QOL, are increasingly important considerations in the formulation of treatment guidelines and shaping overall health policy.

TOOLS FOR THE EVALUATION OF HR-QOL

Patients' perspectives of their general well being have had recognized value for a while.[16,17] What has hindered objective assessments of patients' personal experiences is the lack of valid methods that can be applied easily.[18]

Until recently, assessments performed to define HR-QOL were done with rudimentary, internal institution questionnaires targeted at evaluating clinically observed sequelae after esophagectomy. Inclusion and exclusion were at the discretion of the investigator designing the study. This methodology was obviously disadvantaged by a lack of uniformity and reliability. Additionally, outcomes were often decided by the treating physician. It has now been proven that there are vital differences in patient-versus physician-reported outcomes.[19] Methodically developed, rationally designed, self-reported disease-specific and site-specific questionnaires are giant strides toward uniform evaluation and reporting of HR-QOL data.

The Medical Outcomes Study 36-Item Short-Form Health Survey

The results of the Medical Outcomes Study (MOS) were published in the *Journal of the American Medical Association* in 1989, thus starting a trend toward including patient-oriented outcomes as necessary components to evaluate health care delivery systems and their practices.[20] The 36-Item Short Form Health Survey (SF-36) was developed and validated in 1988 to enable measurement of meaningful MOS outcomes.[21] The survey was developed to be comprehensive yet versatile enough to afford facile applicability across a broad range of clinical and population-based settings. The MOS SF-36 has 1 multiitem scale that assesses 8 health concepts to yield 2 summary measures that include physical and mental health/well-being. It can be self-administered by any person older than 14 years. Alternatively, it can be administered by a trained interviewer, either in person or over the telephone. As opposed to the cumbersome prior questionnaires, the MOS SF-36 can be completed in 5 to 10 minutes. This survey has since undergone rigorous psychometric validation and has been established as a valid and accurate measure of HR-QOL across a broad range of disease states and conditions.[22,23] The MOS SF-20 was developed simultaneously and an even more abbreviated version, the MOS SF-12 was later developed and tested in 1994. Among these, the MOS SF-36 remains the most accurate and therefore the most widely used and reported.

The Functional Assessment of Cancer Therapy System

Driven by the impetus of the MOS results, several other tools were developed in the early 1990s to measure HR-QOL specifically in cancer patients. One of these was the Functional Assessment of Cancer Therapy General (FACT-G) system, introduced in 1993.[24] This 28-item questionnaire covers areas including physical, functional, social, and emotional status and wellbeing. In addition, it contains an evaluation of the patient–physician relationship. Patients can complete the instrument by themselves without assistance in 5 minutes. The results are reported as a summary score. This system subsequently underwent extensive psychometric validation and application on a large scale.[25,26] Its success spawned the development of many disease-specific modules. The FACT–Esophageal (FACT-E) was developed and validated in 2006.[27] The results of the disease-specific module are also reported as a summary score.

The European Organization for the Research and Treatment of Cancer QOL Questionnaires

The European Organization for the Research and Treatment of Cancer (EORTC) reported the development and validation of its core questionnaire (EORTC QLQ C30) in 1993.[28] This questionnaire includes 9 multi-item scales: 5 functional scales (physical, role, cognitive, emotional, and social), 3 symptom scales (fatigue, pain, and nausea and vomiting), and a global health and quality-of-life scale. It also addresses the measurement of several specific symptoms as single items. The EORTC QLQ C30 is perhaps the most rigorously validated and frequently applied tool for the objective measurement of HR-QOL outcomes in existence today.[29–31] Two different esophageal modules (EORTC QLQ OES18 and EORTC QLQ OG25) were designed to be jointly administered in complement with the core questionnaire to provide both a disease-specific as well as overall comprehensive assessment.[32,33]

The 3 tools discussed previously have withstood the test of time and remain the most frequently applied for the contemporary measurement of HR-QOL following esophagectomy (**Table 1**). Multiple other instruments purporting to measure HR-QOL exist, and some of these have been applied toward measurement of outcomes following esophagectomy. These include general scales such as the Gastro-Intestinal Quality of Life Index (GIQLI) and the Profile of Mood States (POMS), as well as disease-specific tools like the Rotterdam Symptom Scale, Spitzer Index, Visick Score, and the University of Washington Quality Of Life (UW-QOL) score.

Disease-specific tools are generally more accurate for the evaluation of outcomes pertinent to that pathology or surgical intervention. To achieve even greater specificity, tools have been designed to assess HR-QOL after specific surgical interventions.[34] Nevertheless, instruments that measure general HR-QOL are vital for an overall health assessment. Besides allowing a more global appraisal of wellbeing, this enables comparison across a variety of disease states and multiple interventions. Thus, optimal HR-QOL research requires combining both general and specific instruments effectively. Ultimately, the development and standardization of objective measurements of HR-QOL facilitates the accrual of meaningful data with cross-cultural reliability and reproducibility.

Table 1
Most common tools for HR-QOL assessment

	Oncology-Specific	Categories	Target Population	Number of Items	Response Categories	Time Recall	Administration	Time to Complete	Results Format
MOS SF-36	No	Physical functioning Role–physical Bodily pain General health Vitality Social functioning Role–emotional Mental health	Adolescents Adults (>14 y)	36	5-point Likert scale	Past 4 wks (standard) Past wk (acute)	Self Interviewer Telephone Computer	5–10 mins	8 scaled subscores 2 summary scores: Physical health Mental health (0–100)
EORTC QLQ C30	Yes	Physical Function/Role Emotional Social	Adults (>18 y)	30	4-point Likert scale	Past wk	Self Interviewer Telephone Computer	10–15 mins	Scaled scores for: Function Symptom Global health status/HR-QOL 6 single items (0–100) No summary score
FACT-G	Yes	Physical Social/family Emotional Functional	4th graders and up (>9–10 y)	27	5-point Likert scale	Past 7 d	Self Interviewer Telephone Computer	5–10 mins	4 subscales: Physical Social/family Emotional Functional (0–24 or 0–28) Overall fact G score (0–108)

SHORT- AND LONG-TERM HR-QOL FOLLOWING ESOPHAGECTOMY
Short Term—up to 1 Year Postoperatively

Blazeby and colleagues[35] studied the short-term QOL in patients undergoing poten-tially curative esophagectomy (**Table 2**). Patients filled out the EORTC QLQ C30 and OES24 questionnaires before treatment, 6 weeks after surgery, every 3 months in the first year, every 6 months in the second year and then annually thereafter. They found a decline in almost all HR-QOL scores after surgery. Interestingly, in the subgroup of patients who survived at least 2 years, the scores improved to preoper-ative levels at 9 months after surgery. The group of patients with survival no more than 2 years did not show similar improvement.

In a separate, prospective study, the same group found marked reductions in phys-ical, role, and social function at 6 weeks after surgery. This was accompanied by an increase in fatigue, nausea and emesis, pain, dyspnea, appetite loss, and coughing. However, the authors reported that most aspects of HR-QOL recovered to preopera-tive levels at 6 months after surgery.[43]

Zieren and colleagues[44] reported very similar results using the EORTC QLQ C30 and the Spitzer Index. Role and physical function, in particular, were found to show significant deterioration. The HR-QOL was restored within 6 months in patients who remained disease free 1 year after surgery. Thus, their study also demonstrated a negative impact of tumor recurrence on HR-QOL.

Brooks and colleagues[45] evaluated the HR-QOL using the FACT-G and FACT-E during the first year after esophagectomy. Subjects answered the questionnaire at diagnosis and then 1, 3, 6, 9, and 12 months after surgery. A decline was found in over-all HR-QOL following surgery, with the patients performing the worst on the functional and physical subscales of the FACT-E. Again, a gradual return to baseline was observed in almost all HR-QOL measures at 9 months postoperatively.

Long Term—More than 1 Year Postoperatively

Donohue and colleagues[46] studied HR-QOL in 132 patients who were alive at least 1 year after surgery without evidence of disease recurrence (**Table 3**). Using the EORTC QLQ C30 and OES18 tools, applied at a median follow-up of 70.3 months, they found that global health status was significantly reduced as compared with the general pop-ulation. The difference persisted, albeit smaller, when comparison was made to age- and sex-matched controls with a diagnosis of esophageal cancer before therapy. On the other hand, in the subset of patients who had baseline scores available for compar-ison, symptoms related to swallowing difficulty, reflux, pain, and coughing decreased over the long term. Swallowing dysfunction correlated highly with poor HR-QOL.

De Boer and colleagues[56] evaluated 35 recurrence-free esophagectomy patients with a minimal 2-year follow-up using the MOS SF-36 and the Rotterdam Symptom Checklist. All 8 SF-36 subscale scores were similar to reference values. The summary physical component score was worse, whereas the summary mental component score was better than the reference value. Although over half of the patients reported symptoms, their global HR-QOL was similar to population controls.

Lagergren and colleagues[52] evaluated 47 patients surviving 3 or more years after esophagectomy using the EORTC QLQ C30 and OES18 questionnaires. These were administered within 6 weeks before surgery (baseline) and then serially at 6 weeks and 3, 6, 9, 12, 18, 24, and 36 months postoperatively. The authors found that most aspects of HR-QOL recovered to preoperative levels by the 3-year assessment, but that scores for physical function, breathlessness, diarrhea, and reflux continued to be significantly worse than at baseline. Conversely, emotional function was improved over baseline.

Table 2
Short-term (<1 year) HR-QOL outcomes following esophagectomy

Reference	n	Survey	Description	Results
Blazeby et al,[35] 2000	92	EORTC QLQ-C30/QLQ-OES24	Compared EG survivors <2 y, EG >2 y and palliative therapy (PT)	Early postoperative-negative HR-QOL; in those surviving at least 2 y, symptoms improved to baseline at 9 mo; in those <2 y never improved; dysphagia improved and maintained after surgery; PT group HR-QOL deteriorated until death
Sweed et al,[36] 2002	23	EORTC QLQ-C30/ESO-24	Reviewed HR-QOL outcomes 3 and 6 mo after esophagectomy (EG)	Global HR-QOL declined slightly over time; this change was not statistically significant; a significant inverse relationship was found between symptom intensity and global HR-QOL
Viklund et al,[37] 2005	100	EORTC QLQ-C30/ESO-24	Swedish nationwide, prospective, HR-QOL at 6 mo	Except for anastomotic strictures, each of the predefined complications (ie, anastomotic leak, infections, cardiopulmonary complications, and operative technical complications) contributed to decreased HR-QOL scores
Cense et al,[38] 2006	92	MOS SF-20/Rotterdam	Prospective study Prolonged intensive care unit stay vs short stay after transthoracic EG for adenocarcinoma	No difference in long-term quality of life or survival between those submitted to the intensive care unit for a short period vs a long period
Rutegard and Lagergren,[39] 2008	355	EORTC QLQ-C30/QLQ-OES18	Hospital/surgeon volume HR-QOL at 6 mo	No HR-QOL advantages of being treated at high-volume hospitals or by high-volume surgeons, as measured 6 mo after esophageal cancer resection
Djarv et al,[40] 2009	355	EORTC QLQ-C30/QLQ-OES18	Preoperative factors associated with poor postoperative HR-QOL	Comorbidity, advanced tumor stage , or a tumor location (upper/middle) had an increased risk of poor HR-QOL Adenocarcinoma had a lower risk of poor HR-QOL than patients with squamous cell carcinoma
Van Heijl et al,[41] 2010	199	MOS SF-20/Rotterdam	Part of randomized control trial–relationship of preoperative and early postoperative HR-QOL on survival	Preoperative (physical symptoms) and 3 mo postoperative (social functioning, pain, and activity level) subscales are independent predictors of survival
Djarv and Lagergren,[42] 2011	401	EORTC QLQ-C30/QLQ-OES18	Relationship of 6-mo postoperative HR-QOL and survival	For each of 9 selected outcomes, poor scores were associated with mortality: global HR-QOL, physical function, social function, fatigue, pain, dyspnea, appetite loss, dysphagia, and esophageal pain

Table 3
Long-term (>1 year) HR-QOL outcomes following esophagectomy

Reference	n	Survey	Description	Results
McLarty et al,[47] 1997	107	MOS SF-36	Evaluated long-term survivors (>5 y) to national norms	Decreased physical functioning but work, activities of daily living (ADLs), social, emotional, health perception and energy similar
de Boer et al,[56] 2000	35	MOS SF-36/Rotterdam	Follow-up of 2 y with no recurrence after transhiatal EG	Over 50% still experienced at least some early satiety, fatigue, dysphagia, heartburn and/or psychological irritability, but overall good HR-QOL
Headrick et al,[49] 2002	54	MOS SF-36	EG for diagnosis of HGD (median follow-up of 63 mo)	For HGD: role–physical and role–emotional scores were better than control; For cancer, the health perception score was worse; scores measuring physical function, social function, mental health, bodily pain, and energy/fatigue were similar
Chang et al,[50] 2006	34	MOS SF-36	Review of EG patients with HGD and cancer while under surveillance	Symptoms present but mild, HR-QOL score equal to or better than controls
Moraca and Low,[51] 2006	36	MOS SF-36	EG for HGD and intramucosal cancer (mean follow-up 4.9 y)	HR-QOL comparable with those of age- and sex-matched controls
Lagergren et al,[52] 2007	47	EORTC QLQ-C30/QLQ-OES18	Survivors for >3 y after EG	HR-QOL recovered to preoperative levels by the 3-y assessment, but scores for physical function, breathlessness, diarrhea, and reflux were significantly worse; however, significantly better emotional function
Djarv et al,[53] 2008	87	EORTC QLQ-C30/QLQ-OES18	Long term outcomes after curative resection (>3 y)	Scores substantially worse than in the reference population with no improvement at 3 y; significantly poorer role and social function, fatigue, diarrhea, appetite loss, nausea, and vomiting
Courrech et al,[54] 2010	36	EORTC QLQ-C30/QLQ-OES18	1 y with no recurrence after EG	Although some symptoms persist, patients who survive 1 y can live satisfactory lives
Gockel et al,[55] 2010	50	EORTC QLQ-C30/QLQ-OES18	HR-QOL in long term survivors (>5 y)	Good overall global score; emotional and cognitive functioning were highest; no dysphagia, but reflux a major problem
Donohoe et al,[46] 2011	80	EORTC QLQ-C30/QLQ-OES18	Long term (>1 y) HR-QOL in disease-free patients	Global health status significantly reduced; symptoms related to swallowing difficulty, reflux, pain, and coughing decreased long term; swallowing dysfunction was highly correlated with a poor HR-QOL

Djarv and colleagues[53] also studied long-term outcomes after curative resection but compared them to a reference population. They evaluated 87 patients who survived a minimum of 3 years after esophagectomy. Patients filled out the EORTC QLQ C30 and OES18 at 6 months and 3 years after surgery. HR-QOL scores following surgery were found to be substantially worse than in the reference population. They detected no significant improvement at 3 years, with patients indicating significantly poorer role and social function. Survivors also reported more fatigue, diarrhea, appetite loss, nausea, and vomiting.

Mc Larty and colleagues[47] studied 107 patients with at least a 5-year survival following resection for stage 1/2 disease using the MOS SF-36. Survivors noted a decrease in physical functioning compared with the national norm. However, HR-QOL scores pertaining to the ability to work, social interaction, daily activities, emotional dysfunction, perception of health, and levels of energy were at par, and mental health scores were actually higher than expected.

Similarly, Gockel and colleagues[55] studied 50 patients with 5-year or longer survival after esophagectomy. Using the EORTC QLQ C30 and OES18 questionnaires administered at a median follow-up of 100.1 months, they discovered that this cohort of patients had good overall global scores. Among individual measures, patients performed especially well on emotional and cognitive functioning. As far as symptom control, dysphagia largely resolved, while reflux posed a significant problem.

Scarpa and colleagues conducted a systematic review summarizing data from the papers by Headrick and colleagues,[49] de Boer and colleagues,[56] and McLarty and colleagues.[47] They concluded that pooled scores for physical role and social function were similar after esophagectomy when compared with an age- and sex-matched US reference population, whereas pooled scores for physical function, vitality, and general health were lower. Interestingly, scores for bodily pain and mental health were higher than relevant norms in long-term survivors.[57]

In a study published in 2012, Derogar and Lagergren[58] provided a longer-term follow-up of the Karolinska Institute experience. One hundred seventeen patients alive at 5 years or longer after esophagectomy were surveyed using the EORTCQLQ C30 and OES18 at 6 months, 3 years, and 5 years after resection. They summarized that for most patients, the HR-QOL remained stable or improved over time. At 5 years, the HR-QOL of the group as a whole was comparable to the reference population. However, there was a small cohort (14%) of patients who deteriorated progressively, and subset analyses of these patients revealed large and clinically significant mean score differences.

TREATMENT MODALITIES AND THEIR IMPACT ON HR-QOL
Neoadjuvant Chemoradiotherapy

Blazeby and colleagues[59] studied the impact of neoadjuvant chemoradiotherapy (CRT) on HR-QOL (**Table 4**). They also compared HR-QOL between patients receiving CRT followed by surgery with those treated by surgery alone. Almost all HR-QOL scores deteriorated during neoadjuvant therapy, but with rapid improvement to baseline before surgery. Global HR-QOL declined significantly at 6 weeks postoperatively, but most aspects recovered to preoperative baseline levels by 6 months regardless of whether they received CRT. Interestingly, patients undergoing CRT reported fewer problems at the 3-month follow-up survey.

Reynolds and colleagues[60] performed a similar investigation using the EORTC QLQ C30 and OES18 at diagnosis, completion of CRT, and 3, 6, and 12 months after surgery. While 147 patients had similar baseline HR-QOL scores, CRT decreased physical and role function despite an associated improvement in dysphagia. Surgery decreased global, functional, and symptom scores at 3 months, but most recovered by 6 months. However, at 12 months following surgery, physical and role function continued to be impaired in the surgery-alone group, while the CRT plus surgery group demonstrated persistently worse social functioning and more financial worries.

HR-QOL Following Esophagectomy Versus Definitive CRT

Avery and colleagues[61] sought to perform a comparative analysis of HR-QOL outcomes between patients receiving definitive CRT versus those who underwent combined modality treatment including esophagectomy. All patients were diagnosed with stage 2/3 esophageal cancer and were asked to fill out the EORTC QLQ C30 and OES18 forms at baseline, at the lowest expected point during each treatment, and then at a point when recovery was reasonably anticipated. They found that both groups reported multiple symptoms and poor function at the worst expected point; however, the decline in HR-QOL was worse for the group undergoing combined modality treatment plus esophagectomy. In addition, while patients in the chemoradiation-only group had significant recovery by 6 months, those in the surgery group had not yet recovered, with deterioration still evident in multiple aspects of general and disease-specific scales.

In another comparison of HR-QOL outcomes between definitive CRT and combined modality therapy, Yamashita and colleagues[64] tested 51 of 66 survivors after a median follow-up of 37.8 months. The surveys were conducted using the FACT-G and FACT-E scoring systems. They reported that the superior disease-free survival for the surgery group was likely a function of the difference at baseline, with the CRT group containing a significantly older population with more advanced stage. Despite this difference, the overall FACT-E scores were significantly worse for the surgery group.

In separate studies, Ariga and colleagues[65] and Teoh and colleagues[67] showed similarly poor HR-QOL outcomes for surgery (without neoadjuvant CRT) as compared with definitive CRT, at least in the short-term. It should be noted, however, that these 2 studies limited their evaluation to patients with squamous histology.

SURGICAL/THERAPEUTIC TECHNIQUES AND QOL

Transthoracic Versus Transhiatal Esophagectomy

In a randomized control trial of transthoracic versus transhiatal esophagectomy, de Boer and colleagues[48] examined HR-QOL outcomes using the MOS SF-20 and the Rotterdam Symptom Checklist (**Table 5**). The surveys were conducted at regular intervals beginning preoperatively and up to 3 years after surgery for a total of 10 evaluations. Global QOL scores showed a small initial decline in both surgical approaches. Thereafter there was continuous improvement approaching to baseline for most aspects by 1 year, with stabilization at 2 to 3 years. The only detected difference occurred at 3 months after surgery, when transhiatal esophagectomy patients had fewer symptoms and better activity.

Egberts and colleagues[81] investigated the difference in HR-QOL among patients undergoing cervical versus intrathoracic anastomosis. Regular evaluations were performed using the EORTC QLQ C30 and the OES18 beginning before surgery and extending up to 24 months after surgery. An initial decline followed by slow recovery was found in both groups, although the authors found that overall HR-QOL never returned to baseline levels. The 2 sites of anastomosis were not significantly different with respect to any of the HR-QOL scales.

Open Versus Minimally Invasive Surgery

Luketich and colleagues[5] looked at the postoperative HR-QOL of patients undergoing minimally invasive esophagectomy. The MOS SF-36 was used to evaluate outcomes

Table 4
Treatment modalities and QOL

Reference	n	Survey	Description	Results
Blazeby et al,[59] 2005	103	EORTC QLQ-C30/QLQ-OES18	HR-QOL with CRT + surgery vs surgery alone	6 wk postoperatively—marked reductions in physical, role, and social function and increase in fatigue, nausea, emesis, pain, dyspnea, appetite loss, and coughing; most aspects of HR-QOL recovered to preoperative levels at 6 mo postoperatively; fewer problems were reported at 3 mo by patients who had CRT
Reynolds et al,[60] 2006	147	EORTC QLQ-C30/QLQ-OES18	HR-QOL with CRT + surgery vs surgery alone	Baseline HR-QOL similar; CRT decreased physical and role function despite improving dysphagia; Most scores recovered by 6 mo in both, but at 12 mo, physical and role still impaired in surgery only, and social functioning and financial worries in CRT + surgery
Avery et al,[61] 2007	132	EORTC QLQ-C30/QLQ-OES18	Locally advanced cancer (stage 2/3) CRT only vs trimodality	CRT patients older, more squamous, and poorer HR-QOL at baseline Worse short-term HR-QOL in combination treatment including surgery; patients preferring early recovery should consider definitive CRT
Van Meerten et al,[62] 2008	52	EORTC QLQ-C30/QLQ-OES18	HR-QOL after neoadjuvant CRT and surgery	Scores of most HR-QOL scales deteriorated during CRT—physical and role–functioning worst; all HR-QOL scores were restored or even improved 1 y postoperatively

Study	N	Instrument	Study Description	Findings
Safieddine et al,[63] 2009	43	FACT-E	Prospective phase 2 study—HR-QOL and trimodality therapy	Decreased HR-QOL with neoadjuvant therapy, but recovery to baseline within 5-7 wk; HR-QOL decreases again after surgical intervention but returns to baseline levels within 3 mo
Yamashita et al,[64] 2009	51	FACT-G+E	Definitive CRT alone vs surgery	CRT was inferior in survival but superior in HR-QOL measures, although the CRT group had a larger number of patients with poorer prognostic factors
Ariga et al,[65] 2009	62	EORTC QLQ-C30/QLQ-OES18	At least 2 y survivors after definitive CRT vs surgery	Almost all HR-QOL scores better in the CRT group; statistically significant for appetite loss, diarrhea, and eating problems; esophageal preservation only independent predictor of global HR-QOL
Hurmuzlu et al,[66] 2011	41	EORTC QLQ-C30/QLQ-OES18	Long-term HR-QOL after high-dose CRT and surgery vs surgery alone	High-dose CRT had significantly worse symptoms and global HR-QOL in almost all functional scales and higher fatigue compared with other 3 groups
Teoh et al,[67] 2011	81	EORTC QLQ-C30/ESO-24	Prospective randomized control trial–surgery or CRT for squamous carcinoma	Surgery worse for physical function and fatigue up to 6 mo; improved at 2 y Dyspnea and coughing worsened 3 mo after surgery; symptoms in the CRT group progressively deteriorated; both had improvements in dysphagia but needed frequent endoscopic intervention

Table 5
Surgical/therapeutic techniques and QOL

Reference	n	Survey	Description	Results
Type of Resection/Reconstruction				
DeBoer et al,[48] 2004	199	MOS SF-30/Rotterdam	Randomized control trial of transhiatal vs extended transthoracic EG	Physical symptoms and activity declined then returned toward baseline within 1 y; psychological wellbeing consistently improved; global HR-QOL initial decline, improved and stabilized in 2–3 y; At 3 mo TH, fewer symptoms and better activity
Cense et al,[68] 2004	14	MOS SF-36/Rotterdam	Reviewed HR-QOL in patients that had colonic interposition	Significantly lower scores in 5/8 subscales (ie, general health, physical role, vitality, social functioning, and mental health); worse satiety, dysphagia, diarrhea, loss of sexual interest, and fatigue
Johansson et al,[69] 2008	32	EORTC QLQ-C30/QLQ-OES18	Gastroesophageal (GE) junction tumors—EG and gastric tube reconstruction vs extended gastrectomy and long Roux-en-Y reconstructions	Global health—no significant difference from reference population Satisfactory results on function and symptom scales. Either technique can be performed with good results
Aghajanzadeh et al,[70] 2009	110	MOS SF-36	Functional outcome and HR-QOL related to EG and type of reconstruction	Colon graft in EG is significantly advantageous compared with other methods because of the ability of patients to gain weight and avoid developing postoperative reflux
Rutegard et al,[71] 2008	355	EORTC QLQ-C30/QLQ-OES18	Swedish population based study—technical factors associated with outcomes and HR-QOL	Extensive surgery not associated with worse outcome; dysphagia similar in handsewn and stapled Colon interposition worse for dyspnea, global, and social role but not statistically significant; technical surgical complications had significant deleterious effects on several aspects of HR-QOL
Wang et al,[72] 2011	97	EORTC QLQ-C30/QLQ-OES18	Minimally invasive EG —retrosternal vs prevertebral reconstruction	2 wk postoperatively—dysphagia and eating worse in retrosternal group; worse global quality of life; at 12 and 24 wk after operation, dyspnea and reflux symptoms better in the retrosternal group and global quality higher

Study	N	Instrument	Purpose/Comparison	Results
Zhang et al,[73] 2011	104	EORTC QLQ-C30/ESO-24	Prospective randomized control trial—narrow gastric tube vs whole stomach for reconstruction	HR-QOL dropped for all patients at 3 wk after surgery; recovery at both 6 mo and 1 y in both groups Gastric tube group significantly better at both 6 mo and 1 y
Minimally invasive esophagectomy				
Luketich et al,[5] 2003	222	MOS SF-36	Reviewed outcomes of minimally invasive EG Half received some form of neoadjuvant therapy	When compared with norms—no difference in physical symptom scores, mental symptom scores slightly lower; comparison of preoperative and postoperative symptoms showed preserved HR-QOL
Leibman et al,[74] 2006	25	EORTC QLQ-C30/QLQ-OES18	Short and long-term outcomes of minimally invasive EG	Significant decrease in physical function, role function, and global health score immediately following surgery, and slow improvement 18–24 mo to approach baseline; dysphagia deteriorated rapidly but improved to baseline at 9 mo
Parameswaren et al,[75] 2010	58	EORTC QLQ-C30/QLQ-OES18	HR-QOL after minimally invasive EG	Deterioration at 6 wk, especially functional and symptoms; improvement at 3 mo; baseline at 6 mo; at 1 y, half of all domains back at baseline
Wang et al,[76] 2010	56	EORTC QLQ-C30/QLQ-OES18	HR-QOL after VATS vs open EG	Scores of global quality and physical functioning were higher in VATS group, with less fatigue, pain, and dyspnea
Montenovo et al,[77] 2011	49	GIQLI	Lap-assisted transhiatal EG of esophagus and GE junction	The mean GIQLI score was 108 (range, 74–138) from a maximum possible value of 144; 71% scored within 2 standard deviations; postoperative symptom scores were worse—diet change, regurgitation, diarrhea, and difficulty swallowing
Sundaram et al,[78] 2012	104	EORTC QLQ-C30/QLQ-OES18	Compare minimally invasive EG to open TTE or THE	No significant difference on any of the scales between the 3 groups
Endoscopic vs surgery				
Rosmolen et al,[79] 2010	91	MOS SF-36, C-30, OES-18, Hospital Anxiety and Depression Scale, Worry of Cancer Scale	Endoscopic therapy (ET) vs EG for Barrett with neoplasia	Surgery worse for eating problems and reflux. ET worse for fear of recurrence; other outcomes similar
Schembre et al,[80] 2010	42	MOS SF-36/GIQLI	EG vs ET for Barrett esophagus with neoplasia	No difference between EG and ET, except for better physical function among EG patients ≥65 y; GIQLI scores were higher among younger ET patients than young EG patients

in patients who had a median follow-up of 19 months. They found that physical component summary scores were not different from the reference population, whereas mental component summary scores were slightly inferior. In a subset analysis using patients for whom preoperative baseline scores were available, physical and mental component summary scores were similar at the 2 time points, indicating preservation of HR-QOL.

Leibman and colleagues also looked at HR-QOL trends in patients following minimally invasive esophagectomy. The EORTC QLQ C30 and OES18 were administered at regular intervals beginning before treatment, then every 3 months for the first year and every 6 months thereafter. They detected a significant decrease in physical function, role function, and global health score immediately following surgery with slow improvement, approaching baseline levels at 18 to 24 months after surgery.[74]

Parameswaran and colleagues[75] performed a similar outcome analysis after minimally invasive surgery and found prompt resolution of symptoms and faster recovery, with almost half of the domains at baseline or better at 1 year after surgery.

Two studies have performed a head-to-head comparison of open versus minimally invasive technique. Wang and colleagues,[76] using the EORTC QLQ C30 and OES18 tools in the short-term following surgery, demonstrated that scores for global QOL and physical functioning deteriorated promptly following surgery in both groups. The pattern of recovery between groups, however, was markedly different. While scores for patients in the minimally invasive group began recovering at 2 weeks and returned to baseline at 12 weeks after surgery, open surgery patients did not begin recovery until 4 weeks and took 24 weeks to return to baseline. The scores for fatigue, pain, and dyspnea were correspondingly better in the minimally invasive group, although this difference was not preserved at the 6-month follow-up.

In a 3-way comparison of minimally invasive esophagectomy with open transhiatal esophagectomy and open transthoracic esophagectomy, Sundaram and colleagues[78] used the same instruments to measure HR-QOL outcomes in patients with a minimum 1-year survival following surgery. There were significant differences between the 3 groups in any of the response categories.

Method of Esophageal Reconstruction

In a small descriptive study of HR-QOL after esophagectomy with colonic interposition, Cense and colleagues[68] evaluated patients alive and disease free 6 months after surgery. The patients scored poorly on 5 of the 8 subscales on the MOS SF-36. Using the Rotterdam Symptom Checklist, they also showed that satiety, dysphagia, diarrhea, loss of sexual interest, and fatigue were frequent and problematic symptoms.

Rutegard and colleagues[71] examined the role of several technical factors on HR-QOL outcomes. They found that patients reconstructed with colonic interposition scored worse for the dyspnea, global, and social role scales; however, these differences did not reach statistical significance. There were no differences in dysphagia scores between hand-sewn and stapled anastomosis.

Wang and colleagues[72] studied the impact of route used to deliver the conduit at the time of reconstruction. They found that patients with retrosternal reconstructions demonstrated worse dysphagia and other eating problems in the early postoperative period (2 weeks) and that this was associated with worse global HR-QOL. However, in the later recovery phase (12–24 weeks), this route was associated with better scores on the symptom scales for dyspnea and reflux and displayed an improved global HR-QOL.

Effect of Postoperative Complications

Viklund and colleagues[37] performed a study to analyze the effect of surgical factors on HR-QOL outcome measures. They evaluated 100 patients who underwent R0 resection using the EORTC QLQ C30 and OES24 forms. They found that the main predictor of a decrease in global HR-QOL 6 months after surgery was the occurrence of complications. Anastomotic leak, postoperative infections, and cardiopulmonary complications all had a negative impact on global HR-QOL 6 months after surgery. Unexpectedly, the occurrence of an anastomotic stricture did not significantly impact the global HR-QOL scores. In a corresponding report, Rutegard and colleagues[39] also showed that technical surgical complications had significant negative impact on several aspects of HR-QOL.

Effect of Volume

Rutegard and Lagergren[39] at the Karolinska Institute studied the effect of surgical volume on HR-QOL outcomes following esophagectomy. Patients in the Swedish national cohort (N = 355) answered the EORTC QLQ C30 and OES18 questionnaires. High-volume centers were defined as those performing 9 or more operations a year, and individuals performing 6 or greater esophagectomies a year qualified as high-volume surgeons. The authors concluded that no clinically significant difference in HR-QOL outcomes was observed between high-volume and low-volume hospitals, or between high-volume and low-volume surgeons.

HR-QOL Following Surgery Versus Endoscopic Therapy

With the concurrent evolution of advanced endoscopic therapies, comparisons are also being drawn between HR-QOL outcomes after esophagectomy versus surveillance endoscopy with or without local therapy for intramucosal carcinoma or high-grade dysplasia. In a small study, Schembre and colleagues[80] evaluated the differences in HR-QOL outcomes following esophagectomy versus endoscopic therapy for patients with early neoplasia in the setting of Barrett esophagus. Using the SF-36 questionnaire at a mean follow-up of 4 years, they detected no significant differences in the HR-QOL scores except for superior physical functioning in patients older than 65 who underwent esophagectomy. Conversely, among younger patients, GIQLI scores were better after endoscopic therapy as compared with esophagectomy.

Rosmolen and colleagues[79] reported slightly different findings in a study using both the SF-36 and the C30/OES18 tools. They reported that the surgery group overall demonstrated worse eating problems and worse reflux. Interestingly, using additional questionnaires, they found that the endoscopic therapy group was likely to exhibit a significantly greater amount of fear relating to their cancer diagnosis.

SUMMARY

Esophagectomy performed in the setting of trimodality therapy remains the best option for potentially curative treatment of esophageal cancer. Despite improvements in operative mortality, it remains a fairly morbid procedure. Reflux, dumping, and dysphagia are the most commonly reported symptoms. However, the impact extends beyond a mere nuisance and can negatively influence the patients' overall physical, psychological. and social wellbeing. Therefore, overall HR-QOL has recently emerged as a parameter of interest in determining outcomes following esophagectomy.

Most studies indicate a global decline in HR-QOL scores following esophagectomy, with a gradual recovery to baseline within 6 to 12 months in the large majority of long-term survivors. Conversely, there are patients who never recover from the initial insult, demonstrate a progressive deterioration in most aspects of HR-QOL, and have worse overall outcomes. This is an important observation for 2 reasons. First, it highlights the need to preoperatively identify accurate predictors of poor postoperative HR-QOL following esophagectomy. Information on expected postoperative HR-QOL would be pivotal for clinical decision making and patient selection and greatly aid in counseling patients about the long-term consequences of surgery. Second, it identifies an added utility for the study of HR-QOL outcomes, as indicators of prognosis during the management of esophageal cancer. Small studies have identified a correlation between HR-QOL and disease-specific recurrence and survival following esophagectomy, but more research is needed.[41,82]

From the surgical perspective, many have tried to demonstrate better QOL after certain esophagectomy techniques. While minimally invasive surgery seems to offer the benefit of an earlier recovery of postoperative HR-QOL scores, type of reconstruction (THE versus TTE), type of interposition, use of neoadjuvant CRT, and volume of operating surgeon/institution have not consistently been shown to influence HR-QOL. There is some evidence supporting better HR-QOL following definitive CRT as compared with surgery with or without CRT; however, one must interpret these data cautiously. First, most of these studies limit their evaluation to patients with squamous esophageal cancer histology.[65,67] Second, studies that include adenocarcinoma have such heterogeneous populations (owing largely to treatment allocation criteria) that they are inherently unsuitable for meaningful analyses.

For early neoplasia detected during the course of surveillance, organ-preserving endoscopic therapies present an attractive alternative to esophagectomy. There is a growing body of evidence to support the equivalence of the 2 modalities as far as overall survival. But prolonged surveillance, coupled with the need for repeated procedures, has its own unique drawbacks, including the fear of cancer recurrence. It can be expected then, that HR-QOL outcomes (to include assessment of such psychological factors), along with cost-benefit analyses, are likely to play an influential role in shaping future research and decision making in the treatment of intramucosal carcinoma of the esophagus.

Although the assessment of HR-QOL as an outcome measure has improved over the last 2 decades, significant limitations remain. The most obvious is the lack of uniform reporting, with multiple tools applied in the various studies. Further, there is lack of consensus as to the best cohort for comparison. Some studies use pretreatment baseline values, while others use population-based controls or matched cohorts of patients receiving no or palliative treatment. Progressive standardization of the assessment tools and reporting of such outcomes will generate evidence that is easier to interpret.

HR-QOL measurement is an underappreciated facet of therapeutic outcomes that might be the most valuable information for the consumer. Acknowledgment of this fact is evidenced by the dramatic increase in number of publications on the subject seen over the past 2 decades. Clearly, much more remains to be learned. The management of esophageal cancer is complex and requires a multidisciplinary team approach. All aspects of therapeutic outcomes, especially QOL, need to be considered to provide the best possible cancer care.

REFERENCES

1. Cameron AJ, Souto EO, Smyrk TC. Small adenocarcinomas of the esophagogastric junction: association with intestinal metaplasia and dysplasia. Am J Gastroenterol 2002;97(6):1375–80.

2. Pera M, Cameron AJ, Trastek VF, et al. Increasing incidence of adenocarcinoma of the esophagus and esophagogastric junction. Gastroenterology 1993;104(2): 510–3.
3. Rouvelas I, Zeng W, Lindblad M, et al. Survival after surgery for oesophageal cancer: a population-based study. Lancet Oncol 2005;6(11):864–70.
4. Walsh TN, Noonan N, Hollywood D, et al. A comparison of multimodal therapy and surgery for esophageal adenocarcinoma. N Engl J Med 1996;335(7):462–7.
5. Luketich JD, Alvelo-Rivera M, Buenaventura PO, et al. Minimally invasive esophagectomy: outcomes in 222 patients. Ann Surg 2003;238(4):486–94 [discussion: 494–5].
6. Orringer MB, Marshall B, Chang AC, et al. Two thousand transhiatal esophagectomies: changing trends, lessons learned. Ann Surg 2007;246(3):363–72 [discussion: 372–4].
7. van Lanschot JJ, Hulscher JB, Buskens CJ, et al. Hospital volume and hospital mortality for esophagectomy. Cancer 2001;91(8):1574–8.
8. Bailey SH, Bull DA, Harpole DH, et al. Outcomes after esophagectomy: a ten-year prospective cohort. Ann Thorac Surg 2003;75(1):217–22 [discussion: 222].
9. Kelsen DP, Ginsberg R, Pajak TF, et al. Chemotherapy followed by surgery compared with surgery alone for localized esophageal cancer. N Engl J Med 1998;339(27):1979–84.
10. Kreder HJ, Wright JG, McLeod R. Outcome studies in surgical research. Surgery 1997;121(2):223–5.
11. Langenhoff BS, Krabbe PF, Wobbes T, et al. Quality of life as an outcome measure in surgical oncology. Br J Surg 2001;88(5):643–52.
12. Parameswaran R, McNair A, Avery KN, et al. The role of health-related quality of life outcomes in clinical decision making in surgery for esophageal cancer: a systematic review. Ann Surg Oncol 2008;15(9):2372–9.
13. van Sandick JW, van Lanschot JJ, Kuiken BW, et al. Impact of endoscopic biopsy surveillance of Barrett's oesophagus on pathological stage and clinical outcome of Barrett's carcinoma. Gut 1998;43(2):216–22.
14. May A, Gossner L, Pech O, et al. Local endoscopic therapy for intraepithelial high-grade neoplasia and early adenocarcinoma in Barrett's oesophagus: acute-phase and intermediate results of a new treatment approach. Eur J Gastroenterol Hepatol 2002;14(10):1085–91.
15. Ell C, May A, Pech O, et al. Curative endoscopic resection of early esophageal adenocarcinomas (Barrett's cancer). Gastrointest Endosc 2007;65(1):3–10.
16. Leplege A, Hunt S. The problem of quality of life in medicine. JAMA 1997;278(1): 47–50.
17. Calman KC. Quality of life in cancer patients—an hypothesis. J Med Ethics 1984; 10(3):124–7.
18. Garratt A, Schmidt L, Mackintosh A, et al. Quality of life measurement: bibliographic study of patient assessed health outcome measures. BMJ 2002; 324(7351):1417.
19. Sneeuw KC, Aaronson NK, Sprangers MA, et al. Evaluating the quality of life of cancer patients: assessments by patients, significant others, physicians and nurses. Br J Cancer 1999;81(1):87–94.
20. Tarlov AR, Ware JE Jr, Greenfield S, et al. The Medical Outcomes Study. An application of methods for monitoring the results of medical care. JAMA 1989;262(7): 925–30.
21. Ware JE Jr, Sherbourne CD. The MOS 36-item short-form health survey (SF-36). I. Conceptual framework and item selection. Med Care 1992;30(6):473–83.

22. McHorney CA, Ware JE Jr, Raczek AE. The MOS 36-Item Short-Form Health Survey (SF-36): II. Psychometric and clinical tests of validity in measuring physical and mental health constructs. Med Care 1993;31(3):247–63.

23. McHorney CA, Ware JE Jr, Lu JF, et al. The MOS 36-item Short-Form Health Survey (SF-36): III. Tests of data quality, scaling assumptions, and reliability across diverse patient groups. Med Care 1994;32(1):40–66.

24. Cella DF, Tulsky DS, Gray G, et al. The Functional Assessment of Cancer Therapy scale: development and validation of the general measure. J Clin Oncol 1993; 11(3):570–9.

25. Fumimoto H, Kobayashi K, Chang CH, et al. Cross-cultural validation of an international questionnaire, the general measure of the Functional Assessment of Cancer Therapy scale (FACT-G), for Japanese. Qual Life Res 2001;10(8):701–9.

26. Weitzner MA, Meyers CA, Gelke CK, et al. The Functional Assessment of Cancer Therapy (FACT) scale. Development of a brain subscale and revalidation of the general version (FACT-G) in patients with primary brain tumors. Cancer 1995; 75(5):1151–61.

27. Darling G, Eton DT, Sulman J, et al. Validation of the functional assessment of cancer therapy esophageal cancer subscale. Cancer 2006;107(4):854–63.

28. Aaronson NK, Ahmedzai S, Bergman B, et al. The European Organization for Research and Treatment of Cancer QLQ-C30: a quality-of-life instrument for use in international clinical trials in oncology. J Natl Cancer Inst 1993;85(5):365–76.

29. Bjordal K, de Graeff A, Fayers PM, et al. A 12-country field study of the EORTC QLQ-C30 (version 3.0) and the head and neck cancer-specific module (EORTC QLQ-H&N35) in head and neck patients. EORTC Quality of Life Group. Eur J Cancer 2000;36(14):1796–807.

30. Groenvold M, Klee MC, Sprangers MA, et al. Validation of the EORTC QLQ-C30 quality of life questionnaire through combined qualitative and quantitative assessment of patient-observer agreement. J Clin Epidemiol 1997;50(4):441–50.

31. Osoba D, Zee B, Pater J, et al. Psychometric properties and responsiveness of the EORTC Quality of Life Questionnaire (QLQ-C30) in patients with breast, ovarian and lung cancer. Qual Life Res 1994;3(5):353–64.

32. Blazeby JM, Conroy T, Hammerlid E, et al. Clinical and psychometric validation of an EORTC questionnaire module, the EORTC QLQ-OES18, to assess quality of life in patients with oesophageal cancer. Eur J Cancer 2003;39(10):1384–94.

33. Lagergren P, Fayers P, Conroy T, et al. Clinical and psychometric validation of a questionnaire module, the EORTC QLQ-OG25, to assess health-related quality of life in patients with cancer of the oesophagus, the oesophago-gastric junction and the stomach. Eur J Cancer 2007;43(14):2066–73.

34. Nakamura M, Kido Y, Yano M, et al. Reliability and validity of a new scale to assess postoperative dysfunction after resection of upper gastrointestinal carcinoma. Surg Today 2005;35(7):535–42.

35. Blazeby JM, Farndon JR, Donovan J, et al. A prospective longitudinal study examining the quality of life of patients with esophageal carcinoma. Cancer 2000;88(8): 1781–7.

36. Sweed MR, Schiech L, Barsevick A, et al. Quality of life after esophagectomy for cancer. Oncol Nurs Forum 2002;29(7):1127–31.

37. Viklund P, Lindblad M, Lagergren J. Influence of surgery-related factors on quality of life after esophageal or cardia cancer resection. World J Surg 2005;29(7):841–8.

38. Cense HA, Hulscher JB, de Boer AG, et al. Effects of prolonged intensive care unit stay on quality of life and long-term survival after transthoracic esophageal resection. Crit Care Med 2006;34(2):354–62.

39. Rutegard M, Lagergren P. No influence of surgical volume on patients' health-related quality of life after esophageal cancer resection. Ann Surg Oncol 2008;15(9):2380–7.
40. Djarv T, Blazeby JM, Lagergren P. Predictors of postoperative quality of life after esophagectomy for cancer. J Clin Oncol 2009;27(12):1963–8.
41. van Heijl M, Sprangers MA, de Boer AG, et al. Preoperative and early postoperative quality of life predict survival in potentially curable patients with esophageal cancer. Ann Surg Oncol 2010;17(1):23–30.
42. Djarv T, Lagergren P. Six-month postoperative quality of life predicts long-term survival after oesophageal cancer surgery. Eur J Cancer 2011;47(4):530–5.
43. Blazeby JM, Metcalfe C, Nicklin J, et al. Association between quality of life scores and short-term outcome after surgery for cancer of the oesophagus or gastric cardia. Br J Surg 2005;92(12):1502–7.
44. Zieren HU, Muller JM, Jacobi CA, et al. Adjuvant postoperative radiation therapy after curative resection of squamous cell carcinoma of the thoracic esophagus: a prospective randomized study. World J Surg 1995;19(3):444–9.
45. Brooks JA, Kesler KA, Johnson CS, et al. Prospective analysis of quality of life after surgical resection for esophageal cancer: preliminary results. J Surg Oncol 2002;81(4):185–94.
46. Donohoe CL, McGillycuddy E, Reynolds JV. Long-term health-related quality of life for disease-free esophageal cancer patients. World J Surg 2011;35(8):1853–60.
47. McLarty AJ, Deschamps C, Trastek VF, et al. Esophageal resection for cancer of the esophagus: long-term function and quality of life. Ann Thorac Surg 1997; 63(6):1568–72.
48. De Boer AG, van Lanschot JJ, van Sandick JW, et al. Quality of life after transhiatal compared with extended transthoracic resection for adenocarcinoma of the esophagus. J Clin Oncol 2004;22(20):4202–8.
49. Headrick JR, Nichols FC 3rd, Miller DL, et al. High-grade esophageal dysplasia: long-term survival and quality of life after esophagectomy. Ann Thorac Surg 2002; 73(6):1697–702 [discussion: 1702–3].
50. Chang LC, Oelschlager BK, Quiroga E, et al. Long-term outcome of esophagectomy for high-grade dysplasia or cancer found during surveillance for Barrett's esophagus. J Gastrointest Surg 2006;10(3):341–6.
51. Moraca RJ, Low DE. Outcomes and health-related quality of life after esophagectomy for high-grade dysplasia and intramucosal cancer. Arch Surg 2006;141(6): 545–9 [discussion: 549–51].
52. Lagergren P, Avery KN, Hughes R, et al. Health-related quality of life among patients cured by surgery for esophageal cancer. Cancer 2007;110(3):686–93.
53. Djarv T, Lagergren J, Blazeby JM, et al. Long-term health-related quality of life following surgery for oesophageal cancer. Br J Surg 2008;95(9):1121–6.
54. Courrech Staal EF, van Sandick JW, van Tinteren H, et al. Health-related quality of life in long-term esophageal cancer survivors after potentially curative treatment. J Thorac Cardiovasc Surg 2010;140(4):777–83.
55. Gockel I, Gonner U, Domeyer M, et al. Long-term survivors of esophageal cancer: disease-specific quality of life, general health and complications. J Surg Oncol 2010;102(5):516–22.
56. De Boer AG, Genovesi PI, Sprangers MA, et al. Quality of life in long-term survivors after curative transhiatal oesophagectomy for oesophageal carcinoma. Br J Surg 2000;87(12):1716–21.
57. Scarpa M, Valente S, Alfieri R, et al. Systematic review of health-related quality of life after esophagectomy for esophageal cancer. World J Gastroenterol 2011; 17(42):4660–74.

58. Derogar M, Lagergren P. Health-related quality of life among 5-year survivors of esophageal cancer surgery: a prospective population-based study. J Clin Oncol 2012;30(4):413–8.

59. Blazeby JM, Sanford E, Falk SJ, et al. Health-related quality of life during neoadjuvant treatment and surgery for localized esophageal carcinoma. Cancer 2005; 103(9):1791–9.

60. Reynolds JV, McLaughlin R, Moore J, et al. Prospective evaluation of quality of life in patients with localized oesophageal cancer treated by multimodality therapy or surgery alone. Br J Surg 2006;93(9):1084–90.

61. Avery KN, Metcalfe C, Barham CP, et al. Quality of life during potentially curative treatment for locally advanced oesophageal cancer. Br J Surg 2007;94(11): 1369–76.

62. van Meerten E, van der Gaast A, Looman CW, et al. Quality of life during neoadjuvant treatment and after surgery for resectable esophageal carcinoma. Int J Radiat Oncol Biol Phys 2008;71(1):160–6.

63. Safieddine N, Xu W, Quadri SM, et al. Health-related quality of life in esophageal cancer: effect of neoadjuvant chemoradiotherapy followed by surgical intervention. J Thorac Cardiovasc Surg 2009;137(1):36–42.

64. Yamashita H, Okuma K, Seto Y, et al. A retrospective comparison of clinical outcomes and quality of life measures between definitive chemoradiation alone and radical surgery for clinical stage II-III esophageal carcinoma. J Surg Oncol 2009;100(6):435–41.

65. Ariga H, Nemoto K, Miyazaki S, et al. Prospective comparison of surgery alone and chemoradiotherapy with selective surgery in resectable squamous cell carcinoma of the esophagus. Int J Radiat Oncol Biol Phys 2009;75(2):348–56.

66. Hurmuzlu M, Aarstad HJ, Aarstad AK, et al. Health-related quality of life in long-term survivors after high-dose chemoradiotherapy followed by surgery in esophageal cancer. Dis Esophagus 2011;24(1):39–47.

67. Teoh AY, Yan Chiu PW, Wong TC, et al. Functional performance and quality of life in patients with squamous esophageal carcinoma receiving surgery or chemoradiation: results from a randomized trial. Ann Surg 2011;253(1):1–5.

68. Cense HA, Visser MR, van Sandick JW, et al. Quality of life after colon interposition by necessity for esophageal cancer replacement. J Surg Oncol 2004;88(1): 32–8.

69. Johansson J, Djerf P, Oberg S, et al. Two different surgical approaches in the treatment of adenocarcinoma at the gastroesophageal junction. World J Surg 2008; 32(6):1013–20.

70. Aghajanzadeh M, Safarpour F, Koohsari MR, et al. Functional outcome of gastrointestinal tract and quality of life after esophageal reconstruction of esophagus cancer. Saudi J Gastroenterol 2009;15(1):24–8.

71. Rutegard M, Lagergren J, Rouvelas I, et al. Population-based study of surgical factors in relation to health-related quality of life after oesophageal cancer resection. Br J Surg 2008;95(5):592–601.

72. Wang H, Tan L, Feng M, et al. Comparison of the short-term health-related quality of life in patients with esophageal cancer with different routes of gastric tube reconstruction after minimally invasive esophagectomy. Qual Life Res 2011;20(2):179–89.

73. Zhang C, Wu QC, Hou PY, et al. Impact of the method of reconstruction after oncologic oesophagectomy on quality of life–a prospective, randomised study. Eur J Cardiothorac Surg 2011;39(1):109–14.

74. Leibman S, Smithers BM, Gotley DC, et al. Minimally invasive esophagectomy: short- and long-term outcomes. Surg Endosc 2006;20(3):428–33.

75. Parameswaran R, Blazeby JM, Hughes R, et al. Health-related quality of life after minimally invasive oesophagectomy. Br J Surg 2010;97(4):525–31.
76. Wang H, Feng M, Tan L, et al. Comparison of the short-term quality of life in patients with esophageal cancer after subtotal esophagectomy via video-assisted thoracoscopic or open surgery. Dis Esophagus 2010;23(5):408–14.
77. Montenovo MI, Chambers K, Pellegrini CA, et al. Outcomes of laparoscopic-assisted transhiatal esophagectomy for adenocarcinoma of the esophagus and esophago-gastric junction. Dis Esophagus 2011;24(6):430–6.
78. Sundaram A, Geronimo JC, Willer BL, et al. Survival and quality of life after minimally invasive esophagectomy: a single-surgeon experience. Surg Endosc 2012; 26(1):168–76.
79. Rosmolen WD, Boer KR, de Leeuw RJ, et al. Quality of life and fear of cancer recurrence after endoscopic and surgical treatment for early neoplasia in Barrett's esophagus. Endoscopy 2010;42(7):525–31.
80. Schembre D, Arai A, Levy S, et al. Quality of life after esophagectomy and endoscopic therapy for Barrett's esophagus with dysplasia. Dis Esophagus 2010; 23(6):458–64.
81. Egberts JH, Schniewind B, Bestmann B, et al. Impact of the site of anastomosis after oncologic esophagectomy on quality of life–a prospective, longitudinal outcome study. Ann Surg Oncol 2008;15(2):566–75.
82. Blazeby JM, Brookes ST, Alderson D. The prognostic value of quality of life scores during treatment for oesophageal cancer. Gut 2001;49(2):227–30.

Palliative Therapy for Patients with Unresectable Esophageal Carcinoma

Richard K. Freeman, MD*, Anthony J. Ascioti, MD,
Raja J. Mahidhara, MD

KEYWORDS

- Esophageal cancer • Palliative therapy • Esophageal stent • Endoluminal therapy
- Dysphagia • Photodynamic therapy

KEY POINTS

- The goals of palliative therapy in patients with esophageal cancer include maintaining the ability to swallow, access for the delivery of nutrition, prevention of hemorrhage, and pain management.
- All patients with symptomatic carcinoma of the esophagus should receive a multidisciplinary evaluation to ensure they are not candidates for traditional multimodality therapy.
- Identifying the most appropriate method of nutritional support for a patient with esophageal cancer must be individualized.
- Which therapy is chosen for the palliation of patients with unresectable esophageal cancer depends on the symptoms requiring attention, the technology available, physician experience and training, and patient desires.

INTRODUCTION

Nearly 17,000 patients were diagnosed with esophageal cancer in the United States in 2011. Unfortunately, only 15% of these patients have a realistic chance of cure with multimodality therapy. Prolonged progression-free survival is possible in some of the remaining patients. However, palliation rather than cure of the cancer is the treatment goal for most patients.

The goals of palliative therapy in patients with esophageal cancer include maintaining the ability to swallow, access for the delivery of nutrition, prevention of hemorrhage, and pain management. The treatment of these patients requires a multidisciplinary approach and can involve the use of a wide spectrum of endoluminal techniques,

Department of Thoracic and Cardiovascular Surgery, St Vincent Hospital, 8433 Harcourt Road, Indianapolis, IN 46260, USA
* Corresponding author.
E-mail address: RFreeman@corvascmds.com

Surg Clin N Am 92 (2012) 1337–1351
http://dx.doi.org/10.1016/j.suc.2012.07.004
0039-6109/12/$ – see front matter © 2012 Elsevier Inc. All rights reserved.

traditional chemotherapy and radiation therapy, and occasionally surgery. This article focuses on locoregional therapy for patients with esophageal cancer who have been found not to be candidates for resection with curative intent.

PATIENT ASSESSMENT

All patients with symptomatic carcinoma of the esophagus should receive a multi-disciplinary evaluation to ensure they are not candidates for traditional multimodality therapy. This includes patients previously designated as "unresectable" and patients with recurrent disease. Such an assessment in conjunction with accepted treatment guidelines, such as those produced by the National Comprehensive Cancer Network, have been shown to improve the treatment and quality of life of these patients.[1,2]

Once a patient is confirmed as not being a candidate for or has failed traditional therapy, a focus on palliation of symptoms can occur. The generation of a summary of a patient's symptoms listed in the context of the previous goals often facilitates multidisciplinary care. Therefore, the use of standardized tools, such as a dysphagia grading scale (**Box 1**), an objective nutritional assessment, and pain ranking scales are useful in planning and coordinating therapy.[3]

PALLIATIVE CARE

Palliative care of patients with malignancy and other serious chronic diseases has emerged as a valuable specialty within medicine. Specialty trained physicians, nurse practitioners, nurses, and social workers have been shown to improve the quality of life of patients while reducing hospital readmissions and nontherapeutic interventions.[4] Almost all patients with symptomatic esophageal carcinoma should receive consideration for an assessment by a palliative care specialist, if available.

NUTRITIONAL SUPPORT

Identifying the most appropriate method of nutritional support for a patient with esophageal cancer must be individualized. The decision is based on the previous therapy the patient has received including surgery, life expectancy, degree of dysphagia, the potential for maintaining adequate oral nutrition, and the patient's wishes. Patients who have not undergone extensive intra-abdominal surgery or esophagectomy are often best served by the placement of a percutaneous endoscopic gastrostomy. These can be placed even with advanced esophageal tumors. Laparoscopic or traditional jejunostomy tube placement is also a reliable method to deliver nutrition to these patients and is preferred if there is any future thought of esophagectomy to protect the blood supply of the stomach.

Box 1
Dysphagia grading system

Grade 0: Able to swallow all solid foods without dysphagia

Grade 1: Able to swallow solid foods with some difficulty

Grade 2: Able to swallow soft or semisoft foods only

Grade 3: Able to swallow liquefied foods and liquids only

Grade 4: Unable to swallow liquids or saliva

The authors' practice has been to mark the site of the jejunostomy on the serosal surface of the jejunum using surgical clips. This facilitates percutaneous access if the jejunostomy tube becomes dislodged or is removed for a time. Patients who undergo abdominal exploration but do not undergo esophagectomy benefit from gastrostomy and jejunostomy placement at the time of surgery.

Parenteral nutrition is a short-term option for patients with esophageal cancer. It is beneficial in anticipation of chemoradiation therapy or endoluminal therapy that would facilitate access for enteral feeding. However, it has generally been considered inferior to enteral nutrition as a long-term nutritional delivery method because of the associated risk of infectious complications, potential electrolyte and liver abnormalities, and expense.[5]

PALLIATION OF DYSPHAGIA

The remainder of this discussion focuses on the available techniques for maintaining a patient's ability to swallow and controlling bleeding from unresectable esophageal carcinoma. The benefits, risks, and possible complications of each technique are discussed.

Surgery

Esophagectomy or esophageal bypass procedures for the purposes of palliating symptoms, such as dysphagia and bleeding from intraluminal tumor, are rarely considered today for patients with locally advanced or metastatic carcinoma of the esophagus. Despite advances in surgical technique and supportive care, the morbidity and mortality remain excessive for such procedures without curative intent especially when these symptoms can often be controlled by currently available nonsurgical techniques.[6–8] Furthermore, patients without metastatic disease lose the opportunity of the potential benefits of definitive chemoradiation therapy.

External-beam Radiation Therapy

Historically, external-beam radiation therapy (EBRT) played an important role in the management of unresectable esophageal cancer for palliation of dysphagia and for maintenance of long-term locoregional disease control. In contrast to the minimal long-term survival benefit of EBRT alone, significant palliation of swallowing is noted in most patients, albeit for a variable period of time.[9,10] In a series that examined the difference before and after EBRT in 127 patients with esophageal cancer by Caspers and colleagues,[11] dysphagia was improved and adequately palliated until death in 71% and 54% of patients, respectively.

However, the duration of benefit may be too short for patients who are expected to survive longer than 3 to 6 months. In a report of 103 patients who underwent EBRT alone by Wara and colleagues,[12] dysphagia was improved for an average of 3 months in 89% of patients. However, only 14% had sustained relief of dysphagia for longer than 12 months. Furthermore, the improvement of dysphagia may take 1 to 2 months after the initiation of radiation therapy.

Chemoradiation Therapy

Combined chemoradiotherapy is considered by many to provide superior palliation for unresectable esophageal carcinoma compared with EBRT. It is generally considered the preferred initial palliative therapy for patients who are suitably fit for combined therapy and who do not have severe dysphagia. Coia and colleagues[13] described posttreatment swallowing function in 120 patients who were treated with different combination regimens. Most patients (88%) noted improvement in dysphagia within an average of 2 weeks. Benefit was maximal by 4 weeks in 86% of patients with all but two reporting they could swallow soft or solid food without dysphagia. Two-thirds of the patients treated with palliative intent had no significant dysphagia until death or their last follow-up examination.

Patients who undergo EBRT alone or as combined therapy are at risk for the development of a tracheoesophageal fistula and postradiotherapy esophageal strictures. Both of these conditions may be benign or malignant and may lead to recurrent dysphagia. Thus, the potential benefits of EBRT or chemoradiation therapy must be carefully considered in the context of the possible complications of EBRT and toxicities of systemic therapy when used purely for palliation. Another consideration for patients is the time required for radiation delivery that may consume a significant portion of some patients' life expectancy.

Endoluminal Brachytherapy

Endoluminal brachytherapy has been reported to produce response rates of up to 70% for patients with esophageal cancer and dysphagia using a 6- or 8-week treatment regime.[14] However, as reported by Rovirosa and colleagues,[15] the mean dysphagia-free interval was only 2.5 months with a significant rate of severe esophagitis. A fibrotic stricture rate of 25% and fistula rate of nearly 10% have also been reported. The short dysphagia-free interval, significant complication rate, time lag to dysphagia relief, and requirement for multiple endoscopies for catheter placement have limited the use of brachytherapy.

Photodynamic Therapy

Photodynamic therapy (PDT) is a nonthermal ablative technique that involves the systemic administration of a photosensitizer followed by the application of light. Because of differences in tumor vascular supply and lymphatic clearance, the photosensitizing agent is preferentially aggregated by malignant cells. When light of the appropriate wavelength is applied to the mucosal surface of the esophagus during flexible esophagoscopy 48 to 72 hours later, a photo-oxidative reaction occurs resulting in cell death. Typically, another endoscopy is performed 2 to 3 days after the initial treatment to assess the tumor response, allow debridement of necrotic tissue, and for a second light exposure, if required. PDT therapy can be repeated to provide optimal tissue ablation.

PDT has been shown to provide significant palliation from dysphagia in patients with advanced disease or locoregional failure after chemoradiotherapy.[16] Luketich and colleagues[17] reported a 91% improvement in dysphagia scores in 77 patients 4 weeks after the initial treatment. In their series, 38% of patients required more than one PDT treatment with seven patients requiring esophageal stent placement for recurrent dysphagia. The mean dysphagia free-interval was 11 weeks with a median survival of 5.9 months. PDT controlled intraluminal bleeding in six of six patients in this series.

An updated series from the same groups found an 85% rate of dysphagia improvement in 215 patients treated with PDT.[18] The mean dysphagia-free interval was 66 days. Stent placement was required in 35 (16%) patients who experienced recurrent dysphagia at a mean interval of 59 days. Intraluminal bleeding was controlled in 29 (93%) of 31 patients.

Complications after PDT include chest pain, odynophagia, transient worsening of dysphagia, fever, leukocytosis, stricture formation, and pleural or pericardial effusion. At present, only one photosensitizing agent, porfimer sodium (Photofrin; Lederle Parenterals, Carolina, PR), is available in the United States. The relatively long half-life of this product results in a 10% rate of skin phototsensitivity reactions despite patients being counseled against sun exposure for 6 weeks after treatment.[19] In the Luketich series, three patients experienced an esophageal perforation after PDT. San Filippo and colleagues[20] have also reported that patients who have undergone previous chemoradiation, radiation, or brachytherapy are at increased risk for serious complication after PDT.

The advantages of PDT are that it is a relatively simple technique that is effective in reducing dysphagia and controlling bleeding in patients with unresectable esophageal carcinoma. It seems to be most effective in patients without significant external compression. Because of fewer alternative therapies, it especially useful in patients with a cervical esophageal malignancy.

Disadvantages of PDT therapy include the high cost of the equipment and photosensitizing agent compared with other endoluminal therapies. Also of concern is the predilection of serious complications in patients who have undergone prior chemoradiation therapy. Photosensitivity requiring the avoidance of direct sunlight, opaque clothing, and sunglasses for 6 weeks also causes some patients to choose an alternative form of therapy.

Laser Therapy

Laser therapy with neodymium:yttrium-aluminum-garnet (Nd:YAG) has been the traditional form of palliative treatment for esophageal cancer.[21] Treatment with the Nd:YAG laser typically requires several sessions. The goal is to fulgurate sufficient malignant tissue to restore luminal patency. The effectiveness of this process varies by the location of the tumor, with mid esophageal lesions being optimal.[22] Treatments can be performed as frequently as every other day and are often completed in three to four sessions.

Luminal patency can be achieved in more than 90% of cases with the Nd:YAG laser, and restoration of swallowing occurs in 70% to 80%.[23] Relief may last for 1 to several months but treatments may have to be repeated. Perforation, the most serious complication, occurs in less than 5% of patients when the procedure is performed by experienced physicians.[24]

Because of the high cost, frequent requirement for multiple treatments, and difficulty treating long-segment obstructions, comparisons of Nd:YAG laser with other forms of palliative therapy have occurred. Marcon[16] compared the use of PDT and laser therapy for the palliation of unresectable esophageal cancer. PDT was found to be more effective for palliation and associated with fewer complications than laser therapy. PDT was particularly superior to laser therapy for proximal esophageal cancers, and was twice as effective at providing longer luminal patency in malignant strictures longer than 8 cm.

Lightdale and colleagues[25] also reported the results of a prospective, randomized trial of 236 patients. PDT and laser therapy showed similar efficacy for the relief of dysphagia. There was a trend toward a more complete response with PDT for tumors located in the upper and middle third of the esophagus and for long-segment tumors. PDT was associated with significantly fewer perforations than with the laser. However, PDT was limited by photosensitivity in 19% of patients. Adverse events forced treatment to be stopped in 3% of PDT patients compared with 19% of patients undergoing laser therapy.

Adam and colleagues[26] compared self-expanding metallic esophageal stent (SEMS) placement with laser therapy in a randomized trial and found a significantly better improvement in dysphagia with stenting. Another report by Dallal and colleagues[24] of 65 patients with inoperable esophageal and esophagogastric cancer who were randomly assigned to stenting or thermal ablation principally with the Nd:YAG laser found median survival was significantly longer in patients who underwent laser tumor ablation. The laser therapy group also had a longer median hospital length of stay and incurred greater costs. Health-related quality of life was impaired in both groups, and deteriorated significantly faster in the stent group. Patients who received a stent more commonly reported chest or abdominal pain.

Endoscopic Alcohol Injection

Injection of absolute alcohol into an esophageal cancer is a chemical method of ablating an exophytic tumor.[27] The advantages of this technique are that it is an inexpensive option, it uses equipment that is readily available, and the method of injecting alcohol is similar to that used during injection of esophageal varices. The disadvantages are that there is relatively little experience with this method and there are potential complications, including chest pain, mediastinitis, tracheoesophageal fistulas, and perforation, which is possibly caused by diffusion of the alcohol along tissue planes.[28] Overall duration of palliation tends to be short and additional endoscopic sessions are often needed.

Endoscopic Injection of Chemotherapy

Another option for the palliation of tumors of the upper aerodigestive tract is injection of tumor with a cisplatnin-epinephrine–containing gel. In two preliminary reports, an objective tumor response and improvement in dysphagia after multiple injections was observed in some patients.[29,30] The use of this approach might be enhanced if used in conjunction with other therapeutic options, such as EBRT, a strategy that requires further study.

Argon Plasma Coagulation

Argon plasma coagulation (APC) is a technique of monopolar, noncontact electrocautery that uses ionized, electrically charged argon gas to cause tissue fulguration and tumor destruction. APC can be delivered through an endoscopic catheter using flexible endoscopy of the esophagus or airway. In a study that included 51 patients with esophageal or esophagogastric junction cancer treated with APC reported by Eikhoff and colleagues,[31] an overall response was seen in 85% of patients with dysphagia improving in 94%. The most common complication in that series was bleeding.

Cryoablation

Cryoablation uses supercooling to cause cryonecrosis of tissue. It is also a catheter-based therapy delivered by flexible endoscopy of the foregut or airway. In a series of 49 patients with esophageal cancer reported by Greenwald and coworkers,[32] a complete intraluminal response was seen in 63% with no serious adverse events reported. Benign strictures developed in 10 patients (13%), all of whom had undergone previous tumor therapy. Cryoablation is also useful for intraluminal bleeding from esophageal malignancies.

Esophageal Dilatation

Esophageal dilatation using a pneumatic balloon or wire-guided bougies can provide the immediate relief of dysphagia in most patients.[33] However, because no attempt is made to reduce the amount of intraluminal tumor or external esophageal compression, recurrence of dysphagia is often rapid and repeat dilatation is usually required. Esophageal dilation is also associated with a small risk of perforation, especially if performed without fluoroscopy or wire guidance or during the course of radiotherapy.[34–37]

Esophageal Stent Placement

The use of an endoluminal esophageal stent to treat esophageal obstruction from tumor is not a new concept to the thoracic surgeon. Esophageal intubation has been used since the nineteenth century when Symonds (1887) described his experience with prostheses made of ivory and silver.[38] In more recent times, various researchers have developed devices for esophageal intubation.[39–41]

Taking advantages of the technology used to make endovascular stents, SEMS became available in the 1990s. These stents could be inserted with flexible esophagoscopy; required significantly less esophageal dilatation; had a lower rate of migration; and provided symptom palliation in patients with locally unresectable or advanced metastatic esophageal cancer, those with poor functional status who cannot tolerate surgery or chemoradiotherapy, or for those with locally recurrent disease after primary treatment.

The subsequent ability to produce a plastic prosthesis coated with silicone has resulted in an esophageal stent with ease of insertion, a minimal requirement for esophageal dilation, and the ability to form an occlusive seal within the lumen of the esophagus. A distinct advantage of these nonmetallic endoprostheses is also their ability to be extracted even after long periods of time without damaging the esophagus, which has allowed their use in a variety of benign and malignant conditions.[42–45]

SEMS and plastic stents are available as uncovered, partially covered, and fully covered. The advantage of covered stents is that they resist tumor ingrowth, but they have a higher migration rate, especially when fully covered.[46] They can also be used in the closure of fistulas and leaks. Partially covered stents are uncovered at their ends, allowing them to be embedded in tissue to prevent migration. Fully covered stents offer the advantage of potentially being removable. Uncovered stents are less likely to migrate, but are subject to tumor ingrowth and obstruction. **Box 2** shows the esophageal stents currently available in the United States.

TECHNIQUE

SEMS and the Polyflex stent can be placed with sedation or general anesthesia using endoscopic guidance. The authors' preference is to also use fluoroscopy (**Fig. 1**). An initial stricture dilation to a minimal luminal diameter of 10 mm to allow passage of the

---

Box 2
Esophageal stents available in the United States

- Wallflex (Boston Scientific, Natick, MA): partially and fully covered nitinol stents
- Esophageal Z stent (Cook Endoscopy, Winston-Salem, NC): partially covered stainless steel stent
- Evolution (Cook Endoscopy): partially covered and fully covered nitinol stents
- Ultraflex stent (Boston Scientific): partially covered and uncovered nitinol stents
- Alimaxx-E stent (Alveolus, Charlotte, NC): fully covered nitinol stent
- Niti-S (Taewoong-Medical Co, Seoul, Korea): fully covered nitinol stent
- Polyflex stent (Boston Scientific): fully covered silicone coated polyester

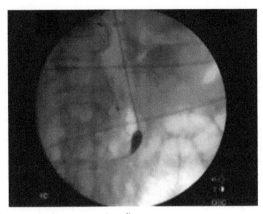

Fig. 1. Esophageal stent deployment using fluoroscopy.

predeployed stent is often required at the beginning of the procedure. After dilatation, the length of the stenosis is measured and a stent size chosen. The authors' practice is to oversize the stent in length and diameter to reduce migration. They also place a percutaneous gastrostomy after dilatation but before stent placement in patients without access for enteral feeding.

Placement is accomplished by endoscopic visualization of the proximal and distal margin of the tumor. These margins are then translated to external markers using fluoroscopy. Stent placement then proceeds under fluoroscopic guidance. After deployment of the stent, flexible endoscopy is again performed to confirm that the stent has fully expanded, is properly positioned, and that there is no distal obstruction.

Patients with large, bulky mid and proximal esophageal tumors and mediastinal tumors should be evaluated for possible tracheal compression after esophageal stent placement. The surgeon should be prepared for the possibility of tracheal compression and the need for endotracheal intubation and stent removal. It is the authors' practice to perform bronchoscopy at the time of esophageal stent placement for patients at risk for tracheal compression. If found, such patients may benefit from airway stent placement.

For proximal esophageal lesions, expandable stent placement can be technically difficult.[47] For stent placement in the distal esophagus, it is important not to leave an excessive length of stent within the stomach because the stent may contact the opposite gastric wall, leading to obstruction, ulceration, and bleeding. As reported, proximal and distal stent placement are associated with a higher migration and failure rate.[48]

After stent placement, patients should be advised to initially avoid bread, large pieces of meat, and uncooked vegetables. In addition, if a stent is placed across the gastroesophageal junction, antireflux precautions and, in most patients, proton pump inhibitors are needed to minimize reflux and aspiration of gastric contents. Most patients can resume a normal diet within a week after stent placement with an acceptable rate of migration.

EFFICACY

More than 95% of patients undergoing stent placement for malignant esophageal obstruction improve to the extent that at least liquids are tolerated especially if vigorous dilatation or a reduction in endoluminal tumor is performed simultaneously.[49–54] In patients with malignant dysphagia in the presence of a tracheoesophageal fistula, closure of the fistula is successful in 70% to 100% of patients.[55–57] However, subsequent tumor ingrowth or overgrowth is common with disease progression and up to 50% of patients require additional interventions for recurrent dysphagia or complications related to the stent.[53]

Studies suggest that esophageal stents are also effective for the treatment of dysphagia caused by compression of the esophagus by extraesophageal malignancies. In a report of 46 patients by Bethge and colleagues,[58] dysphagia scores significantly improved in patients with extrinsic compression. Van Heel and colleagues[59] also reported 50 patients with malignant extrinsic esophageal compression in which stents were placed. Luminal patency was restored in all of their patients.

The type of stent used does not seem to effect palliation. A randomized trial of 101 patients with unresectable esophageal cancer reported by Conio and colleagues[60] found no difference in palliation between the Polyflex plastic stent and the partially covered Ultraflex SEMS. However, stent migration occurred significantly more frequently with the Polyflex stent.

Esophageal stents have been used for the treatment of dysphagia or fistula recurrence after esophagectomy for esophageal cancer. One study examined 81 patients with recurrent esophageal cancer after esophagectomy[61] in which SEMS were placed for dysphagia in 66 patients and for fistula formation in 15 patients. In these patients, SEMS were successful in treating the dysphagia or fistula in 98% and 93% of patients, respectively.

Esophageal stents can also be used for acute perforations in patient with unresectable esophageal malignancies. The authors recently reported a series of 14 patients treated with a Polyflex stent after experiencing an esophageal perforation or fistula associated with an unresectable esophageal or proximal gastric malignancy. Stent placement sealed the perforation or fistula in all 14 patients with no operative intervention required.[48]

Despite initial success, reintervention in the follow-up period because of stent migration, tumor ingrowth, tissue hyperplasia, tumor overgrowth, or food obstruction is necessary in 10% to 50% of stented patients, depending on the type of stent used.[53,56,62,63] Additional stent placement or laser ablation is often needed to treat recurrent obstruction.

The rate of serious complications after initial stent placement is low. However, significant complications can occur with a mortality rate of 0.5% to 2% from a variety of complications.[64–66] **Box 3** lists the more common complications of esophageal stent placement using the categories of intraprocedural, postprocedural, or delayed.

Delayed complications seem to be more frequent in patients who have previously been treated with radiation, chemotherapy, or both, or who undergo subsequent radiation therapy.[67,68] Patients whose tumors invade the aorta may be at particular risk. One report by Sumiyoshi and colleagues[69] included eight patients who had undergone stent placement for progressive or recurrent cancer after chemoradiotherapy and had T4 disease with invasion into the aorta. Six of these patients died suddenly from massive hemorrhage a median of 31 days after stent placement.

The authors have experienced one similar case of an aortoesophageal fistula in a patient with esophageal cancer invading the mediastinum. Although this patient survived emergent surgery to repair the aorta, multiple postoperative morbidities resulted in their death. Based on experience in this patient and another patient with a similar complication with a benign esophageal condition and reports of others, the authors no longer recommend long-term stent placement in patients who have residual or recurrent esophageal cancer abutting the thoracic aorta.

Box 3
Complications of esophageal stent placement

Intraprocedural complications

    Conscious sedation

    Aspiration

    Malposition

    Esophageal perforation

Postprocedural complications

    Chest pain

    Foreign body sensation

    Bleeding

    Tracheal compression

Delayed complications

    Stent migration

    Tracheoesophageal/bronchoesophageal fistula

    Gastroesophageal reflux

    Recurrent dysphagia

    Bleeding

    Perforation

    Stent occlusion

CHOICE OF PALLIATIVE THERAPY IN ESOPHAGEAL CANCER

Which therapy is chosen for the palliation of patients with unresectable esophageal cancer depends on the symptoms requiring attention, the technology available, physician experience, and training and patient desires. When comparing techniques, some objective information does exist and has been discussed in this article. One approach is the algorithm developed by Luketich and colleagues, which reflects their significant experience with these patients (**Fig. 2**).[18] Another resource is the National Comprehensive Cancer Network guidelines for supportive care for patients with esophageal cancer.[2]

It is the authors' preference to consider esophageal stent placement for all patients with a malignant stricture, fistula, or acute perforation as initial therapy because of the ability to provide rapid relief of symptoms (**Fig. 3**). Subsequent ingrowth of tumor is most often treated with endoluminal laser, APC, or cryoablation with or without stent replacement. Removable esophageal stents are also frequently used in patients presenting with significant dysphagia because chemoradiation therapy is initiated. Acute bleeding from intraluminal tumor is most often treated with endoscopic laser, APC, or cryotherapy in the authors' practice. Most of these patients receive long-term palliation from EBRT or chemoradiation therapy if their life expectancy supports further intervention.

A discussion of the choices of palliative therapy for unresectable esophageal cancer is not complete without mentioning the concept of the cost of a therapy that, by definition, has no curative intent. Although several studies exist comparing

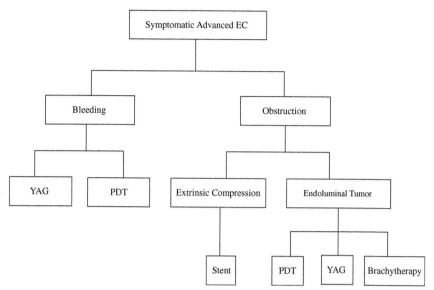

Fig. 2. Treatment selection algorithm for the palliation of dysphagia and bleeding in patients with unresectable esophageal cancer. EC, esophageal carcinoma.

the effectiveness of the treatment options available for these patients as has been discussed, there is a paucity of information indexing effectiveness to cost. Not surprisingly, a similar lack of cost data exists for the treatment of all esophageal cancers as recently reported by Kuppusamy and colleagues.[70] It is important that future studies comparing palliative therapies should measure and compare the costs of initial and subsequent treatment options in patients with unresectable esophageal cancer.

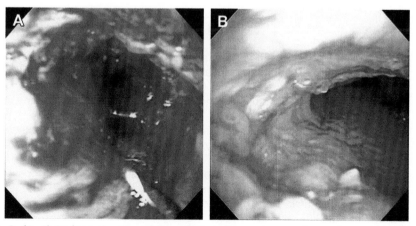

Fig. 3. (*A, B*) Endoscopic view of the midthoracic esophagus of a patient with grade 3 dysphagia (*left*) resulting from unresectable esophageal carcinoma and another endoscopic view at the same level of esophagus after esophageal dilatation, stent placement, and definitive chemoradiation therapy.

REFERENCES

1. Freeman RK, Van Woerkom JM, Vyverberg A, et al. The effect of a multi-disciplinary thoracic malignancy conference on the treatment of patients with esophageal cancer. Ann Thorac Surg 2011;92:1239–43.
2. National Comprehensive Cancer Network Guidelines for the treatment of esophagealcancer. 2011. Available at: http://www.nccn.org/professionals/physician_gls/f_guidelines.asp#site. Accessed May, 2011.
3. Blazeby JM, Williams MH, Brookes ST, et al. Quality of life measurement in patients with oesophageal cancer. Gut 1995;37:505–8.
4. O'Mahoney S, Blank AE, Zallman L, et al. The benefits of a hospital-based inpatient palliative care consultation service: preliminary outcome data. J Palliat Med 2005;8:1033–9.
5. Rivadeneira DE, Evoy D, Fahey TJ, et al. Nutritional support of the cancer patient. CA Cancer J Clin 1998;48:69–80.
6. Orringer MB. Substernal gastric bypass of the excluded esophagus-results of an ill-advised operation. Surgery 1984;96:467.
7. Meunier B, Spiliopoulis Y, Stasik C, et al. Retrosternal bypass operation for unresectable squamous cell cancer of the esophagus. Ann Thorac Surg 1996;62: 373–7.
8. Whooley BP, Law S, Murthy SC, et al. The kirschner operation in unresectable esophageal cancer. Arch Surg 2002;137:1228–32.
9. Van Andel JG, Dees J, Dijkhuis CM. Carcinoma of the esophagus: results of treatment. Ann Surg 1979;190:684–7.
10. Petrovich Z, Langholz B, Formenti S. Management of carcinoma of the esophagus: the role of radiotherapy. Am J Clin Oncol 1991;14:80–4.
11. Caspers RJ, Welvaart K, Verkes RJ. The effects of radiotherapy on dysphagia and survival with patients with esophageal cancer. Radiother Oncol 1988;12:5–19.
12. Wara WM, Mauch PM, Thomas AN, et al. Palliation for carcinoma of the esophagus. Radiology 1976;121:717–21.
13. Coia LR, Soffen EM, Schultheiss TE. Swallowing function in patients with esophageal cancer treated with concurrent radiation and chemotherapy. Cancer 1993; 71:281–9.
14. Sur RK, Donde B, Levin VC, et al. Fractionated high dose rate intraluminal brachytherapy in palliation of advanced esophageal cancer. Int J Radiat Oncol Biol Phys 1998;40:447–53.
15. Rovirosa A, Marsiglia H, Lartigau E, et al. Endoluminal high dose rate brachytherapy with a palliative aim in esophageal cancer; preliminary results at the Institut Gustave Roussy. Tumori 1995;81:359–63.
16. Marcon NE. Photodynamic therapy and cancer of the esophagus. Semin Oncol 1994;21:20–3.
17. Luketich JD, Christie NA, Buenaventura PO. Endoscopic photodynamic therapy for obstructing photodynamic therapy: 77 cases over a two year period. Surg Endosc 2000;14:653–7.
18. Little V, Luketich J, Christie N, et al. Photodynamic therapy as palliation for esophageal cancer: experience in 215 patients. Ann Thorac Surg 2003;76:1687–93.
19. Pass HI. Photodynamic therapy in oncology: mechanisms and clinical use. J Natl Cancer Inst 1993;85:443–56.
20. San Filippo NJ, His A, DeNittis AS. Toxicity of photodynamic therapy after combined external beam radiotherapy and intraluminal brachytherapy for carcinoma of the upper aerodigestive tract. Lasers Surg Med 2001;28:271–81.

21. Reed CE. Comparison of different treatments for unresectable esophageal cancer. World J Surg 1995;19:828–35.
22. Haddad NG, Fleischer DE. Endoscopic laser therapy for esophageal cancer. Gastrointest Endosc Clin N Am 1994;4:863–6.
23. Mellow MH, Pinkas H. Endoscopic laser therapy for malignancies affecting the esophagus and gastroesophageal junction. Analysis of technical and functional efficacy. Arch Intern Med 1985;145:1443–5.
24. Dallal HJ, Smith GD, Grieve DC, et al. A randomized trial of thermal ablative therapy versus expandable metal stents in the palliative treatment of patients with esophageal carcinoma. Gastrointest Endosc 2001;54:549–53.
25. Lightdale CJ, Heier SK, Marcon NE, et al. Photodynamic therapy with porfimer sodium versus thermal ablation therapy with Nd:YAG laser for palliation of esophageal cancer: a multicenter randomized trial. Gastrointest Endosc 1995;42:507–11.
26. Adam A, Ellul J, Watkinson AF, et al. Palliation of inoperable esophageal carcinoma: a prospective randomized trial of laser therapy and stent placement. Radiology 1997;202:344–7.
27. Chung SC, Leong HT, Choi CY, et al. Palliation of malignant oesophageal obstruction by endoscopic alcohol injection. Endoscopy 1994;26:275–6.
28. Moreira LS, Coelho RC, Sadala RU, et al. The use of ethanol injection under endoscopic control to palliate dysphagia caused by esophagogastric cancer. Endoscopy 1994;26:311–7.
29. Monga SP, Wadleigh R, Sharma A, et al. Intratumoral therapy of cisplatin/epinephrine injectable gel for palliation in patients with obstructive esophageal cancer. Am J Clin Oncol 2000;23:386–91.
30. Harbord M, Dawes RF, Barr H, et al. Palliation of patients with dysphagia due to advanced esophageal cancer by endoscopic injection of cisplatin/epinephrine injectable gel. Gastrointest Endosc 2002;56:644–6.
31. Eickhoff A, Jakobs R, Schilling D, et al. Prospective nonrandomized comparison of two modes of argon beam (APC) tumor destruction: effectiveness of the new pulsed APC versus forced APC. Endoscopy 2007;39:637–40.
32. Greenwald BD, Dumot JA, Abrams JA, et al. Endoscopic spray cryotherapy for esophageal cancer: safety and efficacy. Gastrointest Endosc 2010;71:686–8.
33. Boyce HW Jr. Palliation of dysphagia of esophageal cancer by endoscopic lumen restoration techniques. Cancer Control 1999;6:73–7.
34. Heit HA, Johnson LF, Siegel SR, et al. Palliative dilation for dysphagia in esophageal carcinoma. Ann Intern Med 1978;89:629–33.
35. Cassidy DE, Nord HJ, Boyce HW. Management of malignant esophageal strictures: role of esophageal dilation and peroral prosthesis. Am J Gastroenterol 1981;75:173–9.
36. Lundell L, Leth R, Lind T, et al. Palliative endoscopic dilatation in carcinoma of the esophagus and esophagogastric junction. Acta Chir Scand 1989;155:179–83.
37. Hernandez LV, Jacobson JW, Harris MS, et al. Comparison among the perforation rates of Maloney, balloon, and savary dilation of esophageal strictures. Gastrointest Endosc 2000;51:460–3.
38. Symonds CJ. The treatment of malignant stricture of the oesophagus by tubage or permanent catheterism. BMJ 1887;1:870–81.
39. Mousseau M, Forestier J, Barbin J. Place de l'intubation a demeure dans le traitement palliative du cancer de l'oesophage. Arch Fr Mal App Dig 1956;45:208–15.
40. Celestin LR. Permanent intubation in inoperable cancer of the esophagus and cardia: a new tube. Ann R Coll Surg 1959;25:165–72.

41. Atkinson M, Ferguson R. Fiberoptic endoscopic palliative intubation of inoperable oesophagogastric neoplasms. BMJ 1977;1:266–73.

42. Freeman RK, Ascioti AJ, Wozniak TC. Postoperative esophageal leak management with the polyflex esophageal stent. J Thorac Cardiovasc Surg 2007;133: 333–8.

43. Freeman RK, Van Woerkom JM, Ascioti AJ. Esophageal stent placement for the treatment of iatrogenic intrathoracic esophageal perforation. Ann Thorac Surg 2007;83:2003–8.

44. Freeman RK, Van Woerkom JM, Vyverberg A, et al. Esophageal stent placement for the treatment of spontaneous esophageal perforations. Ann Thorac Surg 2009;88:194–8.

45. Freeman RK, Vyverberg A, Ascioti AJ. Esophageal stent placement for the treatment of acute intrathoracic anastomotic leak following esophagectomy. Ann Thorac Surg 2011;92:204–8.

46. Sharma P, Kozarek R. Practice parameters committee of American College of Gastroenterology. Role of esophageal stents in benign and malignant diseases. Am J Gastroenterol 2010;105:258–62.

47. Bethge N, Sommer A, Vakil N. A prospective trial of self-expanding metal stents in the palliation of malignant esophageal strictures near the upper esophageal sphincter. Gastrointest Endosc 1997;45:300–5.

48. Freeman RK, Ascioti AJ, Gianinni T, et al. An analysis of unsuccessful esophageal stent placements for esophageal perforation, fistula or anastomotic leak. Ann Thorac Surg, in press.

49. Acunaş B, Rozanes I, Akpinar S, et al. Palliation of malignant esophageal strictures with self-expanding nitinol stents: drawbacks and complications. Radiology 1996;199:648–51.

50. Saxon RR, Morrison KE, Lakin PC, et al. Malignant esophageal obstruction and esophagorespiratory fistula: palliation with a polyethylene-covered Z-stent. Radiology 1997;202:349–53.

51. Ell C, May A, Hahn EG. Gianturco-Z stents in the palliative treatment of malignant esophageal obstruction and esophagotracheal fistulas. Endoscopy 1995;27: 495–9.

52. Winkelbauer FW, Schöfl R, Niederle B, et al. Palliative treatment of obstructing esophageal cancer with nitinol stents: value, safety, and long-term results. AJR Am J Roentgenol 1996;166:79–83.

53. Rozanes I, Poyanli A, Acunaş B. Palliative treatment of inoperable malignant esophageal strictures with metal stents: one center's experience with four different stents. Eur J Radiol 2002;43:196–9.

54. Siersema PD, Hop WC, van Blankenstein M, et al. A comparison of 3 types of covered metal stents for the palliation of patients with dysphagia caused by oesophagogastric carcinoma: a prospective, randomized study. Gastrointest Endosc 2001;54:145–8.

55. Raijman I, Siddique I, Ajani J. Palliation of malignant dysphagia and fistulae with coated expandable metal stents: experience with 101 patients. Gastrointest Endosc 1998;48:172–7.

56. Morgan RA, Ellul JP, Denton ER, et al. Malignant esophageal fistulas and perforations: management with plastic-covered metallic endoprostheses. Radiology 1997;204:527–30.

57. Verschuur EM, Kuipers EJ, Siersema PD. Esophageal stents for malignant strictures close to the upper esophageal sphincter. Gastrointest Endosc 2007;66: 1082–5.

58. Bethge N, Sommer A, Vakil N. Palliation of malignant esophageal obstruction due to intrinsic and extrinsic lesions with expandable metal stents. Am J Gastroenterol 1998;93:1829–33.

59. van Heel NC, Haringsma J, Spaander MC, et al. Esophageal stents for the relief of malignant dysphagia due to extrinsic compression. Endoscopy 2010;42:536–40.

60. Conio M, Repici A, Battaglia G, et al. A randomized prospective comparison of self-expandable plastic stents and partially covered self-expandable metal stents in the palliation of malignant esophageal dysphagia. Am J Gastroenterol 2007; 102:2667–71.

61. Van Heel NC, Haringsma J, Spaander MC, et al. Esophageal stents for the palliation of malignant dysphagia and fistula recurrence after esophagectomy. Gastrointest Endosc 2010;72:249–53.

62. May A, Hahn EG, Ell C. Self-expanding metal stents for palliation of malignant obstruction in the upper gastrointestinal tract. Comparative assessment of three stent types implemented in 96 implantations. J Clin Gastroenterol 1996;22:261–5.

63. Lagattolla NR, Rowe PH, Anderson H, et al. Restenting malignant oesophageal strictures. Br J Surg 1998;85:261–4.

64. Baron TH. Expandable metal stents for the treatment of cancerous obstruction of the gastrointestinal tract. N Engl J Med 2001;344:1681–3.

65. Baron TH. Minimizing endoscopic complications: endoluminal stents. Gastrointest Endosc Clin N Am 2007;17:83–6.

66. Ramirez FC, Dennert B, Zierer ST, et al. Esophageal self-expandable metallic stents: indications, practice, techniques, and complications. Results of a national survey. Gastrointest Endosc 1997;45:360–5.

67. Kinsman KJ, DeGregorio BT, Katon RM, et al. Prior radiation and chemotherapy increase the risk of life-threatening complications after insertion of metallic stents for esophagogastric malignancy. Gastrointest Endosc 1996;43:196–9.

68. Nishimura Y, Nagata K, Katano S, et al. Severe complications in advanced esophageal cancer treated with radiotherapy after intubation of esophageal stents: a questionnaire survey of the Japanese Society for Esophageal Diseases. Int J Radiat Oncol Biol Phys 2003;56:1327–31.

69. Sumiyoshi T, Gotoda T, Muro K, et al. Morbidity and mortality after self-expandable metallic stent placement in patients with progressive or recurrent esophageal cancer after chemoradiotherapy. Gastrointest Endosc 2003;57:882–7.

70. Kuppusamy MK, Sylvester J, Low DE. In an era of health reform: defining cost differences in current esophageal cancer management strategies and assessing the cost of complications. J Thorac Cardiovasc Surg 2011;141:16–21.

Index

Note: Page numbers of article titles are in **boldface** type.

A

Acid exposure
  adenocarcinoma due to, 1092
Adenocarcinoma, 1081–1085
  absence of *Helicobacter pylori* infection in, 1083
  acid-induced progression to
    reactive oxygen species in, 1093–1094
  age as factor in, 1081–1082
  alcohol consumption and, 1083
  Barrett's esophagus progression to, 1082, 1090, 1093
    biomarkers for, 1094
  causes of, 1155
  chronic acid exposure and, 1092
  development of
    molecular basis of, 1090–1094
  diet and nutrients and, 1083
  epidemiology of, 1090
  gender as factor in, 1081–1082
  GERD and, 1082
  hereditary factors in, 1084
  incidence of, 1156
  NSAIDs. *See* Nonsteroidal anti-inflammatory drugs (NSAIDs).
  obesity and, 1082–1083
  preexisting conditions in, 1084
  prevention of, 1083–1084
  progression of
    molecular basis of, 1090–1094
  race as factor in, 1081–1082
  risk factors for, 1081–1084, 1179–1180
  smoking and, 1083
  treatment of, 1083–1084, 1094–1097
    esophageal cancer–targeted, 1094–1097
Adenocarcinoma of esophagogastric (AEG) junction, **1199–1212**
  advanced
    palliative therapy for, 1206
  causes of, 1200–1201
  diagnosis of, 1201–1202
  epidemiology of, 1200–1201
  incidence of, 1199
  prognosis of, 1199–1200
  Siewert classification of, 1200
  staging of, 1201–1202

Surg Clin N Am 92 (2012) 1353–1367
http://dx.doi.org/10.1016/S0039-6109(12)00178-8
0039-6109/12/$ – see front matter © 2012 Elsevier Inc. All rights reserved.

surgical.theclinics.com

Adenocarcinoma (*continued*)
    survival rate of
        5-year, 1199–1200
    treatment of
        multimodality, 1205–1206
            adjuvant therapy, 1205
            definitive CRT, 1206
            neoadjuvant therapy, 1205–1206
        surgical, 1202–1205
            of Siewert 1 tumors, 1202–1203
            of Siewert 2 and 3 tumors, 1203–1205
Adjuvant therapy
    for AEGs, 1205
    for T2NO esophageal cancer, 1175
AEG junction. *See* Adenocarcinoma of esophagogastric (AEG) junction
Age
    as factor in adenocarcinoma, 1081–1082
    as factor in complications after esophagectomy, 1128
Alcohol consumption
    as factor in adenocarcinoma, 1083
    as factor in squamous cell carcinoma, 1080, 1098
    squamous cell carcinoma related to
        synergism and, 1099
Anastomosis(es)
    gastroesophageal
        creation of
            in thoracoscopic phase of MIE, 1278–1280
Anastomotic leak
    after esophagectomy, 1305–1307
Anesthesia/anesthetics
    for MIE, 1267
Argon plasma coagulation
    for unresectable esophageal cancer, 1342
aStage
    in TNM staging of esophageal cancer, 1120
Autopsy stage
    in TNM staging of esophageal cancer, 1120

B

Barrett's esophagus, **1135–1154**
    bone marrow–derived cells in, 1092–1093
    characteristics of, 1135
    defined, 1137
    diagnosis of, 1137–1142
        biomarkers in, 1141–1142
        described, 1137–1138
        progression predictors in, 1141
        progression risk factors in, 1140–1141
        risk stratification in, 1140–1142
        screening/early detection in, 1138–1140

familial, 1137
GERD and, 1136
management of, 1142–1148
   chemoprevention in, 1147–1148
   endoscopic therapy in, 1144–1147
   fundoplication in, 1147
   surveillance in, 1142–1144
obesity and, 1136–1137
pathogenesis of, 1136–1137
progression of, 1135–1136
progression to adenocarcinoma, 1082, 1090, 1093
   biomarkers for, 1094
risk factors for, 1136–1137
significance of, 1135
by transdifferentiation, 1090–1092
Biomarkers
  in Barrett's esophagus, 1141–1142
    progression to adenocarcinoma, 1094
Bone marrow–derived cells
  in Barrett's esophagus, 1092–1093
Brachytherapy
  endoluminal
    for unresectable esophageal cancer, 1340

C

Cancer(s)
  esophageal. *See* Esophageal cancer
Cardiovascular status
  as factor in complications after esophagectomy, 1128–1130
Cardiovascular system
  esophagectomy effects on, 1302–1303
Cervical esophagus
  management of, 1236
Chemoprevention
  in Barrett's esophagus management, 1147–1148
Chemoradiotherapy (CRT)
  for advanced-stage operable esophageal cancer, 1186–1188
    following resection, 1192
  for AEGs, 1206
  definitive
    for esophageal cancer, **1213–1248**
      clinical trials, 1219–1224
      described, 1218
      future directions in, 1237–1239
      ongoing trials of, 1238
      response-adapted therapy, 1225–1229
      in surgical candidates, 1218, 1225
      toxicity of, 1237
    quality of life after esophagectomy related to, 1323
  neoadjuvant

Chemoradiotherapy (*continued*)
    quality of life after esophagectomy related to, 1322–1325
   for T4 tumors, 1189–1191
   for unresectable esophageal cancer, 1339–1340
Chemotherapy
   for advanced-stage operable esophageal cancer, 1186
     following resection, 1191
   endoscopic injection of
     for unresectable esophageal cancer, 1342
Chylothorax
   after esophagectomy, 1304–1305
Clinical stage (cStage)
   of esophageal cancer, 1111
cM determination
   in TNM staging of esophageal cancer, 1116–1118
cN determination
   in TNM staging of esophageal cancer, 1114–1116
Computed tomography (CT)
   in early esophageal cancer
     in staging, 1157–1158
   in esophageal cancer, 1107, 1109
   in T2 esophageal cancer
     in staging, 1171–1172
Conduit(s)
   esophageal reconstruction with alternative, **1287–1297**. *See also* Esophageal
     reconstruction with alternative conduits
Conduit-related disorders
   after esophagectomy, 1305–1309
CRT. *See* Chemoradiotherapy (CRT)
Cryoablation
   for unresectable esophageal cancer, 1342
CT. *See* Computed tomography (CT)
cT determination
   in TNM staging of esophageal cancer, 1112–1114

D

Definitive chemoradiotherapy (CRT)
   for esophageal cancer, **1213–1248**. *See also* Chemoradiotherapy (CRT), definitive, for
     esophageal cancer
   quality of life after esophagectomy related to, 1323
Diaphragmatic hernia
   after esophagectomy, 1309
Diet
   as factor in adenocarcinoma, 1083
   as factor in squamous cell carcinoma, 1080–1081
Dumping syndrome
   after esophagectomy, 1308
Dysphagia
   after esophagectomy, 1308–1309
   palliation of

in unresectable esophageal cancer, 1339–1343
    argon plasma coagulation, 1342
    CRT, 1339–1340
    cryoablation, 1342
    EBRT, 1339
    endoluminal brachytherapy, 1340
    endoscopic alcohol injection, 1342
    endoscopic injection of chemotherapy, 1342
    esophageal dilatation, 1342–1343
    esophageal stent placement, 1343–1345
    laser therapy, 1341–1342
    photodynamic therapy, 1340–1341
    surgery, 1339

E

EBRT. *See* External-beam radiation therapy (EBRT)
EGFR. *See* Epidermal growth factor receptor (EGFR)
En bloc esophagectomy, 1256–1257
Endoluminal brachytherapy
    for unresectable esophageal cancer, 1340
Endoscopic alcohol injection
    for unresectable esophageal cancer, 1342
Endoscopic evaluation
    in MIE, 1267
Endoscopic injection of chemotherapy
    for unresectable esophageal cancer, 1342
Endoscopic resection (ER)
    in staging of early esophageal cancer, 1157
Endoscopic therapy
    in Barrett's esophagus management, 1144–1147
    in stage 1 esophageal cancer management, 1158–1160
        vs. esophagectomy, 1163–1164
Endoscopic ultrasound (EUS)
    in cT determination in esophageal cancer, 1112–1113
    in staging of early esophageal cancer, 1157
    in staging of T2 esophageal cancer, 1172–1174
EORTC QOL questionnaires. *See* European Organization for the Research and Treatment
    of Cancer (EORTC) QOL questionnaires
Epidermal growth factor receptor (EGFR)
    for esophageal cancer, 1094–1096
ER. *See* Endoscopic resection (ER)
Esophageal cancer. *See also specific types, e.g.,* Squamous cell carcinoma
    advanced-stage operable
        management of, **1179–1197**
            adjuvant therapy in
                following resection, 1191–1192
            chemotherapy in, 1186
            CRT in, 1186–1188
                without surgery, 1188
            lymphadenectomy, 1183–1185

Esophageal (*continued*)

        neoadjuvant CRT *vs.* chemotherapy alone in, 1187–1188

        neoadjuvant therapy in, 1185–1191

            assessment of response to, 1188–1189

        radiation therapy in, 1185–1186

        surgical resection in, 1181–1183

        for T4 tumors, 1189–1191

    CT of, 1107, 1109

    development and progression of

        molecular basis of, **1089–1103**

            adenocarcinoma, 1090–1097

            squamous cell carcinoma, 1097–1100

    diagnosis of, **1105–1126,** 1180–1181

        described, 1106

        in determination of nonanatomic cancer characteristics, 1111–1112

    early

        staging of, 1156–1158

            CT in, 1157–1158

            endoscopy in, 1156–1157

            ER in, 1157

            EUS in, 1157

            PET-CT in, 1157–1158

    epidemiology of, **1077–1087**

        adenocarcinoma, 1081–1085

    geographic predilection for, 1077–1078

    incidence, 1077–1078

    management of

        complexity of, 1214–1215

        definitive CRT for, **1213–1248.** *See also* Chemoradiotherapy (CRT), definitive, for
            esophageal cancer

        EGFR in, 1094–1096

        Her2/neu (ErbB2) inhibitors in, 1096–1097

        radiation therapy in, 1215–1218, 1229–1235

        surgical

            mortality due to, 1127

        VEGF receptor inhibitors in, 1096

    mortality due to, 1179, 1213–1214

    presentation of, 1180

    prevalence of, 1155, 1249, 1337

    small cell

        management of, 1236–1237

    stage 1

        defined, 1158

        management of, **1155–1167**

            endoscopic therapy in, 1158–1160

            esophagectomy in, 1160–1163

                vs. endoscopic therapy, 1163–1164

            for submucosal cancer, 1164

    staging of, **1105–1126**

        classifications in, 1107–1111

        clinical stage, 1111

depth of invasion in, 1107
described, 1106–1111
location in, 1107–1109
modalities in, 1171–1174
    combination of CT, FDG-PET, and EUS, 1174
    CT, 1171–1172
    EUS, 1172–1174
    FDG-PET, 1172
TNM. *See* TNM staging, of esophageal cancer
submucosal
    management of, 1164
superficial
    management of, 1235
survival rates after, 1249
    5-year, 1131, 1213–1214, 1315
T stage, 1170
    nodal metastasis frequency according to, 1170–1171
TNM staging of. *See* TNM staging, of esophageal cancer
T2 stage
    management of, **1169–1178**
        described, 1169–1170
T2NO
    treatment of, 1174–1176
types of, 1179
unresectable
    palliative therapy for, **1337–1351**. *See also* Palliative therapy, for unresectable
        esophageal cancer
Esophageal dilatation
    for unresectable esophageal cancer, 1342–1343
Esophageal reconstruction
    quality of life after esophagectomy related to, 1328
Esophageal reconstruction with alternative conduits, **1287–1297**
    indications for, 1287
    techniques, **1287–1297**. *See also specific techniques*
        long-segment supercharged jejunal conduit, 1287–1293
        short-segment jejunal interposition, 1293–1296
Esophageal stent placement
    for unresectable esophageal cancer, 1343–1345
Esophagectomy, 1128
    complications of, **1299–1313**
        anastomotic leak, 1305–1307
        cardiovascular, 1302–1303
        chylothorax, 1304–1305
        conduit-related disorders, 1305–1309
        diaphragmatic hernia, 1309
        dumping syndrome, 1308
        dysphagia, 1308–1309
        functional conduit disorders, 1307–1309
        predisposing factors for, 1127–1131
            age, 1128
            cardiovascular status, 1128–1130

Esophagectomy (*continued*)
        hepatic dysfunction, 1130–1131
        neoadjuvant chemotherapy/radiotherapy, 1131
        nutritional status, 1130
        pulmonary conditions, 1128
    pulmonary, 1300–1302
    recurrent laryngeal nerve injury, 1303–1304
  contraindications to, 1128
  en bloc, 1256–1257
  Ivor Lewis, 1254–1255
  medical evaluation of patients preparing for, **1127–1133**. *See also* Esophagectomy,
      complications of
  minimally invasive, **1265–1285**. *See also* Minimally invasive esophagectomy (MIE)
  morbidity rates, 1315–1316
  mortality rate after, 1299–1300, 1315
  open
    vs. MIE
        quality of life after esophagectomy related to, 1323, 1326–1328
  quality of life after, **1315–1335**
    evaluation of, 1316–1318
        EORTC QOL questionnaires in, 1317, 1318
        FACT-G system in, 1317, 1318
        MOS in, 1316–1318
    long-term, 1319, 1321, 1322
    postoperative complications effects on, 1329
    short-term, 1319, 1320
    treatment modality effects on, 1322–1329
        definitive CRT, 1323
        neoadjuvant CRT, 1322–1325
        surgical/therapeutic techniques, 1323, 1326–1329
        surgical *vs.* endoscopic therapy, 1329
    volume effects on, 1329
  in stage 1 esophageal cancer management, 1160–1163
    vs. endoscopic therapy, 1163–1164
  traditional techniques of, **1249–1263**. *See also specific techniques*
    described, 1249–1250
    McKeown modification, 1255–1256
    results of, 1259–1261
    three-field lymph node dissection, 1258–1259
    transhiatal esophagectomy, 1250–1254
    transthoracic esophagectomy, 1254–1257
  transhiatal, 1250–1254
    vs. transthoracic esophagectomy, 1259
        quality of life after esophagectomy related to, 1323, 1326–1329
  transthoracic, 1254–1257. *See also* Transthoracic esophagectomy
  vagal-sparing
    technique of, 1161–1163
Esophagogastric junction
  adenocarcinoma of, **1199–1212**. *See also* Adenocarcinoma of esophagogastric (AEG)
      junction
  cancer of

diagnosis and staging of, **1105–1126**
Esophagoscopy
    in cT determination in esophageal cancer, 1113
Esophagus
    Barrett's. *See* Barrett's esophagus
    cervical
        management of, 1236
    thoracic
        mobilization of
            in thoracoscopic phase of MIE, 1276–1278
European Organization for the Research and Treatment of Cancer (EORTC) QOL
    questionnaires
    in quality-of-life evaluation after esophagectomy, 1317, 1318
EUS. *See* Endoscopic ultrasound (EUS)
External-beam radiation therapy (EBRT)
    for unresectable esophageal cancer, 1339

F

FACT-G system. *See* Functional Assessment of Cancer Therapy General (FACT-G) system
FDG-PET. *See* ^{18}F-Fluorodeoxyglucose (FDG)-PET
Feeding jejunostomy tube
    placement of
        in laparoscopic phase of MIE, 1273–1274
^{18}F-Fluorodeoxyglucose (FDG)-PET
    in staging of T2 esophageal cancer, 1172
Functional Assessment of Cancer Therapy General (FACT-G) system
    in quality-of-life evaluation after esophagectomy, 1317, 1318
Functional conduit disorders
    after esophagectomy, 1307–1309
Fundoplication
    in Barrett's esophagus management, 1147

G

Gastroesophageal anastomosis
    creation of
        in thoracoscopic phase of MIE, 1278–1280
Gastroesophageal junction tumors, **1199–1212**. *See also* Adenocarcinoma of
    esophagogastric (AEG) junction
Gastroesophageal reflux disease (GERD)
    adenocarcinoma and, 1082
    as risk factor for Barrett's esophagus, 1136
Gender
    as factor in adenocarcinoma, 1081–1082
    as factor in squamous cell carcinoma, 1078–1079
Gene mutations
    in squamous cell carcinoma, 1099
Genetic(s)
    in adenocarcinoma, 1084
    in squamous cell carcinoma, 1081
GERD. *See* Gastroesophageal reflux disease (GERD)

H

Helicobacter pylori infection
    absence of
        in adenocarcinoma, 1083
Hepatic dysfunction
    as factor in complications after esophagectomy, 1130–1131
Her2/neu (ErbB2) inhibitors
    for esophageal cancer, 1096–1097
Hernia(s)
    diaphragmatic
        after esophagectomy, 1309

I

Ischemia
    conduit
        after esophagectomy, 1307
Ivor Lewis esophagectomy, 1254–1255

L

Laparoscopic phase
    in MIE, 1267–1275
        feeding jejunostomy tube placement in, 1273–1274
        gastric mobilization in, 1268–1270
        gastric tube creation in, 1270–1271
        laparoscopic port placement in, 1267–1268
        patient positioning in, 1267–1268
        pyloroplasty in, 1272
        thoracoscopic phase preparation in, 1274–1275
Laryngeal nerve injury
    recurrent
        after esophagectomy, 1303–1304
Laser therapy
    for unresectable esophageal cancer, 1341–1342
Long-segment supercharged jejunal conduit
    for esophageal replacement, 1287–1297
        complications, 1292
        intraoperative management, 1292
        postoperative management, 1292
        preoperative evaluation, 1287–1288
        results, 1292–1293
        surgical procedure, 1288–1292
            abdomen, 1288
            conduit creation and passage, 1289–1291
            neck, 1289
            reconstruction, 1291–1292
            retrosternal tunnel, 1289
Lymphadenectomy
    for advanced-stage operable esophageal cancer, 1183–1185

extended
    evidence supporting, 1260–1261
Lymphadenopathy
  adequate
    surgical therapy and
      for T2N0 esophageal cancer, 1175–1176

M

McKeown modification, 1255–1256
Medical Outcomes Study (MOS) 36-Item Short-Form Health Survey
  in quality-of-life evaluation after esophagectomy, 1316–1318
MIE. *See* Minimally invasive esophagectomy (MIE)
Minimally invasive esophagectomy (MIE), **1265–1285**
  advantages of, 1265–1266
  anesthetic considerations in, 1267
  described, 1265–1266
  discussion, 1281–1283
  preoperative planning for, 1266–1267
  techniques, 1267–1281
    endoscopic evaluation, 1267
    laparoscopic phase, 1267–1275. *See also* Laparoscopic phase, in MIE
    thoracoscopic phase, 1275–1280. *See also* Thoracoscopic phase, in MIE
  vs. open esophagectomy
    quality of life after esophagectomy related to, 1323, 1326–1328
MOS. *See* Medical Outcomes Study (MOS) 36-Item Short-Form Health Survey

N

Neoadjuvant chemoradiotherapy (CRT)
  for advanced-stage operable esophageal cancer
    vs. chemotherapy alone, 1187–1188
  as factor in complications after esophagectomy, 1131
  quality of life after esophagectomy related to, 1322–1325
Neoadjuvant therapy
  for AEGs, 1205–1206
  for esophageal cancer
    advanced-stage operable, 1185–1191
    clinical stage after, 1118–1119
    pathologic stage after, 1119
    T2N0, 1174–1175
Nonsteroidal anti-inflammatory drugs (NSAIDs)
  in adenocarcinoma prevention, 1083–1084
NSAIDs. *See* Nonsteroidal anti-inflammatory drugs (NSAIDs)
Nutrients
  as factor in adenocarcinoma, 1083
  as factor in squamous cell carcinoma, 1080–1081
Nutritional status
  as factor in complications after esophagectomy, 1130
Nutritional support
  for unresectable esophageal cancer, 1338–1339

O

Obesity
   as risk factor for adenocarcinoma, 1082–1083
   as risk factor for Barrett's esophagus, 1136–1137
Open esophagectomy
   vs. MIE
      quality of life after esophagectomy related to, 1323, 1326–1328

P

Palliative therapy
   for advanced AEGs, 1206
   for unresectable esophageal cancer, **1337–1351**
      choice of, 1346–1347
      described, 1338
      dysphagia-related, 1339–1343. *See also* Dysphagia, palliation of, in unresectable esophageal cancer
      goals of, 1337–1338
      nutritional support, 1338–1339
      patient assessment in, 1338
PET. *See* Positron emission tomography (PET)
Photodynamic therapy
   for unresectable esophageal cancer, 1340–1341
Positron emission tomography (PET)-CT
   in staging of early esophageal cancer, 1157–1158
Proton pump inhibitors
   in adenocarcinoma prevention, 1083–1084
pStage
   in TNM staging of esophageal cancer, 1119
Pulmonary conditions
   as factor in complications after esophagectomy, 1128
Pulmonary system
   esophagectomy effects on, 1300–1302
Pyloroplasty
   in laparoscopic phase of MIE, 1272

Q

Quality of life
   after esophagectomy, **1315–1335**. *See also* Esophagectomy, quality of life after

R

Race
   as factor in adenocarcinoma, 1081–1082
   as factor in squamous cell carcinoma, 1078–1079
Radiation therapy
   for esophageal cancer, 1215–1218, 1229–1235
      advanced-stage operable, 1185–1186
         following resection, 1191

dose and fractionation, 1229–1230
    organs at risk, 1233–1235
    treatment volume and technique, 1230–1233
  external-beam
    for unresectable esophageal cancer, 1339
Reactive oxygen species
  in acid-induced progression to adenocarcinoma, 1093–1094
Recurrent laryngeal nerve injury
  after esophagectomy, 1303–1304
Retreatment stage
  in TNM staging of esophageal cancer, 1119–1120
rStage
  in TNM staging of esophageal cancer, 1119–1120

S

SCEC. See Small cell esophageal cancer (SCEC)
Short-segment jejunal interposition
  for esophageal replacement, 1293–1296
    complications, 1296
    operative technique, 1293–1296
      colon, 1293–1294
    preoperative evaluation, 1294
    results, 1296
Siewert classification
  of AEGs, 1200
Small cell esophageal cancer (SCEC)
  management of, 1236–1237
Smoking
  as factor in adenocarcinoma, 1083
  as factor in squamous cell carcinoma, 1079–1080, 1098–1099
  squamous cell carcinoma related to
    synergism and, 1099
Squamous cell carcinoma, 1078–1081
  alcohol consumption and, 1080, 1098
  causes of, 1155
  described, 1155
  development of
    molecular basis of, 1097–1100
  diet and nutrients in, 1080–1081
  epidemiology of, 1097–1098
  gender as factor in, 1078–1079
  gene mutations in, 1099
  hereditary factors in, 1081
  preexisting conditions in, 1081
  progression of
    molecular basis f, 1097–1100
  race as factor in, 1078–1079
  risk factors for, 1078–1081, 1098–1099, 1179
  smoking and, 1079–1080, 1098–1099
  treatment of, 1099–1100

Statins
    in adenocarcinoma prevention, 1083–1084
Submucosal esophageal cancer
    management of, 1164
Superficial esophageal cancer
    management of, 1235

T

T4 tumors
    management of
        CRT in, 1189–1191
Thoracic esophagus
    mobilization of
        in thoracoscopic phase of MIE, 1276–1278
Thoracoscopic phase
    in MIE, 1275–1280
        diaphragm retraction in, 1276–1278
        esophagogastric specimen removal in, 1276–1278
        gastroesophageal anastomosis creation in, 1278–1280
        patient positioning in, 1275–1276
        port placement in, 1275–1276
        postoperative care, 1280–1281
        preparation for, 1274–1275
        thoracic esophagus mobilization in, 1276–1278
Three-field lymph node dissection
    in esophagectomy, 1258–1259
TNM staging
    described, 1109–1111
    of esophageal cancer, 1105–1106
        aStage, 1120
        cM determination, 1116–1118
        cN determination, 1114–1116
        cStage, 1111
        cT determination, 1112–1114
        described, 1106–1111
        determination of nonanatomic cancer characteristics in, 1111–1112
        examination selection in, 1118
        pStage, 1119
        rStage, 1119–1120
        ycStage, 1118–1119
        ypStage, 1119
Transhiatal esophagectomy, 1250–1254
    vs. transthoracic esophagectomy, 1259
        quality of life after esophagectomy related to, 1323, 1326–1329
Transthoracic esophagectomy, 1254–1257
    en bloc esophagectomy, 1256–1257
    Ivor Lewis esophagectomy, 1254–1255
    left transthoracic approach, 1256
    McKeown modification, 1255–1256
    vs. transhiatal esophagectomy, 1259

quality of life after esophagectomy related to, 1323, 1326–1329
Tumor(s). *See specific types*

V

Vagal-sparing esophagectomy
    technique of, 1161–1163
Vascular endothelial growth factor (VEGF) receptor inhibitors
    for esophageal cancer, 1096
VEGF receptor inhibitors. *See* Vascular endothelial growth factor (VEGF) receptor inhibitors

Y

ycStage
    in TNM staging of esophageal cancer, 1118–1119
ypStage
    in TNM staging of esophageal cancer, 1119

United States Postal Service

Statement of Ownership, Management, and Circulation
(All Periodicals Publications Except Requestor Publications)

1. Publication Title
Surgical Clinics of North America

2. Publication Number
5 2 9 - 8 0 0 0

3. Filing Date
9/14/12

4. Issue Frequency
Feb, Apr, Jun, Aug, Oct, Dec

5. Number of Issues Published Annually
6

6. Annual Subscription Price
$339.00

7. Complete Mailing Address of Known Office of Publication *(Not printer) (Street, city, county, state, and ZIP+4®)*
Elsevier Inc.
360 Park Avenue South
New York, NY 10010-1710

Contact Person
Stephen Bushing

Telephone *(Include area code)*
215-239-3688

8. Complete Mailing Address of Headquarters or General Business Office of Publisher *(Not printer)*
Elsevier Inc., 360 Park Avenue South, New York, NY 10010-1710

9. Full Names and Complete Mailing Addresses of Publisher, Editor, and Managing Editor *(Do not leave blank)*

Publisher *(Name and complete mailing address)*
Kim Murphy, Elsevier, Inc., 1600 John F. Kennedy Blvd. Suite 1800, Philadelphia, PA 19103-2899

Editor *(Name and complete mailing address)*
John Vassallo, Elsevier, Inc., 1600 John F. Kennedy Blvd. Suite 1800, Philadelphia, PA 19103-2899

Managing Editor *(Name and complete mailing address)*
Barbara Cohen-Kligerman, Elsevier, Inc., 1600 John F. Kennedy Blvd. Suite 1800, Philadelphia, PA 19103-2899

10. Owner *(Do not leave blank. If the publication is owned by a corporation, give the name and address of the corporation immediately followed by the names and addresses of all stockholders owning or holding 1 percent or more of the total amount of stock. If not owned by a corporation, give the names and addresses of the individual owners. If owned by a partnership or other unincorporated firm, give its name and address as well as those of each individual owner. If the publication is published by a nonprofit organization, give its name and address.)*

Full Name	Complete Mailing Address
Wholly owned subsidiary of	1600 John F. Kennedy Blvd., Ste. 1800
Reed/Elsevier, US holdings	Philadelphia, PA 19103-2899

11. Known Bondholders, Mortgagees, and Other Security Holders Owning or Holding 1 Percent or More of Total Amount of Bonds, Mortgages, or Other Securities. If none, check box ☐ None

Full Name	Complete Mailing Address
N/A	

12. Tax Status *(For completion by nonprofit organizations authorized to mail at nonprofit rates) (Check one)*
The purpose, function, and nonprofit status of this organization and the exempt status for federal income tax purposes:
☐ Has Not Changed During Preceding 12 Months
☐ Has Changed During Preceding 12 Months *(Publisher must submit explanation of change with this statement)*

PS Form 3526, September 2007 (Page 1 of 3 (Instructions Page 3)) PSN 7530-01-000-9931 **PRIVACY NOTICE**: See our Privacy policy in www.usps.com

---

13. Publication Title
Surgical Clinics of North America

14. Issue Date for Circulation Data Below
August 2012

15. Extent and Nature of Circulation

			Average No. Copies Each Issue During Preceding 12 Months	No. Copies of Single Issue Published Nearest to Filing Date
a. Total Number of Copies *(Net press run)*			2407	2038
b. Paid Circulation (By Mail and Outside the Mail)	(1)	Mailed Outside-County Paid Subscriptions Stated on PS Form 3541. *(Include paid distribution above nominal rate, advertiser's proof copies, and exchange copies)*	995	886
	(2)	Mailed In-County Paid Subscriptions Stated on PS Form 3541 *(Include paid distribution above nominal rate, advertiser's proof copies, and exchange copies)*		
	(3)	Paid Distribution Outside the Mails Including Sales Through Dealers and Carriers, Street Vendors, Counter Sales, and Other Paid Distribution Outside USPS®	783	812
	(4)	Paid Distribution by Other Classes Mailed Through the USPS (e.g. First-Class Mail®)		
c. Total Paid Distribution *(Sum of 15b (1), (2), (3), and (4))*		▶	1778	1698
d. Free or Nominal Rate Distribution (By Mail and Outside the Mail)	(1)	Free or Nominal Rate Outside-County Copies Included on PS Form 3541	98	94
	(2)	Free or Nominal Rate In-County Copies Included on PS Form 3541		
	(3)	Free or Nominal Rate Copies Mailed at Other Classes Through the USPS (e.g. First-Class Mail)		
	(4)	Free or Nominal Rate Distribution Outside the Mail (Carriers or other means)		
e. Total Free or Nominal Rate Distribution *(Sum of 15d (1), (2), (3) and (4))*		▶	98	94
f. Total Distribution *(Sum of 15c and 15e)*		▶	1876	1792
g. Copies not Distributed *(See instructions to publishers #4 (page 63))*		▶	531	246
h. Total *(Sum of 15f and g)*		▶	2407	2038
i. Percent Paid *(15c divided by 15f times 100)*		▶	94.78%	94.75%

16. Publication of Statement of Ownership

If the publication is a general publication, publication of this statement is required. Will be printed ☐ Publication not required
in the October 2012 issue of this publication.

17. Signature and Title of Editor, Publisher, Business Manager, or Owner

Stephen R. Bushing — **Date:** September 14, 2012

Stephen R. Bushing - Inventory/Distribution Coordinator

I certify that all information furnished on this form is true and complete. I understand that anyone who furnishes false or misleading information on this form or who omits material or information requested on the form may be subject to criminal sanctions (including fines and imprisonment) and/or civil sanctions (including civil penalties).

PS Form 3526, September 2007 (Page 2 of 3)

Printed and bound by CPI Group (UK) Ltd, Croydon, CR0 4YY

03/10/2024

01040440-0013